PAIN AND THE SURVIVAL BRAIN

Kieran McNally

Disclaimer

The content and guidance provided in this book stem from the author's research, as well as their personal and professional experiences. It is essential to note that this information is not a replacement for seeking advice from a qualified healthcare professional. The author and publisher disclaim any responsibility for any negative effects or outcomes arising from the application of the recommendations, preparations, or procedures outlined in this book. It is imperative to consult with a healthcare professional for all matters related to your physical health.

Dedication

I would like to dedicate this book to my parents Anne and Louis. In particular, my mother Anne who always supported and believed in me. My partner Arlene for doing an amazing job of raising our two kids. And finally, our kids Ada and Bobby that mean everything to me, and who I love so much.

I hope this book can inspire them to finding a career in something that they love.

Acknowledgements

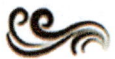

When you are self-publishing, you have to learn everything on your own. You will make many mistakes along the way, and when you are trying to source help, finding the right people can be a challenge. When you finally come across people that make your life a lot easier and can provide guidance, it is something that is welcomed. I was lucky enough to find these people.

Firstly, I would like to acknowledge my editors, Hugh Barker and Tom Feltham, for the editorial advice throughout this book. They both helped me develop my vision and enhance this book without taking away my writing style or the personality I tried to give it.

Secondly, I'd like to thank my illustrator, Roderick Brydon, for his contribution to this book. He was able to turn my words into images without any revisions. To work with someone like this is a very satisfying process.

I would also like to thank my beta readers, Aine Moran, Derek Wheatley, and Brian Jewell, for reading my manuscript and providing me with invaluable feedback before publishing.

Last but by no means least, a special mention to Phil Greenfield, who was another beta reader but from an academic perspective. I think Phil was the perfect person to beta read this book for me. Firstly, because he is himself a published author and, secondly, he is very knowledgeable on this subject. I also asked Phil if he would write the foreword, which he did beautifully. This was also greatly appreciated.

For me, writing a book was a huge challenge, but I wouldn't have done it without the help and guidance of all that are mentioned above. For their help, I will be eternally grateful.

Table of Contents

Dedication iii

Acknowledgements iv

Foreword ix

Introduction 1

Chapter 1: The Chronic Pain Crisis 5

Chapter 2: What Is Pain? 21

Chapter 3: Stress 47

Chapter 4: Biological 79

Chapter 5: Psychological 139

Chapter 6: Social 192

Chapter 7: Sleep 254

Chapter 8: Your Pain Map 275

Chapter 9: Putting It All Together 286

Chapter 10: Optimise Yourself for Recovery 296

Review 345

About the author 346

Notes 347

Foreword

by Phil Greenfield

The world has changed.

Back in the day, if we wanted to source reliable information on a particular subject, we'd consult a parent, or a teacher, or we'd visit the library. Now, in the internet age, we are presented with more information than we might possibly be able to consume in a lifetime, much of it conflicting. In cyberspace, we might regularly explore all sorts of fruitless cul-de-sacs, and find ourselves going down a multitude of energy-sapping rabbit holes in search of what is both useful, and accurate.

Also back in the day, there were pioneers... those who went out on a limb and travelled far in order to explore new territory, and who then went on to produce maps of their discovery. This, so that those of us who did not possess such a call to adventure might more easily navigate that new territory should we ever pass that way in the future.

There's probably no more difficult terrain to traverse in life than the landscape of pain and suffering. Our popular narratives about the unpleasant sensation that we call 'pain', have been rapidly altering over the last decade. What was once viewed as a phenomenon which arose purely from bodily tissue damage is now known to have multiple factors upon which it depends for both its appearance and its persistence. The help offered by clinicians and others, to those who are in pain, has also changed to reflect this development, resulting in a blurring of lines between professions, and the arising of a greater emphasis on 'coaching' styles of intervention for pain sufferers.

These two worlds - the old and the new - are colliding right now, and as often happens in these situations, there's polarisation, as those who are called to help people with pain are falling into two camps - one group doubling down on the old biomechanical, 'damage'-based model, and the other rejecting everything that has gone before and tossing out the biomechanical baby along with the bathwater.

A truth is that we have come to understand much about the basis for our pain experience from the classical biological sciences, and the newer, more contemporary thinking serves to add an extra and helpful dimension. But to find language to easily describe this synthesis is something that clinicians are finding notoriously difficult, and in that respect may currently result in greater confusion being experienced by those sufferers who are approaching practitioners for help.

In this context, we now need pioneers and map-makers more than we ever did; those who are willing to wade through the swamps and scale the cliff faces of what's out there on the information superhighway and make some sense of this rapidly unfolding brave new world, for the good of clinicians and sufferers alike.

I believe that in this fine book, Kieran McNally has done exactly this, and produced an impressively committed piece of work. The information presented in 'Pain And The Survival Brain' is comprehensive, well organised, well-referenced, and extremely accessible, striking an excellent balance between technical explanation and the world of everyday life. There's humour and hope aplenty in here, but also appropriately uncompromising guidance for those who wish to take the often arduous journey of attempting to resolve the kind of chronic pain problems suffered by so many modern people.

Also in this book, I get a strong sense of the man behind the words... a practical but compassionate fellow whose mission it has been to both educate and inspire those who show up at his clinic for help, and who is now reaching out into the wider world through his words in this impressive volume.

Pain is complex. Our long-held ideas that pain is a 'thing' that can be imaged, measured, and hopefully deleted, have not resulted in the kind of spectacular outcomes that either those working in the field, or the general public, would have hoped for. Those who are now assimilating modern thinking into their practice have realised that to enter into the world of helping those in pain is to appreciate that every little piece of a personal pain puzzle may contribute to the big pain picture, and only by taking a multi-faceted approach will each contribution to that picture be acknowledged, assessed and addressed, and hopefully lead to some degree of resolution for the sufferer.

I am sure that by way of this book, Kieran's understanding will be appreciated by many as providing a useful contribution to their ability to safely find their feet as they walk across the face of this ever-changing world, and that his style of guidance will empower and build resilience in those who are taking their first tenuous steps on the journey beyond the confines of chronic pain.

Introduction

*P*ain and the Survival Brain serves as a comprehensive guide to how I see chronic pain. It's everything that I currently comprehend about pain: its influences and causes; how we experience it and why it persists; why pain is helpful and why it can become unhelpful.

We are going to cover a vast amount of information in many key areas that could be contributing to your pain, but before we get into any of those areas, I want to spend a bit of time building a foundation so you can learn why we have pain. I will refer back to our evolution and our ancestors quite a lot. I do so because I am trying to demonstrate that much of why we are the way we are is based around survival. How we process information, think, act and behave is based around the brain's priority of staying alive. I chose to name the book *Pain and the Survival Brain* for that reason. The brain had to develop into this survival organ because of the hardships we endured and the adversity we overcame to get to where we are today. But life has changed greatly since the time of our ancestors, especially in the last fifty years. This is mainly due to technology and the rapid advancement of our civilisation. But our brains are still in survival mode.

I believe that this book compiles information about pain in a way that isn't done in any pain book that I am aware of. We will go deeper than the usual surface level information regarding pain, injuries and their causes. All of this will be done in an easy to understand and logical way. For me, it needs to be made simple because it's for your everyday reader. Too often when it comes to pain and injuries things get confusing, complicated and scary. It's important to me that you interpret the words I use the way they are intended, as opposed to them getting lost in translation. I am a firm believer that this information is easier to digest and comprehend if it's done in a conversational way.

I have written the book in a way that will make this journey unique to each pain sufferer who reads it. It doesn't focus on a specific type of pain or pathology. Usually this is not a good thing because when you try to cater to everybody, it will end up resonating with nobody. But I hope this will be the exception to the rule.

My hope is that what you learn from this book is how personal pain is. That you reach an understanding that pain isn't a singular entity that needs fixing or turning off. When we experience pain, it's not the same as anyone else's, even if the pain experience seems the same.

If you are a chronic pain sufferer then you may be familiar with some of this information. It is my hope that even if you know some of this information there will still be plenty of information that will be new for you, which will give you many areas to explore.

Ultimately, the aim is to provide you with a profound understanding and empower you to navigate your pain journey. There is no one-size-fits-all solution to chronic pain, and my hope is that this book equips you with the tools and knowledge to find your unique path towards relief and recovery.

So, let's get started.

Chapter 1

The Chronic Pain Crisis

When I say there is a chronic pain crisis, I don't say this lightly. This is a worldwide crisis with one in five people suffering from persistent pain. That's 20% of the population that is living with persistent pain every day. Chronic pain has become such a problem that even the World Health Organization (WHO) now considers chronic pain a public health epidemic. You may wonder how it has come to this; given the advances in modern technology, surgical procedures and new pharmacological approaches, it should perhaps be expected that persistent pain would be on the decline. But on the contrary, the amount of people who are suffering every day is increasing all the time. In fact, chronic pain has risen by up to 10% since 2002.[1]

This chronic pain crisis not only has devastating consequences on quality of life, mental health, function and activities, but it also costs the American medical industry 100 billion dollars every year for treatment related to pain management. This is more than cancer, diabetes and heart disease treatments combined.[2]

It affects the workforce, with many millions of hours lost per year. A fifth of patients surveyed with chronic pain reported having lost their job and a third reported a reduction in the hours they worked because of their pain. Furthermore, 71% of people with chronic pain consider themselves disabled.[3] Not only that, but as many as 14% of chronic pain sufferers have made suicide attempts,[4] and one in five chronic pain sufferers have considered suicide.

Yet despite these harrowing statistics, chronic pain remains somewhat overlooked in mainstream discourse. Its invisible nature sets it apart – unlike a visible broken leg, chronic pain doesn't present itself on the surface. The lack of visibility fuels stigma, judgment, invalidation, disability, poverty and a compromised quality of life. The chronic pain crisis doesn't just affect healthcare; it affects the individual, the family, the workforce and the economy. It's a multifaceted problem that is just getting worse. It truly is a worldwide epidemic and I think it's time we modified our approach.

Why I have written this book

After helping people with pain for the best part of a decade, and having seen thousands of pain sufferers coming through my clinic, I started to see a pattern. Time after time, patients would come in and tell me similar stories about their pain. The common thread was how uneducated people are on the subject of pain. Many of them didn't understand why they were in pain, even though they had been suffering for years. They felt confused, hopeless, lost, afraid and anxious. They felt doomed because they felt broken and thought that their body was wearing out on them. It bothered me that this information hadn't just been constructed in their own head, but it had also been reinforced by other health professionals. To be honest, I wasn't surprised this was happening. In general, I believe there is a poor understanding of pain.

The main consensus is that it's only due to tissue health. Many health professionals believe this is the case, and, as such, their approach and advice are in line with this. This was also my thought process, even after college. I began practicing with the belief that I knew it all. I have always been very passionate about my work and always wanted to provide the best treatments for my clients.

Sometimes, clients of mine weren't getting the results I had been expecting. This frustrated me as I had always followed the protocols that I had learned through my education. But still people were suffering. I needed to know why. I began to research and learn as much as I could about the process of pain. I am a curious, logical person by nature. I don't just accept information for what it is. I want to know the "why" behind something that works or doesn't work. It needs to make sense to me before I accept information as the truth. It wasn't until I read a book by Professor Lorimer Moseley and Dr David Butler, *Explain Pain,* that my eyes started to open. I could see that pain was a much more complex and fascinating process. I realised how little I knew and how much I had to learn. Anyone who has read the book will tell you that it's an easy read, mainly because it's written for the patient and not the practitioner. So, for the practitioner to be learning from a "novice" pain book like this, something must have gone wrong. The more I researched pain, the more rabbit holes I went down, which led me to research areas such as psychology, neuroscience, sociology, strength and conditioning, human movement and even some evolutionary biology. Researching these fields gave me new perspectives on how pain and the brain worked. Looking at pain through this new lens answered a lot of unanswered questions for me. It helped me understand why some of my clients in the past hadn't gotten the results I had been expecting. It helped me understand why treatments hadn't worked, why my advice wasn't always appropriate and even how the words I had been using could have been confusing, frightening and ultimately more damaging.

To me, for someone in this industry to be instilling fear and worry, even unintentionally, was neglectful. But it happens every day: from doctors to physios and from chiropractors to sports therapists, and even massage therapists.

It sounds ironic but a study published by the *British Medical Journal* found that chronic pain was partly iatrogenic. This means that healthcare actually contributes to the development and exacerbation of chronic pain. The scientific study doesn't suggest that a patient is getting physically harmed in a healthcare provider's establishment. It's alluding to the language that is used by healthcare professionals. Patients' poor understanding of scans. Inaccurate or outdated advice and treatments provided can give the patient a pessimistic outlook on life and recovery.

This in turn further disables the pain sufferer, leading them to adopt postures that are rigid and guarded out of fear; this leads to avoidant behaviours, increasing anxiety, depression and withdrawal from things that give meaning in their life. All of this increases their pain and disability.

The first rule in healthcare is "first, do no harm." I'm not suggesting that healthcare providers are intentionally causing harm to their patients but if you're treating someone with pain and you don't understand pain yourself, then it's neglectful, regardless if your intentions are good or not. And yes, I would have been part of this unintentional neglect. I would have given out information to people that could be disabling them further; this would have been due to my own poor understanding and education. I recognise this now. This is one reason why I have written this book.

It's our duty as healthcare providers to stay up to date with the newest information, especially if it's our niche. People trust us and come to us for advice. Often, they spend their hard-earned cash for this information. It's our responsibility to provide the most up-to-date and accurate information as possible. We cannot just relay the information that we received in school and universities. Sometimes information taught in curricula can be outdated; even if it is not, science can move very quickly, which is why we need to move with science. We need to stay on top of the new research that is published in the scientific journals and convey this information to our clients in the simplest way possible. There is no excuse not to be up to date nowadays. It's never been easier to access information. Gone are the days where you needed to go to the local library and check out a book. Today we have an incredible amount of information at our fingertips.

Now don't get me wrong, I'm not suggesting that I am a guru and I know it all, because I don't. I still have a lot to learn and I am hungry to keep on learning. But given a deeper understanding of pain, I believe that there will be fewer people who come into my clinic who end up more disabled than they came in.

You may question my choice to use the word "disabled." But if you ask people suffering with persistent pain, 71% of them consider themselves to be disabled. Disability in its essence is defined as "a physical or mental condition that limits a person's movements, senses, or activities." This is exactly what chronic pain does. It creates limitations in movement, senses and activities.

Our healthcare system

I believe there is a big problem in how we treat pain in the West. I also don't believe that our health systems are adequately equipped to address the sheer number of people experiencing persistent pain. Its design seems more tailored to acute problems rather than chronic ones. As many as 40% of individuals dealing with chronic pain feel they do not receive sufficient treatment within primary care settings.[5]

One main contributing factor to this is how much time is allocated to pain management during training. Interestingly, this varies across regions. In Europe, the median hours dedicated to this topic is around twenty, while in the US, it's just twelve hours. Shockingly, in Romania, a mere four hours are spent on pain management education. The curricula mainly focus on neuroanatomy, neurophysiology, and pharmacology, often neglecting crucial areas like clinical assessment and non-pharmacological approaches.

Unsurprisingly, newly qualified doctors frequently express a sense of "unpreparedness" to handle pain management.[6] In US medical school, the average hours allocated to pain education was a mere eleven hours whilst the UK was slightly better with an increase to thirteen hours.[7]

This is in spite of the fact that a third of appointments with general practitioners involve patients suffering from chronic pain, with many having endured this discomfort for more than six months. Reflecting on the numbers, with just eleven to thirteen hours dedicated to pain education training and a notable 20% of the population struggling with chronic pain, logically, the equation doesn't seem to add up.

My goal

In March 2020, Covid-19 came along; unfortunately, I had to close my business for a number of months due to lockdown, so, rather than getting bogged down in being unemployed I took the opportunity to start writing this book. Little did I know that, almost four years later, I would still be writing it.

This book aims to help you comprehend the multifaceted nature of pain, its various origins, and the factors contributing to its persistence. Many individuals out there, perhaps even you, believe there's no way to escape this agony. While this may hold true for a fraction of those experiencing pain, I firmly believe that proper education and guidance presents a genuine opportunity for transformative change.

My goal is to try to give you a deeper understanding of pain: what influences it, why you have it and more importantly what I believe is the best way to resolve it. Some of this information may be controversial or may challenge your beliefs. Some of it might be hard for you to understand or digest as it goes against everything you know or have been taught. This is partly because the majority of the industry still hasn't caught up with the best ways to treat pain.

Conventional treatment is devoted to the symptom, pain, rather than the reason the pain is there in the first place: this often involves medication and/or rest. Although we're slowly shifting away from the conventional approach to treating pain, it's still too slow, with the vast majority still using a deeply outdated approach.

It is well established that pain has much more complex causes than tissue damage or tissue health. However, regardless of this knowledge, the diagnosis and treatment of pain is greatly influenced by it. Pain is deeply complex and the longer you have it, the more complex it is.

It's my hope that I can give you new belief that your pain can be improved. At the very least, I can give you a different understanding which will help you think differently. Perhaps this will even empower you to find the best practitioner for you in your area by being more informed and educated enough to ask better questions. Finding the right healthcare provider is crucial.

For too long, our focus has been on treating the symptom of pain. There actually needs to be a radical shift across the board in the way we view and treat pain. But this can't happen until there is a radical shift in our level of understanding of what causes pain. It's time to move away from the conventional approach to treating pain, which we can call the biomedical model.

The conventional approach

"A purely biomedical approach is at its best suboptimal"
– George Engel

Throughout history there has been an overreliance on the biomedical model. I'll explain a bit more about the model soon, but it's essentially assumed that pain is derived from a single cause – i.e. an injury, illness or disease – and removal of this will result in reduction of the symptom. As such, any treatment that is provided is designed to remove or restore the pathology (illness, disease, injury), which will equate to a reduction in the symptom i.e., pain. This is the theory anyway.

For example, if you sprain your ankle and you go to your GP, they will assess you, prescribe something for the pain, refer you for an X-ray to rule out a broken ankle and then refer you for some physiotherapy if necessary. As the ankle heals this is essentially the removal of the pathology, which in turn reduces the pain. This approach has been tried and tested and will work fine for many acute problems. This is why it's such a popular approach. However, it is also limited. As you will learn throughout this book, it is a simplistic way of viewing or treating pain and doesn't work with many types of pain, especially pain that has become chronic. So, there are a great deal of patients who will slip through the net.

This conventional approach doesn't take into consideration the many other aspects that contribute to pain beyond the biomedical model. We will discuss these in due course. You might wonder how healthcare providers differentiate between those with physical injuries and those experiencing pain due to other factors. It demands a deeper comprehension of pain and its origins, improved interviewing skills, and, most importantly, time – a resource often scarce in the healthcare domain.

It is critical that the right questions and language are used from the beginning. I don't care who you are. Whether you're a doctor, chiropractor, physiotherapist, the early stages of someone's pain experiences are the most important ones.

I want to clarify that I'm not criticising doctors or healthcare professionals in any way. Quite the opposite – I hold them in high regard. They operate under overwhelming workloads and limited staffing, tasked with mastering an extensive range of knowledge across various fields and referring patients as needed.

But the biomedical model is solely designed to find the cause of the pain and removal of the pathology. This could for example mean referrals for investigation in orthopaedics, rheumatology or neurology. Each of these will look through their lens to find the source of the problem. However, the source of the pain is not always a single entity nor is it always a physical problem, which is why the system for treating pain is dysfunctional as a whole. The biomedical approach to pain has been shown to be less successful, cost more and potentially it exacerbates pain and healthcare utilisation. It entails excessive imaging, medication over-prescription and surgeries with poor outcomes.[8]

As we progress through the book, I will show that there are many reasons why we experience pain. The general consensus among people today is that, if you have pain, it must mean that something is damaged. This is not true. In this book it is my goal to help you understand why.

My consultations

"If you can't explain it simply, you don't understand it well enough"
– Albert Einstein

My clinical consultations are very clear and simple to understand. In the past, I have made the mistake of throwing too much information at clients, overloading them with fancy words that overwhelm and confuse them. When I was in my accountant's office recently, and he was speaking to me about figures, I thought to myself he might as well be speaking Chinese to me. It was horrible to feel like I should know what he was talking about. And I was too afraid to say, "I don't understand." I just nodded and left more confused than I had gone in. I realised this could be what a client feels like if they don't understand what I'm saying. Afraid to speak and say they're not following. Nobody wants to come across as stupid so they say nothing.

So, I vowed to change my approach. I now aim to keep things in line with the fundamentals of what I believe to be important but explain it on a need-to-know basis and in a comprehensible way.

When you understand why things hurt, implementing strategies to change whatever is influencing your pain is easier. Simply being given a program of exercises without much context behind it can leave a person not respecting the rehab and consequently not implementing it. People need to know and understand why they are implementing the strategies.

I feel you need a logical explanation why you may be in pain. When there is a logic behind the pain then the rehab seems more reasonable. Doing your exercises with the WHY in mind motivates you. So with that being said, let's get started.

Who is this book for?

The obvious answer to this is anyone who is suffering with pain, or anyone who cares for someone suffering with pain. But the people who will probably benefit the most out of this book are in the chronic pain category. This is anyone who has been suffering with pain for three months or more. Usually, these people will have tried many avenues and have seen many different types of healthcare professionals, to no avail. When they finally come to me, I usually hear, "I've been to everyone." But in truth they have seen lots of the same type of person: a practitioner who views pain in one way and one way only.

On a daily basis, I hear the words, "Wow, I haven't ever heard it explained like this before." It's nice to hear this but it's also sad. It's nice in the sense that I get to see their face when I explain to them what pain is and potentially give them new hope of resolving it. But it is sad on the other hand that they "have been to everyone" and yet no one has ever explained it like this to them before. This just reinforces to me how far we still have to go before pain is treated in the correct way.

I don't just look at pain from a structural viewpoint; I want to find a logical explanation for why you may be suffering, while taking into account what influences pain. Very few practitioners out there look at pain from a physical, psychological, emotional, social, and lifestyle point of view. And chronic pain often connects with many of these areas.

How to get the most out of this book

Throughout this book you will be given a chance to take notes about the areas that are specific to your individual story. Pain is unique to each individual and the best way to figure out your pain is to write it down on paper. I will be talking about a vast number of areas that influence pain; I encourage you to use the notes section at the end of each chapter to write down whatever you feel resonates with your story. This information will be important later in the book when we try to map out your pain. So please take the time to jot this information down.

It's best to put some thought into your notes. The more detailed the better. Being too vague may leave you forgetting what you were thinking about at the time of writing when reflecting later. There will be many topics covered; some will be relevant to you and your life and some won't be.

I will also suggest further reading and more detailed information on specific topics I'm covering. To keep things simple, I will be drawing a line on the level of complexity in order to give you a good enough level of the science while not getting bogged down in the nitty gritty of the terminology.

What is your story?

First, we need to figure out how you got into pain. This will be your individual story. Everybody's story is different. We all have different lives, we all think differently, have different beliefs, experiences, fitness levels, genetics, and behaviours. We move differently, and have different lifestyles, diet, nutrition, sleep and stress levels. If you have ever compared your pain to someone else's pain, it is time to leave that behind. From now we are going to start to map out your own specific pain.

I often get referrals from clients; when they come in, they say, "I have the same problem as Mary." In most cases they may have very similar symptoms but rarely the same influencers. Their pain may be in a similar area and feel the same while being driven by totally different things. So, when you are thinking about your story, forget about what other people have told you about their pain and how it connects to your story.

Having a better understanding of pain in general can help make sense of pain, but having a better understating of "your pain" specifically can give you back control. And I say "your pain" for a reason, because this pain is yours and nobody else's. It's specific to you; it's your experience, and it belongs to you.

Previous diagnosis

Before we begin with the main bulk of the content, I want to talk a little bit about previous diagnoses. If you've been experiencing persistent pain for a considerable duration, it's likely you've received a diagnosis, or possibly even multiple diagnoses. This is completely understandable and it has its merits. Diagnoses serve various purposes, aiding in the explanation of issues to patients and facilitating efficient communication among medical professionals. They can open doors to tailored treatments and specialised healthcare facilities. A diagnosis often provides a sense of reassurance, as it offers clarity regarding the problem at hand. This can be particularly comforting, as being left in the dark about your condition can evoke fear. Furthermore, a diagnosis imbues your situation with meaning, potentially revealing a path towards resolution.

However, alongside these benefits, there are potential drawbacks to consider. A diagnosis attaches a label, and labels tend to come with inherent limitations. These restrictions can sometimes exacerbate fear and anxiety, ultimately impacting behaviour. All of this can increase pain.

While acknowledging the importance of diagnosis and its role in healthcare, it's essential to emphasise that this book is primarily geared towards aiding the individual rather than focusing solely on a specific diagnosis or pathology.

So, with that being said, let's dive in.

Chapter 2

What Is Pain?

One recent advance in medicine is that, along with temperature, blood pressure, respiratory rate, and heart rate, pain is now considered the fifth vital sign when it comes to assessing patients. But what is pain? It's generally something we feel or experience but is there ever any thought to what this phenomenon really is?

The official definition from the International Association for the Study of Pain (IASP) describes pain as an unpleasant sensory and emotional experience associated with, or resembling that associated with, actual or potential tissue damage.

This not a definition that rolls off the tongue. I like to think of pain in more simple terms. Pain is a form of communication. The nervous system has many ways it likes to communicate to us to motivate us to undertake some sort of behaviour. When you feel hungry, you eat. When you feel thirsty, you drink. When you feel tired, you'll listen to the communication and sleep. These are a few ways your body tries to communicate something to you. Pain is just another way it does this. When you feel pain, you'll stop what you are doing and change something.

Pain's primary focus is to keep you alive. It does this by creating an unpleasant feeling when there is some actual danger or perceived threat of danger. So pain can't be a nice warm fuzzy feeling. The feeling has to be unpleasant, otherwise it would be less likely to get our attention.

Classifications

Pain is classified in two ways. First you have "acute" pain. Acute pain is pain that is present from 0–3 months. This is common with tissue damage, illness or fatigue. It's usually short-lived, specific to an area and often associated with tissue health (although not always).

The second is "chronic pain." Chronic pain is more complex because it's less to do with tissue health. Chronic pain is pain that lasts for three to six months or longer. If it lasts beyond this period, most tissue damage will have healed by then so it can't be driving the pain anymore. More things need to be considered. All of which we will discuss as we go through the book.

The alarm system

Pain is like a home alarm system. Every good alarm system will have sensors to detect any potential danger or damage, such as cameras, smoke alarms, carbon monoxide alarms and sensors around the doors and windows to protect against burglaries or break-ins. These sensors are continuously detecting changes in and around the house and sending messages to the alarm panel for interpretation.

The sensors represent the nerves in your body and the alarm panel is the spinal cord in this analogy. As the alarm panel receives the info it transfers it up to the monitored alarm system in the alarm company's head office. This is the brain. The head office is the brains of the operation (excuse the pun) and any changes or decisions will be made from here. Within a normal functioning alarm system there is constant communication between the sensors, control panel and the monitored alarm system. This ensures that there is safety within the house and if there is any danger or potential danger the alarm can go off to get your attention.

We'll use this analogy to help explain the different classifications of pain because not all pain is the same. Many people are being treated for one type of pain when they have another. A good place to start is to decipher which type of pain you have.

The three types of pain are nociceptive pain, neuropathic pain and nociplastic pain.

Nociceptive pain

Just as with an alarm system, your body has different sensors that try to detect changes that could be harmful to it. These sensors are called "nociceptors." Nociceptors are sensory nerve endings that detect signals from damaged tissue or the threat of damaged tissue. We have nociceptors everywhere within the body except in our hair and fingernails. (This is why it's easy to bite our nails or get a haircut without any pain.) Nociceptors detect changes in pressure, touch and temperature as well as chemical changes internally or externally and send that information up to the spinal cord which then relays the messages up to the brain to be analysed.

Nociceptors are not your regular type of receptor. They have a threshold that needs to be breached before they fire off. Just like any alarm system it takes a certain amount of stimulus before a signal is sent to the control panel. Just as lighting a match doesn't set off a smoke alarm and knocking on the window doesn't set off the house alarm, there needs to be a certain amount of threat before any sensor is activated. When the nociceptive threshold has been breached, the nociceptors fire a message via the spinal cord, informing the brain of the damage or potential damage. This process is called "nociception."

I'm sure at some point in your life you stood too close to the fire and your arm started to burn. This is a process in which nociceptors are being stimulated, and then sending a message, warning the brain of the potential danger of the fire. Your brain acts accordingly and you experience pain to get your attention as the burning pain sensation motivates you to move away from the fire. Nociceptors are very clever and they become active before there is any tissue damage as a protective measure. Once you move away, and the threat of the fire has ceased, then the nociceptors stop firing messages up to the brain and the brain reduces the level of pain.

Another example of this is if you have gone for a really long walk and your muscles and joints become tired and achy. Again, this is nociception at play, warning you or encouraging you to take a rest because your muscles are getting fatigued. If nociceptors didn't act this way and become excited before injury the human race could have never survived the harsh evolution we have endured. If humans navigated or hunted the land with no warning system, we could more easily have got injured and then become easy prey for predators that would love to see an injured human limping around. This is why it's essential that nociceptors try to warn us of potential danger first. But they don't always get the chance to warn us of danger, as injury to the body can occur abruptly. Twisting and spraining an ankle doesn't give your nociceptors much time to warn you of potential danger.

Similarly, a smoke alarm is designed to detect smoke before there is any fire in the house but sometimes a fire can blaze up without warning and there is nothing the alarm system can do about it.

When injury occurs, the nociceptors become highly active, telling our control panel (the spinal cord) that there is an injury. The panel relays that information up to the monitored alarm system (the brain) where a decision is made. The brain can decide to create movement, stiffen up, trigger inflammation or create pain depending on what would be best for survival. If you touch a thorn the reaction may be a withdrawal reflex; if you sprain your ankle, it will be very sharp pain, followed by some inflammation. And if you sit in one position for too long, then you will feel an uncomfortable ache.

These are all different types of pains created for specific motivations and behaviours. It wouldn't make sense to get a dull ache if you prodded a thorn because it's important to get your hand away from the sharp object quickly. Likewise, it wouldn't make sense to get a sharp pain if you were sitting in one position for an extended period of time.

Different sensors around the house can set off different types of alarms. Whether it's the house alarm, smoke alarm or carbon monoxide alarm they are all alerted by their respective sensors. And the human body's sensors are nociceptors.

Nociceptive pain is the most common way we feel pain. It's mostly short lived but not always. We'll look more closely at this type of pain in the next chapter.

Neuropathic pain

Neuropathic pain is pain resulting from damage or disease to the nervous system. Pain felt from neuropathic pain is different to nociceptive pain. It usually presents itself as burning, numbness, tingling, pins and needles or pain evoked from light touch and temperature change.[2] There can also be a dead feeling or a feeling of loss of function within a joint. Lack of feeling within a joint can cause people to trip or lose balance because of the adaptation of their senses. Neuropathic pain can result from cancer, stroke, diabetes, repetitive strain, or injury to tissue. Using the alarm system analogy, it's like a sensor wire has been damaged so the alarm system has become sensitised or faulty. With a faulty alarm system, it is hard to predict what is setting the system off.

Nociplastic pain

Nociplastic pain refers to changes to the pain system because of an injury, disease or trauma. Let's go back to the house alarm analogy. Say there was a fire in the house. The alarm system went off. The occupants woke up in the middle of the night and realised what was happening. The parents ran into the bedroom to grab the kids and get them out of the house. Everybody was scared and there was a lot of commotion and panic before they all got out of the house safely. The fire brigade and ambulance eventually came, the fire was put out and the family were treated for some minor injuries and some smoke inhalation.

Roll on a few months. Everybody made a full recovery, thank God. The house insurance covered all of the damage and the house looked brand new again – on the surface anyway. Things were a little different on the inside. First of all, the family were on high alert. Mammy and Daddy would wake up a few times throughout the night and go in and check on the kids. They would lie awake and worry about a fire happening again.

The monitored alarm system isn't working as it used to either. Imagine that, when the fire started, the person who was supposed to be monitoring the alarm system was having a toilet break. When she got back, she noticed that the house had been on fire for five minutes without her sounding the alarm. For this she feels very guilty. As a result of this she is now overcompensating and constantly ringing the police to report break-ins when it's just people like the postman or milkman routinely calling by. She is constantly calling the house and neighbours' houses to make sure that everything is okay.

This is nociplastic pain: pain that is experienced when there is no physical danger to the tissue anymore. The brain and nervous system have changed and become more sensitised, experiencing pain when there is no longer any threat. The fear of movement and injury becomes paralysing and all of this feeds the problem. Over time, other factors start to contribute to the pain. Sleep is affected, stress levels remain elevated, work, social life, sports, and hobbies are all impacted. This creates negative changes within the brain. The alarm system becomes highly sensitive and hypervigilant and this increases the likelihood of pain.

Neuroplasticity

For years scientists believed that, once we became adults, our brains were hardwired and couldn't change. Now we know that the brain is forever changing. It changes to learning new skills, having new thoughts, forming new habits and changing behaviours. It's continually remodelling itself until the day we die. Neuroscientist Jerzy Konorski named this process "neuroplasticity," meaning "changeable brain," way back in 1948.

The brain is filled with billions of neurons. Neurons are messengers carrying information. Each neuron can have up to 10,000 connections with other neurons.[10] This means there are trillions of connections in the brain. New connections between neurons are formed from new thoughts and experiences that start as early as in the womb.

There are billions of pathways lighting up in our brain every time we think, feel or do something. When you learn something new, neurons connect together, creating new pathways in the brain. Repeating that new skill strengthens the new connections between the neurons. We can imagine a new pathway between neurons as being like a trail in a forest. The first time you walk down this forest trail the terrain isn't going to be very good. You may need to hack away bushes that are in your way and stamp down some long grass until a new trail is formed. Moving this way is slow and unpredictable. New forest trails can be winding and sometimes it is not too clear which direction the trail is headed.

Similarly, learning any new task can be slow and imprecise. Repetition improves any skill just as repeatedly walking down the forest trail improves the trail. As your new trail becomes busier and more people start to use it, the trail widens and is upgraded to a pathway. Pathways are clearer. You can move more freely down a pathway. Multiple people can move down the pathway at the same time.

Pathways are a great way to travel, but not always the most efficient. They are still limited. But pathways that are continuously used will eventually be upgraded to roads. When a pathway becomes a road, messages are able to travel faster and more efficiently with less chance of getting lost along the way. When these neural connections are widened and upgraded to a road in the brain the messages are able to travel much more easily, making you much better at the task.

This is true for any new skill. We'll use basketball for an example. Let's imagine that you started to take some free throws, having never played basketball before in your life. You're obviously not going to be very good at it to begin with. When you first shoot the ball, your brain's neurons make connections with other neurons, creating a new forest trail in the brain. These connections won't be very strong at first and why would they? They are new and haven't been stimulated in that way before. But if you go out into your garden every day and continue taking the free throws, these connections start to strengthen. Now you're getting better at throwing the ball, more and more shots are going into the basket.

You often hear people talk about muscle memory. Muscle memory isn't in your muscles. It's actually in your brain.[11] It's a series of connections that are created when you learn a skill. The more you practice that skill, the more refined the connections get until ultimately you get better at the skill. The skill is memorised by the brain and the muscles are told what to do when you need to perform the skill. The brain does all the work but the muscles get all the credit.

As the pathway improves, things start to become second nature. You don't have to think about the technique as much. Throwing the ball just becomes natural and effortless. If somebody was to ask you where your hand was when you threw the ball, you wouldn't really be able to say as you're not even consciously thinking about the movement. When things become second nature, the road in your brain is now a highway. Highways are the best quality road you can get. The connection between A and B on a highway is so much better than on a road or a trail. The connections between the neurons in your brain are so conditioned to lighting up in the brain that it's now done on autopilot.

This is neuroplasticity. Your brain has changed. It's different to how it was before you started to throw free throws. It has formed new movements, new connections and now a new habit. Now that it's a habit, throwing a ball requires less energy. These connections are encoded so well in your brain that even thinking about shooting the ball will light up the same connections when viewed in an MRI scanner.[12]

The brain is a conditioning machine that forms habits to save energy. Consciously thinking about how to do things is taxing on the brain and requires a lot of energy. So, the brain has to figure out a way of expending less energy. You could even argue the brain is lazy. It doesn't want to waste energy. It wants to do things using the least amount of energy possible. It can thus save the energy for more physically demanding things like evading a predator or hunting. This is why it learns things and forms habits. Habits consume less energy because you're doing them on autopilot. The connections in your brain are so used to firing that way that they fire effortlessly. It's an amazing system to have; it helps us learn, remember to navigate, spell, play instruments, play sports, paint and pretty much anything else you can think of.

But here's the catch. It can be devastating too. Neuroplasticity can also lead the brain to making connections that influence unwanted pain. The longer this goes on, and the more the brain rehearses pain, the better you get at doing it. Even rehearsing negative thoughts and fears associated with pain can strengthen connections that affect the pain experience.

For a lot of you reading this book, this will be the case. There could have been an initial injury that started the process of pain. Then your behaviours, thoughts, lifestyles, beliefs, fears, worries, and sleep were all affected. This effectively changes your brain through neuroplasticity, and ultimately how your pain is influenced. Now you experience pain through different influencers but the pain experienced can still feel the same even if the original injury has healed.

There is some good news though. For most people this is reversible. As Professor G. Lorimer Moseley says, "Your brain has got you into this situation but it can also get you out of it too."

This is the point of this book. I want you to take a look at what changes the plasticity of the brain that makes it have such a profound influence on your pain experience, then help you find ways to change the plasticity of the brain so you no longer experience unhelpful pain. We can do this by creating new and more positive connections that actively change your brain for the better.

But first we need to figure out what is influencing your pain. What has got you here today? What initially happened and subsequently happened after you first started experiencing pain? The way you can figure this out is by understanding all the things that influence pain. This is where the "biopsychosocial model" comes into play.

The biopsychosocial model

"If someone has a pain in his hand, one does not comfort the hand, but the sufferer" – Ludwig Wittgenstein

The biopsychosocial model is the most up to date and well-supported pain theory today. This model gives us a structure to help us reach a logical explanation for why a person may be suffering with pain.

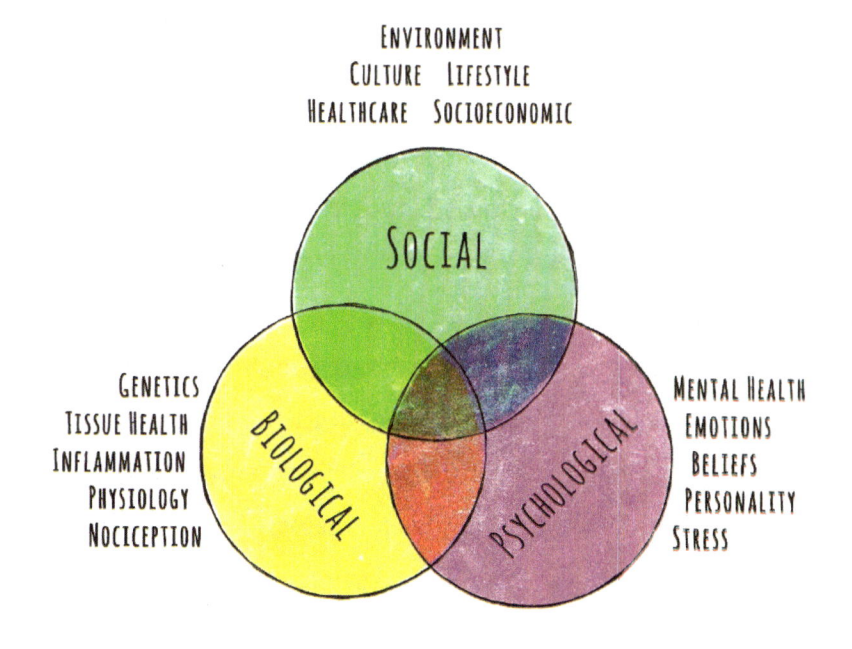

THE BIOPSYCHOSOCIAL MODEL

Traditionally, it was assumed that the "bio" or "biological" portion of this model was the sole contributor to pain; the amount of pain felt was proportionate to the amount of biological damage. Although this concept was widely accepted, it didn't really explain many types of pain. If the concepts behind the biomedical model were true, then the phenomenon of "phantom limb pain" (pain felt in an amputated limb) would not exist, for example. Despite the limitations of the biomedical model, many people, including healthcare professionals, still view pain through this linear model. While the biomedical model does a reasonable job of explaining certain types of tissue-related pain, it doesn't explain a large proportion of pain that is experienced. It certainly doesn't explain chronic pain. When there is no tissue damage, threat of tissue damage, disease, or infection within the body, the biomedical model struggles.

Today the much more sophisticated biopsychosocial model is becoming more accepted as the best theory among pain scientists and many healthcare professionals – but frustratingly the application of the model still has a long way to go. Despite the biopsychosocial model gaining so much attention of late, it doesn't stop healthcare professionals examining patients solely through a biomedical lens. I'm sure many of you reading this book can testify to sometimes feeling like the person assessing you thinks that the pain is all in your head because there is no obvious injury.

To break down the biopsychosocial model:

- Bio – Biology – Tissue health, inflammation, nociception, genetics

- Psycho – Psychology – Your thoughts, beliefs, worries, expectations and actions

- Social – Work, family, friends, hobbies, healthcare, culture

The biopsychosocial model gives chronic pain sufferers hope because it gives us so many more areas to explore than the conventional approach.

Throughout this book I will discuss all areas of the biopsychosocial model that can influence your pain to the point where the brain has changed where you experience excess pain.

"The biopsychosocial model gives us a deeper meaning to pain"
– Greg Lehman

The pain is in your head

To begin to explain how pain works, I have to tell you that the pain you are feeling is in your head. And no, I'm not being insensitive, unempathetic or unprofessional. I'm just telling you the truth. All pain is in your head because all pain is influenced by the brain, no matter where you feel it, no matter how it happens. Whether you fall down the stairs and break your leg, have a toothache or have a sore tummy after eating some dodgy food, all pain is influenced by the brain. So technically the pain is "in your head," because your brain is in your skull. But this is not to say that your pain is imagined or made up.

All pain is created by that fascinating organ between your ears. As we go through this journey of explaining pain, I will speak about the brain and survival many times. This is because it's first and foremost a survival brain. Keeping you alive is paramount. That's it. Procreation second, but survival is the priority. The brain has many protective and survival mechanisms with which to achieve that. Hunger, thirst, fear, anxiety, and memory are all mechanisms designed to keep you alive. Without these, you might die of thirst or starvation, you could walk out in front of a car or you could try to pet a lion. The brain has developed over millions of years so that things like this don't happen. So you know you should be careful of a lion and you can learn how to find your way home. You know when it's time to eat and drink.

Pain lets us know if there is any damage, potential damage, illnesses, infection or disease. Pain teaches us things. It helps us learn about things that are harmful or that are potentially dangerous. Pain interrupts everything that goes on in your life so you can attend to what's going on right now. If you're making a sandwich and you cut your finger, you don't continue making the sandwich. You attend to your painful finger.

Pain educates us too. I have two young kids under four at home. The house is filled with noise, as you can imagine. Every ten minutes you can hear a child cry in one form or another. They are tripping, banging and falling all over the place, but learning at the same time. Pain gives us a learning opportunity. Pain is our friend and our teacher. Maybe it is like one of those teachers that you didn't like in school, but when you look back and think about it, that same teacher taught you a lot. This teacher has taught us that touching a hot kettle will damage our skin, tripping over a curb could cause injury and that knives are dangerous.

On a number of occasions in my consultations I have had clients who said, "I wish I could not experience pain." Without thinking too deeply about this topic you might think this could be a good idea. Would it be beneficial not to feel pain? The answer is a resounding no!

There are some unfortunate people in the world with a rare condition called Congenital Insensitivity to Pain (CIP). These people cannot feel pain. Ironically their pain-free life is very much pain-full. Not in the physical sense of course. This condition is so dangerous that most people with the condition die in their childhood due to unnoticed injuries, infections or diseases going undiagnosed or them never learning about things that are harmful to themselves.

I recently watched a documentary on the condition; the parents of kids with CIP were under enormous stress as their kids would just be running around banging into walls, giving themselves concussion because they thought it was fun. There was even one ten-year-old girl who had been walking around with a broken leg for weeks unnoticed. Think about any time you went to the doctor throughout your life, whether it was due to sickness, injury or infection. The most likely motivator for your trip to the doctor's office was pain. Pain is a teacher, motivator and survival mechanism, and we should be glad we experience it.[13]

But pain isn't flawless. Sometimes pain can become unhelpful and you can experience it even when it doesn't serve a purpose anymore.

Unnecessary pain can be felt even without any potential threat or damage to the tissue. You'll see many examples of this as we go through the book.

How pain works

The receptor system is a subsystem of the nervous system. Receptors are sensory nerve endings that detect changes in our internal or external environment and then relay that information up to the brain, so it can make sense of them. There are many types of receptors throughout the body that pick up various types of stimuli. These include light, temperature, sound, smells, pressure and touch as well as noxious stimuli that are deemed potentially harmful by the brain.

The brain can decide what is useful or important information and what's not. Then, it can make changes accordingly. When the brain receives this information, it makes sense of it. Not all of this information will be conscious. In fact, most of the information that is picked up by these receptors won't be. You will only be made conscious of a stimulus if there is a threat to survival or if the brain is trying to motivate some behaviour, such as needing to go to the toilet, finding a way to modulate your temperature, or trying to swat away a mosquito.

If every piece of sensory information that the brain received was conscious, you would be bombarded with all sorts of sensory inputs. Imagine walking down the road and being consciously aware of the feeling of clothes on your back rubbing over your skin, while noticing every temperature change, all your bowel movements, every breath you take and so on. It would be a sensory overload that you wouldn't be able to consciously process. So, the brain filters what's useful to you and what's not.

The hen house

My uncle owns a hen house which is occupied by hundreds of hens. If you have ever walked into a hen house you will know how foul the smell is in there. At first the smell is so strong it makes you want to gag. But over the course of a couple of minutes you don't even smell the hens anymore.

Why is this happening?

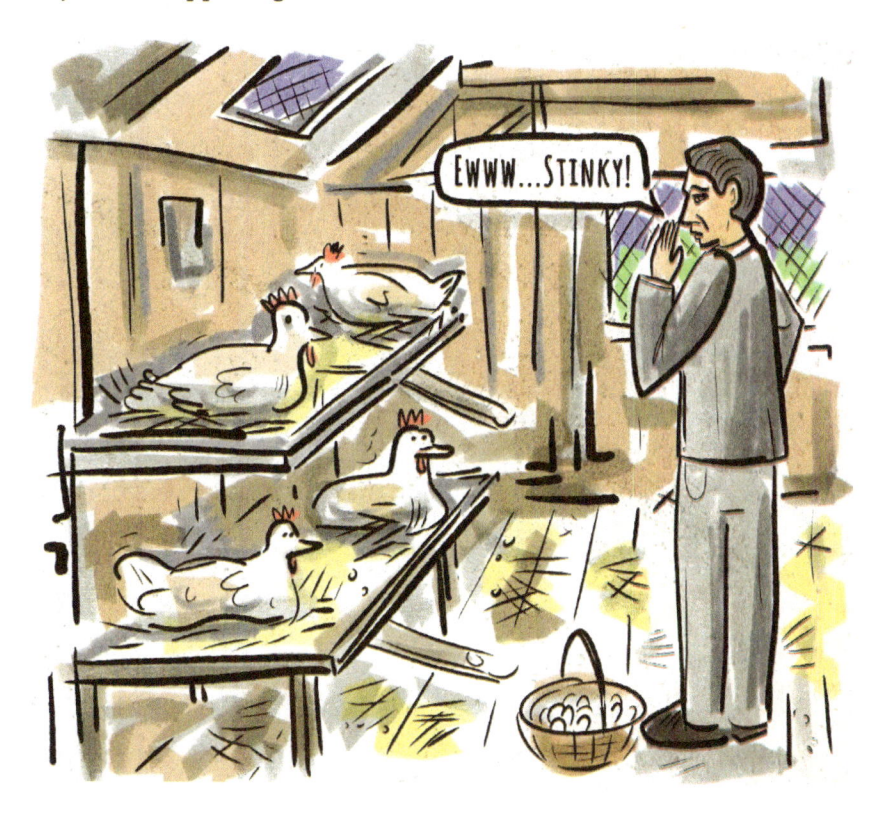

When I first walked into the hen house the olfactory nerves in my nose picked up the smell and relayed it to the brain for the brain to make sense of that stimulus. The brain made me aware of the foul smell because it was novel to me. Once I had been made aware of the smell and made sense of it after a few minutes, there is no real advantage to smelling it anymore, so, the brain reduces my awareness of the smell in order to use its resources to detect other, potentially more important things. The sensory receptors are still picking up the smell of the hens, but the brain doesn't make me aware of it anymore.

This process is called desensitisation and it is happening all the time, even to you right now. While you're sitting there reading this book, I want you to notice the pressure of your shoe around your foot. Up until now, I bet you hadn't been aware of it, had you? Now concentrate on your foot and everything that's around it. Now I bet you notice that there is a pressure or feeling of some kind around your foot.

This survival mechanism's aim is to disregard the familiar in order to detect any stimulus that is out of the ordinary. You don't feel the weight of your clothes on your back but you do feel a mosquito when it lands on your hand. The mosquito poses a threat but your clothes do not; that's the difference. Comprehension of this process helps you to begin to appreciate how pain and the brain works.

Does threat exist?

The fundamental question for the brain when it comes to experiencing pain is not how much tissue damage exists; it's how much threat there is to the body. In fact, pain doesn't correlate well with tissue damage. Most of the time when you experience pain on a day-to-day basis there isn't tissue damage. Think about when you're bursting to go for a wee, have a headache, have been sitting for too long in one position or put your hand under hot water. On all these occasions, pain is experienced in the absence of tissue damage.

You can also have no pain even with the presence of tissue damage. Take a broken leg for example. If you break your leg, I think we can all agree it would be painful. You get a cast on and after approximately two weeks the pain is gone. The leg is still broken but the threat has subsided because the healing process has begun and the cast is giving some added protection.

In a 2004 paper a study was conducted on asymptomatic tennis players. Researchers took MRIs which showed that 85% of these players had abnormal findings on their scans, but they were experiencing no pain.[14] This was due to the fact that there was not enough perceived or actual threat. The brain felt it was able to manage whatever number of workloads the tennis players were under without feeling threatened. In cases like these, if there is no threat, there is no pain.

It can work the other way: a cut on a violinist's finger causes more pain than a cut on a non-violinist's finger.[15] This is crazy but when you think about it, to a violinist, a cut is more of a threat to the system as their finger is their livelihood, so of course their nervous system would want to protect them.

There are many areas of the peripheral and central nervous system that communicate together to decide whether pain should be experienced. There isn't one pain region in the brain that decides to create pain. It's actually a collective effort by many areas of the brain. These areas communicate together and decide whether it is worth creating a pain experience. You could consider them to be like a boardroom in a big company. No decision for a large company is going to be made by one department on its own. The CEO will gather all department managers together in a boardroom meeting so they can have their own say. There will be the managers from finance, production, transport, sales and marketing, research and development, and human resources. Together with everyone's input any decision about the company is made with all inputs counting to at least some degree.

The human brain is like this. The receptor system can send up information that there is potential danger or damage but there has to be a decision at the boardroom level that no pain is required.

The brain evaluates everything from a biopsychosocial standpoint and then makes a decision. Is there enough threat to me that I have to create pain to motivate some sort of behaviour? If the brain feels you are under threat, then it can create pain to warn you to either take a rest or get some medical attention.

Amazingly, pain scientists have discovered that pain can be experienced without any physical stimulus. The pain can be felt independent of nociception. It's as if the nociception department has gone on annual leave and all other departments have decided to create pain without nociception. (One example is that spouses have reported labour pains, even with no physical stimulus, when in the delivery room as their loved ones are giving birth. This is due to a high level of activation in the prefrontal cortex and insula.)[13]

This will become clearer as we go through the book.

The biopsychosocial model teaches us not just to focus on tissue damage but many more areas that can influence pain. In this book, I'll talk a lot about the influencers of pain, because that's what I am always trying to chase, the influencers. Not the pain itself. Why is pain there in the first place? Why is the brain perceiving threat? If you can get to the bottom of this, then it's a lot easier to change. If you only focus on your pain, then you'll be forever searching for the cure or magic silver bullet that doesn't exist.

Throughout this book we will be breaking down each influencer into how it can play its part in your pain. Some of this may not be applicable to you but some of it will be. Everybody's story is different so their influencers will be different.

Same symptoms, different influencers

Mary was a client of mine who had been suffering with sciatica for two years. She was an office worker who spent eight hours a day sitting in front of the computer. Her fitness levels weren't great; she would sometimes walk two kilometres to work and she would class that as exercise. Her pain started when she decided to do a 10K walk for charity. She had an achy back that night but thought nothing of it. This achy back started to fester and get more irritated over time until she was suffering all day at work. She was finding it hard to sit, and the pain had started to creep down her leg.

This is a common story and in Mary's situation it wasn't hard to figure out the problem. It was a classic case of overuse and sensitisation, followed by poor movement habits; this meant that things became more sensitive over time. It was a case of getting her to move better and change her daily habits. She was delighted with everything so she sent in her friend Paul who had the "same problem."

Paul came into the clinic with the same complaint. He had sciatica pain which was travelling down his leg into his foot. But Paul's story was totally different. He had a fall over a year earlier. Up until his accident he had loved the gym. He was an anxious person by nature and had always felt he needed the gym to keep his "emotions in check" and let off steam. After his accident he had gone to speak to his local GP who had examined him for two minutes and told him he had the back of a seventy-year-old. After that, he had stopped exercising and begun "minding himself" as "he didn't want to wear away his back." His sleep had been affected because he wasn't able to blow off steam and he was worried that he might soon need back surgery.

What can we take from these stories? They both had the same symptoms but they had been influenced by totally different things. If you just treat the symptom of pain, especially when it becomes chronic pain, the results are limited.

The experience of pain is very personal so the treatment has to be personalised. This is the beauty of the biopsychosocial model because it gives us the opportunity to treat the pain sufferer on a deeper level.

You'll be glad to know Paul is back at the gym.

What, nociception and no pain?

The same principles apply to nociceptors too. Just because we have nociception doesn't mean we will have pain. Nociceptors can get excited and the brain can still decide not to create pain.

Your brain can decide to dampen down or care less about the nociceptive signals from the nociceptors once it deems they are not threatening enough. Likewise, the brain can care more and thus amplify the signals and make the pain more intense if it perceives the nociceptive information to be threatening enough.

Imagine you get into a hot bath. These nerve endings act quickly by telling your brain, "HEY, BRAIN! You're in a very hot bath here." Your brain instantly takes this information on board, evaluates it, and, if it deems there to be enough of a threat, pain is experienced. This makes you consciously aware that the bath water is very hot, but once the brain realises that it's not a threat to the body it desensitises and you can enjoy your nice relaxing hot bath. The nociceptors don't suddenly stop sending up the information about the temperature of the bath. They are still active but the brain has decided to overwrite the information arriving from the nerves.

Research from pain scientists shows that thermal nociceptors get excited at approximately 43 degrees Celsius but on average pain isn't usually felt until the temperature is raised to approximately 45–46 degrees.[16] So just because these nociceptors send the information about the water temperature, it doesn't mean that pain will be experienced.

To summarise, pain perception is a subjective experience, influenced by complex interactions of biological, psychological, and social factors.

Chapter 3

Stress

If you asked most people on the street what stress is, the vast majority of them would define it as something to do with emotion: the feeling of being overwhelmed or stressed out. Stress is a term that is coined for someone who is under some sort of emotional pressure. But there is more to stress than "feeling stressed out." Stress plays a vital role in life and it is ironically essential for health. The fact of the matter is that Mother Nature didn't just give us this ability to feel stress for the sake of it. It's part of our physiology for a reason.

Stress is your body's way of responding to any kind of demand, perceived danger or actual danger. But in order to properly define stress, we need to talk about what stress *isn't*.

Homeostasis is the body's ability to maintain balance and harmony within itself. It's a self-regulating system that is designed to adapt to changes from our internal or external environment, then make appropriate changes to maintain that balance within the body. For example, we cool down by sweating in the heat, or generate heat by shivering in the cold. This is your body trying to maintain homeostasis. An injury disturbs the tissue's homeostasis which activates the immune system to start the healing process to bring back order and balance to the body. Similarly with exercise, physically stressing the tissue activates immune cells to build and repair tissue to restore homeostasis within the body. Homeostasis is like a default setting whereby the body is programmed to know when things are just right: your "Goldilocks zone" if you will. Anything that moves your body away from homeostasis is a stressor.[17]

If you can get your head around the concept that the brain's objective is always to maintain order and balance or "homeostasis", then you're well on your way to becoming pain-free. However, a high proportion of people who are suffering with pain can't achieve this. Not being able to achieve homeostasis for any sustained period of time puts a tremendous amount of stress on your body.

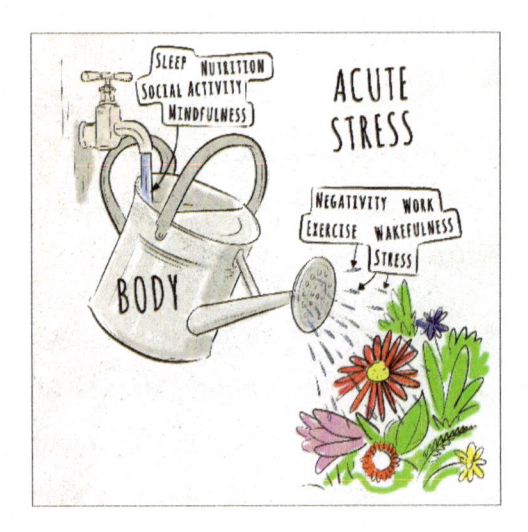

Short bursts of stress over minutes or hours with adequate recovery time is called acute stress. This type of stress is good for you and has been shown to build resilience, physical and emotional strength and wellbeing.[18] Acute stress can keep you stimulated, motivated and alert. It can help you grow, and build resilience both physically and psychologically. It has also been shown to help with memory and learning. When you are exposed to a stressor you are asking questions of your body. As a result, your body adapts to be more capable of managing that stressor the next time. Once the stressor is dealt with, your body works to return to homeostasis.

Let's say you're lifting weights in the gym. If you're comfortably able to do an exercise then you are not physically stressing your body enough to make a change. Your body won't need to adapt because you're not stressing your body's tissues enough to force a change. But if you lift heavy enough weights your body says to itself, "Right, I want to be more capable of managing this the next time." So, it adapts to the stressor and is better prepared the next time.

Have you ever started a new job where, at the end of the first day, you get home and fall asleep on the couch because you're so exhausted? Then after a couple of weeks you're well able to do the job and even do some overtime if required. Or maybe you started to train for a 5K run and for the first few runs you struggled to even run 1K? A couple of months later you were able to do 5K without any problem! This is possible as a result of the human body being so good at responding and adapting to stress.

It's well documented how important physical stress is to health. But exposure to emotional stress is just as important to health. Think about anything that was challenging for you in your life so far, be it public speaking, school assignments or work challenges that you overcame. At first, they may have felt like impossible tasks and you may have been stressed about doing them. But how much better off were you after you completed the task? If you were asked to do a similar task a second time you would be more prepared and confident, and less likely to get overwhelmed. Again, this is because of your body's response to emotional stress. You adapt to the stressor, and learn.

There are people who argue that members of "Gen Z" have been sheltered, overparented and protected from being exposed to any stressors in real life. Kids get participation medals even when they lose to avoid the feeling of failure or disappointment. Parents complain to teachers about bad grades and teachers give better grades to avoid the conflict or hassle from parents. Kids supposedly get what they want when they want it, and don't have to do any chores or work for their allowance. This has supposedly led to a generation with a weaker mentality who suffer from low self-esteem, higher anxiety levels and higher depression rates than previous generations.[19]

If this is partially true, this didn't happen because a generation of bad parents came along. They just wanted to give their kids the best opportunity and perhaps give them the things that they never had. But when these kids grew up and realised that their parents couldn't get them the job or that promotion they wanted, or they didn't get anything for failing, it was difficult to cope with.[20] Life is full of disappointments and not being exposed to acute levels of emotional stress early on doesn't help them build the resilience they need for the inevitable stresses of real life. This is because the brain feels it doesn't need to build that resilience as life is easy and safe. The reality is that life is not easy and you need to be prepared for the challenges of real-life stresses that we have to deal with on a daily basis. G. Michael Hopf said it perfectly: "Hard times create strong men. Strong men create good times. Good times create weak men. And, weak men create hard times."

Our stress system is there for a reason. Being exposed to acute levels of stress can be hard in the short term, but in the medium to long term it builds a better and more prepared version of you. Just as not exercising your muscles weakens you physically, acute levels of stress can be a good thing that will develop a level of physical and mental resilience that will serve you in the future when you need it.[21]

We are all different when it comes to how we respond to stressors. You may find something like public speaking acutely stressful, while another person enjoys it and feels no stress about it. The experiences you have will play a big part in how you respond to stress but there are also other factors to be considered such as genetics, education, cultures, learned behaviours and developmental factors. And for this reason, everybody's stress response will be different.

Two competing systems

Now let's talk about what happens when we have a stress response as we have moved away from homeostasis. Within our autonomic nervous systems, we have two subdivisions: the sympathetic nervous system and the parasympathetic nervous system. These systems are automatic (hence "autonomic nervous system"), running in our unconscious. Our sympathetic nervous system is typically called our "fight-or-flight response." This is a response to any demand, danger or perceived danger, like when we are confronted with the threat of a lion. When we are in this state our central nervous system moves us away from homeostasis, increases the functions of systems including the respiratory system, and elevates our heart rate to get more blood to our muscles so we can fight or run away. It also increases glucose levels to give us an energy boost and dilates our pupils so we are more alert. It also decreases function in other systems that don't serve a purpose for the immediate danger like the reproductive, immune and digestive systems. This is in order to conserve energy.[22]

When you have evaded the lion and there is no more danger or perceived danger, there is no more use for the sympathetic nervous system. Staying in it is taxing on the body. It uses up an abundance of resources, which is why when the immediate threat has gone, it's important to move to its counterpart, the parasympathetic nervous system. This is more commonly known as your body's "rest-and-digest" phase. The parasympathetic nervous system promotes a "rest-and-digest" response, promotes calming of the nerves, and a return to regular function, restoring the immune function and enhancing digestion. When you are relaxing at home and digesting your food it is important to be in this state. This state is essential for relaxing, sleeping and repairing or recovering tissue.

These two systems can be pictured as continually fighting over who gets to be used. The more you are in the sympathetic part of your nervous system, the more stress hormones such as adrenaline and cortisol that will be produced. When you are in your parasympathetic nervous system you will produce less arousal hormones and instead produce calming hormones like acetylcholine, which lowers the heart rate.

For many different reasons your brain can perceive any regular daily life interactions as a threat and activate the fight-or-flight response as a result. This is normal and not a problem. Moving into a fight-or-flight response can be beneficial even if there is no physical threat at hand.

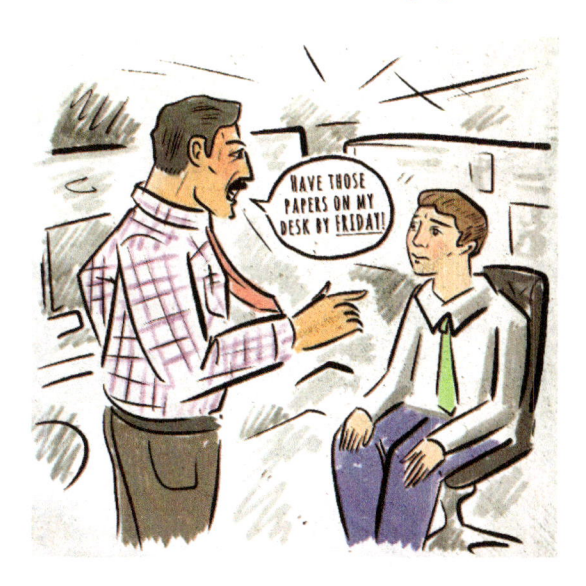

For example, if your boss says that, if you don't work harder, you're going to lose your job, you may perceive this as a threat. Although the threat isn't physical the stress response is appropriate because it motivates you to work harder and achieve what you need to get done!

It only becomes an issue if the stressor doesn't go away or is never resolved. This is when acute stress becomes chronic.

Chronic stress

Imagine there was a bear following you wherever you went. When you went into work, he was there growling at you as you read through your emails, when you were driving home, he was sitting in the back seat of your car sniffing your ear, and, as you were trying to sleep, he would be standing at the end of your bed. All day, the fear of being eaten at any moment would be unbearable (excuse the pun). For that reason, you would be living in a fight-or-flight response all the time. At any moment the bear could attack you so your body needs to be ready to fight it off or run away. All day cortisol and adrenaline are being produced, your heart rate is elevated, and your muscles are engaged just waiting for this imminent attack. Now let's replace the bear with your boss, mortgage payments or fear of movement. This perpetual state of stress without adequate breaks, recuperation or recovery is chronic stress.

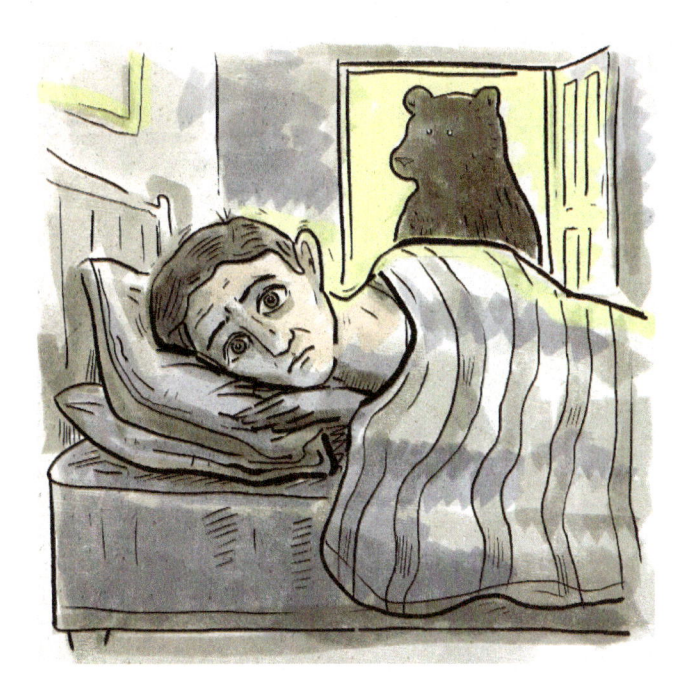

Regardless of whether it's a physical or perceived threat the same stress response is turned on. Activating our sympathetic nervous system is our only way of dealing with threat.

When you are chronically stressed in any way your nervous system deems there to be a threat all the time. Your brain is anticipating danger that doesn't exist. Having this bear follow you around all the time without you ever being able to lose him keeps that stress response turned on all the time. But there are only so many resources you have to fuel the energy required for the fight-or-flight response until eventually your body exhausts itself. Chronic stress restricts the body's ability to restore homeostasis. Your body wants to restore balance but can't and this prolonged chronic stress contributes to development of disease.[23]

The bottom line: chronic stress puts too many demands on the body and doesn't give you enough time for nutrition, emotional first aid and sleep so you can recover both physically or emotionally.

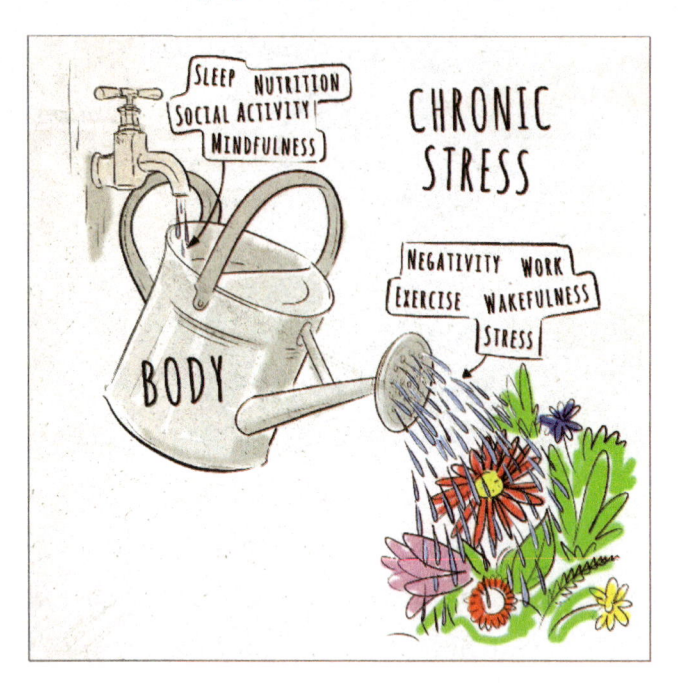

My stress is normal

Some people feel comfortable in stressful environments for varying reasons. They may have grown up this way, always on the go. Perhaps their parents were the same. A stressful lifestyle is normal to them. However, just because you feel normal in this state, it doesn't mean this is healthy.

In my consultations I often ask, "How are the stress levels"? Sometimes I get the answer, "No worse than usual." To which I reply, "What does that even mean?" To some, living in a world of stress is normal, so when they are in pain, they will never consider the possibility that their pain could be influenced by stressors, as their stress levels are the same as usual.

When you are driving your car and you need to overtake the vehicle ahead you would signal (I hope), accelerate, take the car to approximately 7,000 revs and overtake the vehicle ahead. Once you have overtaken, you switch back into fifth gear and bring the car back to under 3,000 revs. But what if you constantly drove around at 7,000 revs? For a period of time your car would be fine. It would be able to cope with this constant demand that you are putting it under. But with continuous driving at 7,000 revs there will come a time where things suddenly start to fail. You may get an oil leak or a noise in the fan or the car begins to stall because it can't cope with this constant demand. When you bring it to the garage and the mechanic asks if you have been driving the car hard, your answer is, "No more than usual." What does that really tell the mechanic about the car and what it's been through?

The evolution of our brain

Over the course of time, animals have evolved for survival purposes. Some animals evolved to have a better sense of smell while others have developed better eyesight for hunting or evasion purposes. As humans, we haven't evolved as much in these areas because we haven't needed to. When we were more like chimpanzees, approximately three million years ago, food became scarce so we had to start to travel between forests to find different sources of food. Because of these new journeys away from the familiar forest we had many more threats than we had previously had in the safety of our forest. If a lion came along, we couldn't just climb up a tree to safety anymore. To cut a long story short, we needed a more complex brain to help us navigate, imagine, communicate, problem-solve, think ahead and plan our journey. So, Mother Nature saw fit to begin to evolve us in a different way.

Humans have had the greatest evolution of all. We as a species have become extremely intelligent in comparison to the rest of the animal kingdom (although you probably wouldn't think this after watching an episode of *Love Island*). This is due to an enlargement of an area of the brain called the cerebral cortex. This is the outermost layer of the brain. If you saw a brain outside the skull, the wrinkly looking bit is the cerebral cortex. Ironically this wrinkly looking part is the newest part of the brain. Most animals have a cerebral cortex, but in humans it's larger in comparison to our body and more complex, with trillions more synaptic connections. This more advanced cerebral cortex allows us to be consciously aware, imagine, develop complex emotions, problem-solve, think, plan ahead, speak and understand language. The cerebral cortex is a mouthful so let's just call it our "new brain" to make it easier.

Before we became really smart and able to be consciously aware of things around us, we had a brain similar to most animals in some senses. Our older brain's job was all about survival and reproduction. This area of our brain is called the limbic system. The limbic system is the part of the brain which is involved in our behavioural and emotional responses, especially when it comes to behaviours we need for survival such as feeding, reproduction and caring for our young.[24] It's sometimes easier to think of our limbic system as our "old brain." Our old brain sits underneath the new brain and is made up of some areas that are crucial to understand when you are suffering with pain.

As I said in previous chapters I don't want to get too scientific and use words that may lose or confuse you but, in this case, I will sometimes need to make an exception, because the limbic system is one of the main drivers when it comes to pain. The limbic system is our primal survival part of the brain and is home to three areas I want to focus on, called the hippocampus, amygdala and hypothalamus.

We will begin with the hippocampus.

The hippocampus

Brain parts often have odd names, the hippocampus being one of them. Early neuroscientists didn't fully understand the functions of parts of the brain so they named the parts by what they looked like. The hippocampus means "seahorse" in Greek, as it resembles a seahorse. As neuroscience progressed, more areas of the brain instead became known for their functions. In 1952, in one of the most famous cases in neuroscience history, a patient named Henry Molaison or H.M. as he became known, had both his hippocampi surgically removed due to ongoing seizures after he was involved in an accident as a kid. William Scoville, a neurosurgeon known for experimental surgeries, offered H.M. this risky procedure. What resulted from this surgery would make H.M. the most studied person in neuroscience history; he would change our understanding of how memory is formed. Upon waking up from his surgery, the initial assessment looked promising. H.M.'s seizures had stopped, but one thing was different: H.M. wasn't able to form new memories,[25] specifically explicit or declarative memories. An example would be remembering what you had for breakfast or learning how to spell a new word. The hippocampus doesn't save the memory, it just consolidates the memory from its respective areas of the brain, sort of like a librarian. If you need a book, the librarian knows where to find it – when you need to retrieve the memory, the hippocampus knows where to find it.

In H.M.'s case he couldn't create new memories because he didn't have a hippocampus to consolidate them anymore. All he had was a window of approximately fifteen minutes before he completely forgot what he had just learned. So, he would sit and watch the same movies over and over again and never remember a thing about them. But oddly he could still remember things from the past. This is because, if a memory is important enough, the hippocampus replays it over and over, areas of the brain where memory is stored communicate to each other independently of the hippocampus. This is how a short-term memory is transferred into a long-term memory.[26]

This mostly happens when you're asleep. The hippocampus seems to be involved in the replaying of the memory over and over in your brain, almost as if it's burning the memory into a hard-drive.[27] This may also explain why some traumas turn into nightmares; this is because the memory is replaying because of its significance or importance. Storing bad memories or traumas may not be pleasant but, to the brain, they are important as they help us to avoid or be better prepared for something similar. Emotional memories are stored more vividly. Think of 9/11 or when Princess Diana died. Everyone knows where they were when they heard that news, because there is a lot of emotion stored with memories like this. The more emotive the memory, the more likely it is to be remembered. And this brings us to the amygdala.

The amygdala is the area of the brain that is most active in processing negative emotions such as worry, anger and most notably fear. It translates to the name "almond" because, you've guessed it, it is shaped like an almond. The amygdala forms associations to memory with emotions and triggers responses. For instance, if you get bitten by a snake, the significance of this information will be stored in the amygdala for future reference.[28] In the future, if you heard a hiss, this would provoke a fear response from the amygdala and it would initiate a fight-or-flight response as a result. Before the bite, the hissing sound alone wasn't enough to create a fear response but after the bite the amygdala learned that a hiss spells potential danger so it associates fear with a hiss. Now the hiss on its own is enough to activate a fight-or-flight response. This process is called classic conditioning and it's the most commonly understood way that conditioning happens in humans.[29]

The amygdala gets direct sensory information, stores it and learns it on its own.[30] It doesn't have to learn what emotion is. The emotion is hard-wired in the amygdala. It just learns what causes the reaction. For example, we don't have to learn how to be scared, we just learn what to be scared of. Once the trigger is enough to provoke a response from the amygdala, the amygdala sends a message to an area of the brain called the **hypothalamus**, which is the control centre of the endocrine system and nervous system when it comes to regulation of homeostasis.[31] From here there is a release of specific hormones that activate our fight-or-flight response and further release of cortisol and adrenaline from the adrenal glands.[32] This stress response system is called the hypothalamic-pituitary-adrenal axis or HPA-axis for short. Now bear with me for a second, because there is a reason why I'm going into so much detail here. We have already spoken about the role of the hippocampus, which is largely about memory consolidation, but another of its roles is to inhibit or control the activity of the HPA-axis.[33]

Sustained chronic stress actually reduces the size of the hippocampus. This not only makes it harder to form new memories but also, when the hippocampus deteriorates due to chronic stress, its ability to control the stress response weakens.[34] This feeds back into the stress response by limiting the control of the stress response and increasing the efficiency of the stress. Hypothetically speaking, something that wouldn't have caused a stress response in the past is now more likely to as the hippocampus's ability to control the stress response has diminished.

These three areas of the brain have been critical for our survival, because, if you were attacked by a lion the memory would be consolidated by the hippocampus and the associated fear would be stored in the amygdala. The hippocampus would retrieve information about the experience that might be useful, for example the associated environment, weather, sounds, and smells. All of these can be linked to the emotion of fear. If in the future you went into an area that was similar or you smelled something that was similar to the lion, your body's protective responses would kick into gear, and you would become more alert and prepare yourself for fight or flight. So, thank God we have a system like this.

Past experiences

So, it's pivotal for the brain to store memories from the past to keep you safe in the future. This has been a key survival tool that has served us very well throughout our existence.

In everyday life, this system works well. For instance, let's say you injured your back while lifting a basket of washing. Fast forward a couple of weeks, the pain in your back has gone away and life has gone back to normal. When you go to lift the basket the next time your brain remembers that you injured your back before and it doesn't want you to injure yourself again. So, it will use the information it has stored to avoid that. Because of the stored negative experience, a symptom of pain or tightness can be produced before, during or after lifting the basket just to remind you to be extra careful doing it. In fact, if the pain was sufficiently bad, just the thought of doing it may trigger a pain response.

Your brain has retrieved the negative experience and associated emotion. As a result, it can provoke a protective response such as fear, pain, anxiety, elevated heart rate, or tightness. Or maybe the memory alone is enough to make you more diligent. In more extreme cases, even an inflammatory response can be triggered. This will be explained in greater detail in Chapter 10 when we are speaking about "the pain barrier line." But note that memory is stored for protective purposes and the brain is preparing for potential threat because of the past experiences that have been stored.

The limbic system (old brain) is comprised of many more areas than just the amygdala, hippocampus and hypothalamus, but for the purpose of explaining this system, it's easier just to mention these three areas.

The old and new brain

About 50,000 years ago, having an old and new brain working together was giving us a better chance of survival. We had to constantly predict whether there was a predator out there waiting to harm us. If we didn't predict this well enough, we were dead. So, the areas of the old brain would consolidate memories and related emotions from previous experiences in order to use that information to help us in the future.

The main differences between the old and the new brain is that the old brain's main priority is survival of the species. The old brain thinks in simple black and white facts. It doesn't like grey areas. Something is either threatening or it's not. Much of the time the old brain will dominate the new brain. This makes sense because our survival instincts are the priority. Once the old brain perceives there may be a threat it will take over and activate its fight-or-flight response, even if there isn't any real danger. The danger can be just perceived. Back when we lived in caves, there were many more dangers to be aware of: not just vicious animals, but also other tribes, weather, rough landscapes and terrains. Many of the perceived dangers were justified and the fight-or-flight response was appropriate. Nowadays we don't have these types of threats in the western world. "Tribes" are governed by law. You cannot just decide to kill someone without consequences. Vicious animals aren't just roaming the towns and cities hunting for food; we live in secure homes and we don't have to walk through dangerous terrain to get from A to B (for the most part, anyway).

The new brain thinks logically and wants to find the meaning in things. Sometimes the new brain can calm the old brain down with reassurance and logical thinking, for instance if there is a sound of rustling in the bushes the logical new brain would say, "Don't worry, I saw a family of rabbits around the bushes. If there was a lion there the bunnies wouldn't be there." This may calm the old brain down so it moves back into the rest-and-digest phase. In other cases, the new brain backs up the old brain and logically says, "I saw some lions around that bush yesterday," thus pushing the old brain further into the fight-or-flight response, and for good reason.

You're probably thinking, "So what the hell have bunny rabbits and lions got to do with my pain?" Don't worry; I'm getting to the point, I promise.

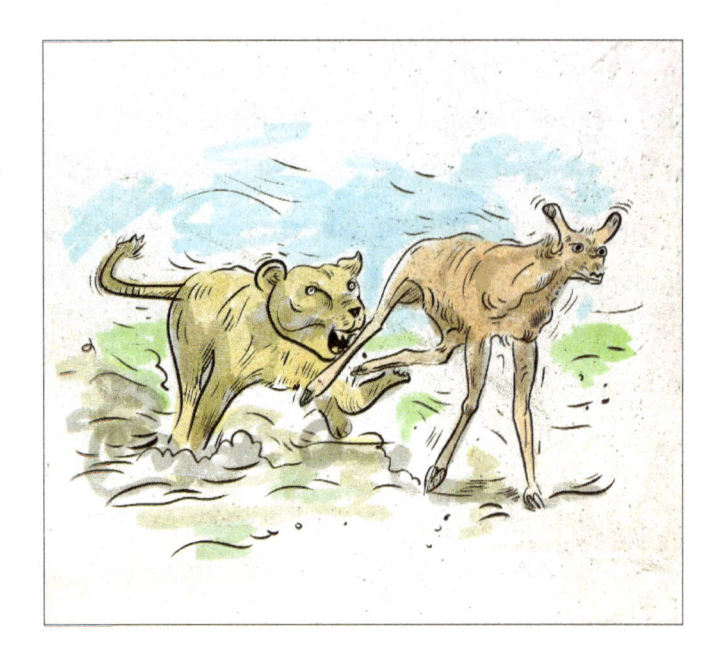

Deer and lion

If you've ever watched *Animal Planet*, you will have seen a lion chase after a deer. If the deer was lucky enough to get away, you may have seen the deer eating some grass a few minutes later. This is a perfect example of the deer's old brain kicking into its fight-or-flight response mode in order to get away from the lion. If the deer was lucky enough to escape, it doesn't take it long before it goes back into rest-and-digest mode and starts eating grass again.

Can you imagine if you were attacked by a lion and, as soon as you got away, you sat down and ate a Sunday roast? This would never happen because our more sophisticated new brain would be evaluating what had just happened. The new brain would process what happened and imagining what could have happened if the lion had managed to get its claws into you.

The shock, fear, worry, anxiety and stress of running this scenario over and over in your head would be relentless. You would be telling everyone you saw that you were almost eaten by a lion. The last thing you would be thinking about is food. This is a classic example of how the new and old brain do work and, arguably, don't work together. The new brain would be reliving the incident using memory and imagination. What's fascinating is that the brain doesn't know the difference between real and imaginary.[35] As you keep imagining what a catastrophe it would have been if the lion had had you for dinner the brain Is reliving the incident over and over, thus strengthening the memory. Your heart rate is still elevated, muscles are engaged and you are prepared for fight or flight. Consequently, stress hormones are still being released even though the incident has long passed. So, because of your emotional image of what might have happened, you physically react too.

In our distant past, it was useful to go over the memories of being attacked by a lion. This is a healthy system if you live in the wild and need to replay dangerous incidents in your head so you are better prepared for the next time. By being able to do this you increase your survival chances, as you can plan what you are going to do the next time if a similar situation arises. You might think to yourself... if a lion runs at me this is what I am going to do. Today, the same might be true if you make a mistake driving and narrowly avoid a serious accident.

But twenty-first-century life has changed dramatically while our brains haven't. We have inherited this system but we often misuse it in the modern world. We replay incidents that are not threatening over and over in our heads, even if there is nothing useful to take from them. We go on thinking about things like what somebody said to us at work or imagining worst-case scenarios about our pain, injuries or surgeries. This process of reinforcing negative memories increases fear, worry and anger and keeps you in fight-or-flight mode, ultimately changing the brain for the worst.

The new brain can be a bad influence

As humans, we worry and catastrophise about injuries and pain.

Our new brain is trying to find the logic and meaning of the pain. It is asking, "Is it because of my arthritis, my bulging disk or a trapped nerve?" It will use its inquisitive nature to try and find the answer. We live in an information-packed world where we can often find the answer to whatever we want at the click of a mouse. Though I say "the answer" loosely, because most of the time the place where we find "the answer" isn't the right place to get "the answer."

Poor knowledge of pain can allow the new brain to reinforce the old brain with what you believe to be true. This is where the old brain and the new brain may be technically working together but in reality, it's self-sabotage. It can be a case of the blind leading the blind.

The new brain is using its logic, based on negative beliefs and wrong information. This will reinforce the old brain's decision to go into fight-or-flight. But the reinforcement by the new brain can be based around poor or wrong information that you may have retrieved from a Google search, a friend or even a healthcare practitioner. For example, you may have injured yourself picking up that basket of washing. This information will be stored for the future in case the same situation arises. But in the meantime, you read somewhere that a bulging disc has similar symptoms to what you are experiencing. Now, your new brain's logical thought is that the reason you injured your back is because of a bulging disc. If you combine this with the information that is saved by the old brain you are creating a perfect storm which is going to push you into an overly protective response anytime you go to pick something up.

It's important to note that this is not your fault. This is just the way our brains have evolved over time. Your brain's job is to keep you safe and avoid any danger; it is doing that job, but in some cases, it's overdoing it without us being aware of it. This brain of ours has arguably been like this for hundreds of thousands of years and it's unlikely our brain's evolution will ever catch up with the modern world given the speed of technological advancement. All we can do is try to educate ourselves as best as possible. Having a better understanding of your stress response is a great start to understanding yourself and how you respond to stressors.

Remember; stress is a good thing. It's healthy and necessary for growth. Our stress response system was only designed for short term stress, not long-term stress.

Danger = Deal with immediate threat

Safety = Relax and recuperate

But we live in a world where our stress response is never switched off. Mortgage payments, work, family life, relationships, the news, health concerns are all things that keep our body in a state of fight-or-flight, a state of readiness for a lion that isn't in the bushes.

Breathing

Breathing is the most necessary function of life. Every living creature needs to breathe to survive. It's the first thing any mammal that has ever lived has done when they came out of the womb and it's the last thing they did before they died. It's so necessary that, after not doing it for approximately three minutes, the average human will lose consciousness and die. But for something that is so essential to life, why is it taken for granted?

Unless of course if you're a yoga teacher, deep sea diver or a Buddhist, you probably never think about how you breathe. And why would you? First of all, breathing is done automatically. The air you breathe is all around you in abundance and you don't really have to look for it. We don't ever really have to look for some air so it's not really on the top of our priority list. It's not as if you have to write it down on your to-do list. So, for those reasons alone, it can be taken for granted. It's only when something becomes scarce that we become concerned or start to take notice. If for some reason there was a shortage of oxygen, it would become top of the priority list. But this doesn't really apply to the average person.

However, although air is all around us in abundance, there is a large portion of the population that doesn't breathe very well. This is probably an understatement. Today people tend to take too many breaths. It's estimated that on average we take twice the number of breaths that we did one hundred years ago. As well as that, in some studies up to 50% of people breathe through their mouth.[36] You might question what's wrong with this. Well, it's true there is still oxygen going into your lungs but James Nestor, author of *Breath*, summed this up nicely by saying "breathing through your mouth is going to allow you to survive but it doesn't mean it's healthy."

Let's just sort through the differences between mouth breathing and nasal breathing. Your nasal cavity is not just a hole in your face. Your nose is a complex organ that serves a purpose. Not only does breathing through your nose filter out chemicals, bacteria, dust and pollution. It also humidifies and heats the temperature of the air arriving, which helps increase oxygen absorption by up to 20% within the lungs. Nasal breathing also increases the production of nitrous oxide, a gas that travels with the air to the lungs, which helps dilate the blood vessels in the lungs.[37] This vasodilation helps with oxygen absorption. If there is more oxygen absorbed with each breath, fewer breaths will be required.

There is a resistance when breathing through your nose. This nasal resistance slows down the breath in order to allow all of the above to happen; the slower breathing also allows time for the gas exchange between the oxygen arriving and the carbon dioxide leaving.

A mouth breath on the other hand takes in non-filtered, non-humidified air with up to six times less nitrous oxide. As a mouth breath meets no resistance, the breath is faster so there isn't enough time for your lungs to maximise the amount of oxygen absorption before it has to leave again. It seems counterintuitive, but the slower the breathing, the more oxygen is absorbed.

A mouth breath also tends to be shallower and more chest-dominated. According to the textbook *Respiratory Physiology* (West, 2000), the lower 10% of the lungs transport more than 40 ml of oxygen per minute, while the upper 10% of the lungs transport less than 6 ml per minute.

So, you could say that shallow chest breathing is starving yourself of oxygen, which is why you take more chest breaths per minute. Some studies show that the average person takes twenty breaths per minute.[38] That's a breath cycle every three seconds. This amount of breathing is a form of hyperventilation. I know when we think of someone hyperventilating we tend to think of somebody who is panicking and is given a brown paper bag to breathe into to calm down. But hyperventilating really just means over-breathing. This over-breathing affects up to 50% of the population.[39]

There are several reasons why someone could develop this way of breathing, for example through living or working in a stressful environment, obesity or overeating, poor physical fitness, anxiety,

PTSD, pain or genetics. Another interesting reason is because of evolutionary changes we have been through. Human beings' jaws have become smaller over the last 400 years due to the fact that we eat softer foods. This smaller jaw reduces the size of our airway, which can promote mouth breathing.[40]

Hyperventilation and your fight-or-flight response go hand in hand. Think about being scared, panicking or exercising. Your heart rate is elevated and your breath becomes shallower and more chest-dominated. This is okay when you are in an emergency but not when you're reading through emails, worrying about mortgage payments or even watching television. Like anything we do as humans the more we do it, the more conditioned we become to doing it until this is how we breathe normally.

Considering we breathe 25,000 times per day this constant state of stress compounds and uses up a lot of unnecessary resources. This can affect recovery, cell growth, sleep quality, immune function, digestion and of course pain.

Bracing and holding your breath

Imagine having to be reminded to breathe. It sounds strange but this is something that I have to remind my clients to do on a daily basis. During my initial assessment with my clients, one of the first things I get my clients to do is to ask them to pick up a tiny foam wedge that's in my office; I strategically leave it lying in the middle of the floor. Most of them are clever enough to figure out that this is a cheeky but subtle way to assess what type of posture they are adopting during the lift. And yes, that is something I will be looking out for but it's not the only thing. Another key aspect I am looking out for is how they are breathing during the movement. Are they gasping for air and holding their breath during the movement? More often than not, when someone is in pain and asked to perform a movement, if there is an expectation that something is going to hurt, they will take in a big influx of air, hold their breath, brace and then perform the movement.

This bracing and breath holding is an attempt to "protect" themselves from pain. This is normal behaviour for someone who is in pain. Nobody wants to feel pain so they adopt a bracing posture in an attempt to mitigate their pain. Ironically this protective bracing does everything but mitigate pain. Certainly, over the long term anyway.

The reason why this test is important is because I believe that, if somebody feels the need to hold their breath when picking up something as light as this foam wedge, then they are most likely holding their breath when they are doing any physical daily task. If that is the case then we could be talking hundreds of times per day, from picking up the letters from the postman to putting a glass in the cupboard.

Let's take a look at what we do when we hold our breath. We hold our breath when we feel we need to guard something or if we anticipate danger. Again, most of the time this is done on an unconscious level and it usually starts when pain begins to manifest in the first place. Nobody likes the feeling of pain during movement, so the thought of doing something that may be painful will trigger these protective responses.

Tensing up, holding your breath and guarding is common with pain sufferers to whom it may seem the most logical thing to do.

In the short term, bracing may provide you with some protection. Or at the very least it will give you the sense that you are protecting yourself. However, in the long term, it becomes part of the problem. Bracing, especially if you're bracing because you don't feel safe doing the movement or if there is a history of injury in that position, can enhance sympathetic nervous system (fight or flight) response. It's not something that you would be paying attention to and you often wouldn't even realise you're doing it.

If you're holding your breath when making a specific movement, on a subconscious level, you're telling your brain that you don't feel safe making this movement. So, the perception is danger.

So, if you don't feel safe putting a glass in a cupboard or picking up the wedge, you hold your breath in anticipation of pain. This anticipation of pain will arouse pain-creating regions and actually contribute to pain, ironically. The expectation that this could hurt feeds itself and can make pain worse. The more often you do this the more it becomes wired in the brain and it can become another paired association due to neuroplasticity changes.

How much do you breathe? (An exercise)

A simple way to find out how much you breathe is to count your breaths. You can do this now by lying down on a bed or sitting upright on a chair.

Put one hand on your chest and one hand on your belly. Set a timer on your phone to one minute and just breathe as normal. One inhale and one exhale equate to one breath cycle. Count how many breath cycles you complete in one minute. On average we should take about six to ten breaths per minute under normal stress-free circumstances. The further you are above the average, the harder your body is working and the less efficient it is.

And also take into consideration that, if you're reading this book, you should be as relaxed as you probably ever will be on a normal day. What if you're in the office trying to get work done or if you're in an environment where there is a lot of stress? Then you would expect that it will be much higher. So, I would recommend trying this in a few settings. Test yourself in the morning, at work and in bed before sleep.

There is another thing I want you to pay attention to. You can do this after your breathing test. Lie back down and put one hand over your belly and the other over your chest again. During your breath cycle, if the hand over your belly isn't rising first and your chest is, then you are not accessing the deeper part of your lungs. This is something we will work on improving later. For now, just take note of this in the notes section.

It doesn't have to be pain that is causing this dysfunctional breathing. Poor knowledge, fear of movement or being self-conscious of weight can also promote sucking in your belly when breathing.

Don't worry if your breathing rate is high now. Your body is capable of managing under stressful circumstances. In fact, it thrives under stress. It's only when there is no break from the stress, when your breathing is constantly elevated, that it starts to become pathogenic and problems start to arise. If you notice that your breathing is elevated during the day, then don't get bogged down thinking this is a negative. Think of it as a positive because it's one thing that hasn't been identified before that we can start to change straight away.

NOTES

Chapter 4

Biological

Pain that is disproportionate to the stimulus

I will start this biopsychosocial model explanation with the "bio," or biological, part of this model.

The biological aspect of pain used to be treated as the exclusive cause of pain, but now we know that pain is a complex multifactorial experience involving biological, psychological and emotional processes. With that being said there can be a misconception that the biological aspect doesn't matter as much when it comes to chronic pain.

I want to be clear here. Just because the biopsychosocial model has gained some traction and we're moving away from the conventional biomedical model, I have seen a tendency to dismiss the bio part of this model and focus more on the psychological and social aspects.

I want to quash this right now. All of these areas are important, especially the biological aspect. Just because I suggest the biological aspect isn't the sole cause of pain doesn't mean that it can't be the primary cause of pain. And when we speak about pain being disproportionate to tissue health don't take that to mean that we should disregard the biological aspect of this model when dealing with chronic pain.

It can certainly be argued that the biological aspect is the most important aspect of the model when dealing with acute pain, while there are more complex processes to consider when dealing with chronic pain. But there still is a large biological factor when dealing with chronic pain.

What people most associate with the biological aspect of the biopsychosocial model is the state of the body's tissues. But the biological aspect of the biopsychosocial model is about more than just tissue.

Here we will go through all the relevant biological aspects and how they influence pain. Remember to take note of whatever you think is relevant to your situation and write it in the notes area at the end of this chapter.

Let's begin

In Chapter 2 I explained what a nociceptor is and how important its role is. Now I want to just dive into this a little more. Nociceptors are important when it comes to the majority of pain, so I guess it's important that you know more about them.

First off, nociceptors becoming sensitised is a normal physiological process. This is essential when it helps avoid injury or helps your tissues to heal. However, prolonged sensitivity to nociceptors beyond the healing phase can become unhelpful and can lead to disability, fear of movement, weakness and, you guessed it, chronic pain.

Just to recap, nociceptors are stimulated in three ways:

Mechanical – pinching, pressure, stretch, strain

Chemical – chemical changes within the body, lactic acid, corrosive chemicals, or venom

Thermal – changes in temperature (too hot or too cold)

Each area has its own respective nociceptive threshold. Nociceptors are not your regular type of receptor. They don't just pick up any stimulus that passes by. Nociceptors are specialised receptors that only detect a stimulus indicating actual or potential danger. For that reason, in order for a nociceptor to be stimulated, the stimulus has to be strong enough to pass a threshold. It's a prerequisite. Otherwise, the nociceptor will not take any notice.[41]

For a mechanical nociceptor (mechanoreceptors) to be stimulated, there needs to be a certain amount of pressure or strain on the tissue. For a thermal nociceptor (thermoreceptors), the immediate environment has to reach a temperature that is either too hot or too cold, and for a chemical nociceptor (chemoreceptors) there needs to be enough changes in such things as CO_2 or Ph level in the blood, or corrosive chemicals for the nociceptor to fire off its message.

When I talk in this book about nociceptors, I am mainly talking about the mechanical receptors in the periphery. These nociceptors innervate your muscles, ligaments, bones, organs and all other soft tissue.

Peripheral sensitisation is the result of a nociceptor in the periphery becoming sensitised, which results in them becoming excited with less stimulation. There can be a number of reasons why a nociceptor cannot only become sensitised but also stay sensitised.

Tissue damage – The first and most obvious way for a nociceptor to fire is if there is tissue damage. After an injury, nociceptor thresholds are lowered, making it easier for them to become excited and send information up to the brain. This is just a protective measure to warn you that there is tissue damage, to help avoid further injury and to allow your tissue to heal.

Recently, my friend Mary was out walking when she tripped and went over on her ankle, spraining it. Today she needed to get down to the shops to buy some groceries. As she walked out her door and down her driveway, she was experiencing pain in her ankle. Every step she took, the pain was getting worse and worse. A common belief is that because Mary continues to try to walk on it and the pain increases, she is causing more and more damage. Although this sounds reasonable, it's unlikely to be true.

Obviously before the ankle sprain, she was able to walk to the shops without pain, but due to the tissue in her ankle being injured, the threshold of the nociceptors in her ankle has lowered, making them more excited faster than before her accident. This is a great system, by the way. We want this to happen because, if it didn't happen, Mary would continue to do things that could further damage the injured tissue and disrupt the healing process. So, the nociceptors fire off information up to the brain to warn the brain that there is still tissue damage. The brain evaluates the information and makes pain to communicate this to Mary. So, Mary listens to her body, goes home and rests her ankle and allows the healing process to do its thing.

Inflammation is the second way nociceptors can become excited more easily. Where there is tissue damage, there will be inflammation. When there is tissue damage the immune system releases substances called inflammatory mediators. These inflammatory mediators lower the threshold of the nociceptors, making them more excitable so that they fire off with less stimulation.

Inflammation reduces the threshold of the nociceptors around the areas that are infected or injured. The reason for this is that, because the healing process is underway the brain wants you to be aware of it so you don't try to do too much too soon. Inflammation can also reduce the threshold of neighbouring nociceptors to the site of injury even if there is no injury to that area. This is why, when areas are inflamed, there can be widespread pain initially but, as the inflammation reduces, the pain becomes more localised to the site of injury.

Here's the kicker. This can happen even if there is no tissue damage. But more about this in a little while.

Repetitive stimulation to nociceptors over a sustained period of time can also lower the threshold of the nociceptor. You don't even have to be injured for this to happen. Just consistently crossing over the threshold of nociceptor is enough to reduce the threshold so that it takes less to set it off the next time.[42]

A few months after Mary sprained her ankle, all of the tissue that was previously damaged has healed, but she is still experiencing pain. One reason that she's still in pain is that she's been constantly using her ankle while it was injured. She continuously crossed over the reduced threshold line of the nociceptors, which allowed them to fire off messages to the brain more easily. The constant over-stimulation of the nociceptors in her ankle resulted in her ankle becoming sensitised. Soft tissue heals within a three-to-six-month period. But even if the tissue has healed, the nociceptor threshold can stay lowered in this way. This is very common with chronic pain sufferers.

Weak tissue – Tissue that is weaker is more likely to contribute to nociceptors getting excited much sooner than stronger or more conditioned tissue.[43] If tissue becomes deconditioned after prolonged inactivity or injury, it is more susceptible to injury or re-injury, due to the tissue being less physically capable of actions that were previously habitual. Also, if tissue is weak, you're more likely to get injured.[44]

In Mary's case she has been in pain for a few months with her ankle injury. Pain motivated her to undertake less physical activity and because of this reduced physical activity, her tissue became deconditioned compared to what it was like before the injury. So, the injury to the tissue was the primary cause to the reduction in the nociceptor threshold but, since then, the injury has healed. However, now, because of Mary's inactivity, the tissue there has become deconditioned and now that is the primary cause of her nociceptor threshold remaining low.

If you don't work them, muscles get smaller. If they are smaller, they will be able to do less activity. This will lead to pain sooner than if they were strong and conditioned.[45]

When people take time away from activity due to injury, work, or family commitments, I find that many of them compare themselves to who they were two, five, or even ten years ago. Humans by nature are ego-driven and we compare ourselves to who we were when we were at our peak fitness. So, when we return to activity we want to get as close as possible to how we were when we were at our peak. This often results in people doing too much too soon and sensitising their nociceptors, especially if the reason for the inactivity was a previous injury. This is something that I am going to help you avoid in your recovery plan (Chapter 10). We will have a step-by-step process to reduce the chances of doing too much too soon.

Weak tissue can include an unstable joint. If muscles or ligaments are not strong enough to stabilise the joint then they could be considered weak. Again, going back to Mary's ankle sprain, another potential reason why she was experiencing prolonged pain was that her ankle wasn't strong enough to stabilise itself. Think about it, if a joint is unstable and there is an increased potential for injury then you want these nociceptors active, to warn you that something still isn't right. But a lot of people just misinterpret this message and assume that it's still injured or it hasn't healed right. It's another reason not to self-diagnose. A reputable trained professional should figure this out in no time.

How much of this do you, "the patient," need to know? Honestly, not a whole lot. It should be the practitioner that figures this out. But the mere fact that you've resorted to buying this book suggests you haven't found answers to why you're in pain.

How can you help figure out if your nociceptor threshold has been lowered?

Ask yourself these questions:

- Are you injured? Remember tissue heals within three to six months so if it has persisted beyond that it is unlikely to be due to injury, unless of course you are unlucky enough to keep injuring yourself. Humans are very adaptable and resilient so to keep injuring yourself over and over is unlikely but not impossible.

- Have you ever been diagnosed with an autoimmune condition such as type 1 diabetes, rheumatoid arthritis, psoriatic arthritis or lupus?

- Is your tissue deconditioned or has it become deconditioned? This could be because of injury or inactivity. Muscles not getting stimulated get smaller and bones become less resilient. It's simple science. Avoidance of activity because of pain can end up contributing to further pain, because of your tissues becoming deconditioned. This is very common in pain sufferers. So, a question to ask yourself is how conditioned are you? Do you work out or do a physical job, and do you feel strong?

- Are you doing too much activity? Overtraining and prolonged activity such as standing, walking, or repetitive movements can all contribute to nociceptor thresholds being lowered. Constantly repeating the same movements over and over can sensitise the receptors.

- Is there inflammation? You may have higher inflammatory markers in your blood or there could be visible acute inflammation in the tissue.

If any of these are related to your situation, write them down at the end of this chapter and we will come back to them later.

Central sensitisation

Central sensitisation is a condition that affects many chronic pain sufferers. It's a process where the nociceptors in the periphery continuously bombard the central nervous system with impulses.

The nociceptive threshold can be breached and start to produce these nerve impulses due to injury, surgery, illness or a repetitive strain. Once the impulses reach the spinal cord, this is where the sensitivity happens.

What should happen in a non-sensitised system is that, when nerve impulses reach the spinal cord from the periphery, the nerve impulses are sent up to the brain to be interpreted. But once central sensitisation starts to occur, the nerve impulse that arrives at the spinal cord becomes augmented. Imagine you have a microphone and an amp. If you speak into the microphone, the sound of your voice travels through the microphone to the amp where the sound of your voice is augmented. Suddenly everybody can hear you speaking at a louder volume. When central sensitisation occurs, the nerve impulses arriving at the spinal cord are amplified before being sent up to the brain. The brain processes the information arriving as more of a threat due to the amplified nerve impulse, which results in even the lightest touch on the skin being perceived as if you have been hit by a hammer.

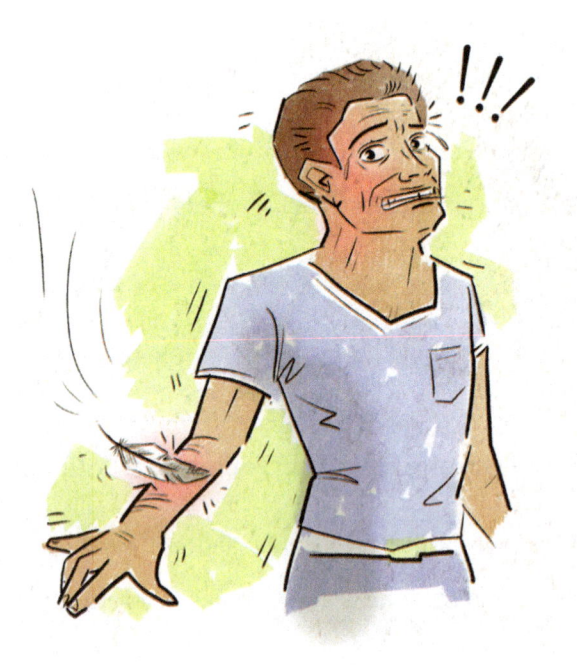

As it gets more and more sensitised it reacts more vigorously to less input. This process is called "Wind Up." Because this process has happened before, the spinal cord remembers the pattern, so this information isn't even sent to the brain for interpretation. The spinal cord does all the work and pain is experienced at this level. Other senses can become sensitised too. You may become sensitised to light, sound, taste or smell.

The key aspect of central sensitisation is purely a sensory problem. The plasticity of the nervous system has altered to influence pain by way of amplification of nerve stimuli, reduction of inhibitory molecules and an increase of synaptic efficiency, meaning it's an ever-changing complex condition. Central sensitisation is involved in a large proportion of chronic pain conditions.[46]

Inflammation

Inflammation is a biological miracle. But we often don't look at it this way. We look at inflammation as if it's something evolution has got wrong that we need to eliminate. As soon as inflammation occurs, the priority is to reduce or remove it. Throughout my sporting life if I ever had any injuries and there was some noticeable inflammation, my first instinct was to reduce it. To me it was a nuisance that I wanted to minimise if I could. I would take measures such as applying ice, heat, elevating the body part, having a massage, or taking some anti-inflammatories. And this thought process was common with athletes in any sport I was involved with. It still is today.

Often, I would go to the doctor's office, where I would be prescribed stronger anti-inflammatories, which I would gladly take. It never occurred to me what inflammation's purpose was and why it was there in the first place. It wasn't until I became involved in healthcare that I started to question the logic of why we would try to get rid of something that our body produces when there is an injury. Surely to God, Mother Nature hasn't made a big mistake in producing inflammation when we are injured. The more I researched and questioned this logic, the more I learned that I had been making a mistake.

It definitely gets an unjustified bad reputation. Maybe we just don't like inflammation because it hurts. It may hurt, but it serves a vital purpose. Inflammation is the process whereby the immune system recognises and removes harmful and foreign stimuli and begins the healing process.

Like pain, there are two ways we classify inflammation: acute or chronic inflammation. We're all familiar with acute inflammation. We will have all experienced this at some point in our life. When inflammation occurs, you may experience redness, heat, swelling, pain or loss of function to the inflamed area. Acute inflammation is short-lived and it's generally involved when there are infections, viruses, bacteria, or injuries to the body.

A typical immune response

If there are any intruders in your body, inflammation is the first line of defence. When an inflammation occurs in your body, many different immune system cells get involved. The immune system releases various substances known as inflammatory mediators. These include the hormones bradykinin and histamine which cause the small blood vessels in the tissue to dilate, allowing more blood to reach the injured or infected tissue. For this reason, inflamed areas turn red and feel hot. [47]

The immune system works better at higher temperatures – it's harder for viruses to grow at 40 degrees. The increased blood flow also allows more immune system cells to be carried to the injured tissue, where they help remove damaged tissue components so that the body can begin to heal.

Inflammation is required for growth. We have already spoken about homeostasis and how the body is always trying to restore balance. Inflammation is a part of this too. When there is an injury, inflammation helps to restore the body's tissues. For example, if you go for a long walk or run and you feel stiff or sore the next day. This stiffness and soreness is inflammation working to heal microscopic tears from your exercise. The presence of inflammation sensitises the nociceptors, which increases sensitivity in the areas that have been worked out.

Let's go back to the house alarm analogy. Inflammation can be the fire service, police and the paramedics. Inflammation does a number of things. If there is a house fire, inflammation is sent down immediately, just like the fire service, to help put out the fire and help stop the damage getting worse. If there are any intruders in the system like a virus or bacteria, inflammation acts like the police service and is sent down to get rid of them. If there is any tissue damage, inflammation acts like the paramedics, the first responders on the scene, to start the healing process.

Swelling beyond the injured area is another way of restricting movement in your joint. Inflammation can make a joint feel heavier, and have less strength or loss of function. That feeling of loss of power or heaviness grabs your attention and makes you feel like you don't want to use the joint. These are clever ways in which your immune system protects you from further injury and encourages healing.

The inflammatory nociception feedback loop

So, both nociceptors and inflammation act as protective mechanisms. But in some cases, inflammation that is left untreated can create a negative feedback loop cycle. Inflammation that is produced sensitises the nociceptors, which in turn increases the inflammation being produced. This cycle can continue: the inflammation lowers the threshold of the nociceptors; the nociceptors fire off messages, which cause an inflammatory response.[48] It's as if the monitored alarm system is getting calls to say that there has been a break-in and as a response the police are sent over to the house to make sure everything is okay. As the police break in the back door to check, this sets off the alarm again, and more police officers are sent as a result and the cycle continues.

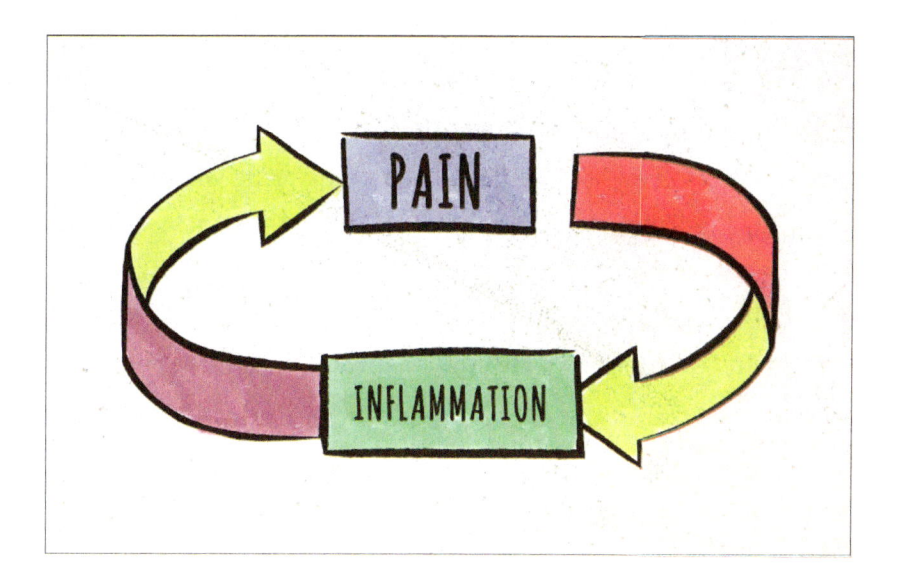

The immune system can also learn to react independently without the help of the nervous system.[49] It can start trying to sense danger on its own. This is like the police randomly turning up to your house without being called by the alarm system, because they had a hunch that things weren't okay. This learned response by the immune system is not a helpful inflammatory process.

An inflammatory response can be triggered by movements that previously caused injury, overuse, fear of movement, poor sleep or elevated stress levels. In some studies, just thinking about movement has been shown to be sufficient to trigger an inflammatory response.[50] So there are two sides to inflammation. Acute inflammation restores, protects and regenerates tissue. It's like a wonder fluid cure and we should be glad we have it. But just like pain, inflammation isn't without its flaws. This is especially true when it comes to chronic inflammation.

Chronic inflammation

Chronic inflammation is inflammation that persists beyond a period of several months to years.[51] It's like that annoying uncle who overstays his welcome or just calls in unannounced.

Chronic inflammation diseases are the most significant cause of death in the world. In fact, the World Health Organization (WHO) ranks chronic diseases as the greatest threat to human health. Worldwide, three out of five people die due to chronic inflammatory diseases such as stroke, chronic respiratory diseases, heart disorders, cancer, obesity and diabetes.[52]

Chronic inflammation is distinct from acute inflammation because, when it becomes chronic, the immune system can become inflammatory and produce inflammation when there is no threat to the body or healing to be done. An immune system that is inflammatory is not a healthy immune system. Chronic inflammation can manifest as acute inflammation or recurrent episodes of acute inflammation that can eventually end up becoming chronic. In some cases, chronic inflammation is an independent response that doesn't develop after acute inflammation, for example, in diseases such as tuberculosis and rheumatoid arthritis. In cases like these the body perceives normal tissue as a foreign object (a thorn or a virus for example) and attacks it in a protective response, resulting in pain and more acute inflammation.[53] From the perspective of the body, it's under attack, so the immune system keeps on fighting.

Chronic inflammation can be difficult to identify because it's often invisible and doesn't show the tell-tale signs that acute inflammation causes (redness, heat, swelling and pain).

Acute vs systematic inflammation

Let's get back to the house alarm analogy. Imagine every now and again the monitored alarm system calls out the fire, police and ambulance services. The police arrive and start grabbing the occupants of the house, throwing them on the ground and putting them in cuffs, assuming that they have broken into the house. In all the commotion lamps are being knocked over and broken. Tables are being overturned, the front door has been kicked in. The house is getting messed up for no reason and has been turned upside down in order to get all the occupants out of the house, only to find that that there had been no break-in or intruders.

Chronic inflammation is like this. The immune system is primed and ready for an attack. But this primed readiness can be costly as, if left untreated, it can cause further damage or disease in the body's tissue.[54]

The protection is sent down to "protect" the part of the body that the brain or immune system feels requires it. But this protection causes collateral damage. As more tissue damage is caused, the immune system's own "protection" pain is amplified.

Should you get rid of inflammation?

Well, it's a difficult question. For acute injuries my personal view is that acute inflammation serves a vital purpose. So, you shouldn't be too quick to get rid of it straight away. In fact, more recent studies have shown that using non-steroid anti-inflammatory drugs (NSAIDs) too early can actually interfere with the healing process and affect how strong the tissue is when it heals.[55]

Even Dr Gabe Mirkin, MD, the creator of the Rest Ice Compression Elevation (RICE) approach, has since come out and said that he no longer endorses this method as it delays recovery by disrupting the natural inflammatory process. But again, this is for acute inflammation, when there is tissue damage to be resolved. Most of you reading this will have been suffering with pain for a long time, so you are less likely to have tissue damage. This suggests there is no benefit to your inflammation. If the inflammation isn't serving a purpose, then why keep it?

Sometimes it's not so easy to know if there's inflammation there at all.

Often, there are no obvious signs of inflammation when it's chronic. You can get bloods taken by your GP but even the tests can still sometimes be inaccurate. The best thing you can do is to take matters in your own hands and take steps that reduce pro-inflammatory cell production. Don't wait for a flare-up to take action. Prevention is always better than the cure. There are many areas that initiate the pro-inflammatory system. Here are some risk factors to watch out for:

Age. Increasing age is positively correlated with elevated levels of several inflammatory molecules. The age-associated increase in inflammatory molecules may be due to mitochondrial dysfunction or free radicals.

Obviously, you cannot change this, but it's important to note it's a risk factor.

Smoking. If you're a smoker it's probably not a shock to you that smoking is bad for your health. You're also probably sick of listening to people preaching to you that you need to quit. I'm not here to give you a lecture on quitting because you've probably heard it all before and may have attempted to stop many times. I actually did smoke myself for a few years. I started because, like many teenagers do, I thought it was cool. I'm probably hanging myself out to dry here, because I denied it to my parents for years. Luckily for me, I did manage to quit when I was around twenty years old. But as a twenty-year-old it would have been a lot easier to quit than your average chronic pain patient who is thirty-five plus. Most people start smoking in their teens, so by the time they reach their mid-thirties they could have been smoking for more than twenty years. This means it's harder than just putting down the cigarette and putting on a patch. Often it is ingrained in their identity. It's not just a habit. There's a physical craving but it can also be a short-term, unconscious coping mechanism for stress and pain relief.

But here is just how smoking interferes with the inflammatory process. And while I'm on the topic, I may as well explain how it interferes with pain in general.

Firstly, cigarette smoking is associated with lowering the production of anti-inflammatory molecules and inducing inflammation. This means that at times of physiological stress, poor sleep, or too much or too little physical activity, there can be an increase of a pro-inflammatory response and a lowered anti-inflammatory response. Whenever your body feels the need to produce inflammation it will be produced sooner, there will be more of it and it will stay for longer. In fact, smoking is the strongest risk factor for the inflammatory disease rheumatoid arthritis.[56]

Smoking and pain appear to be bi-directional, with pain increasing smoking behaviours and smoking increasing pain. Pain sufferers find it extremely difficult to quit because, in the early stages of quitting, any symptoms of pain increase, which encourages them to smoke again in order to help reduce the pain – chronic pain patients abstaining from smoking for 12–24 hours rated their pain 3.5 times higher than people who didn't abstain. This increase in pain will incentivise smoking as a coping mechanism and reduce the chances of giving up.[57]

Smoking also offers an opportunity for distraction. When you smoke there is a release of endorphins and dopamine in reward centres of the brain. This makes smoking pleasurable, which also offers a short-term analgesic effect. This seems to perpetuate smoking as a coping strategy for pain,[58] but the pain reduction is short-lived, as "Smokers with chronic pain have worsened overall symptoms of pain as well as worse sleep, and psychological and mood outcomes compared to non-smokers."

Generally speaking, smokers with chronic pain feel pain more intensely and take more opioid medications to mitigate their pain compared to non-smokers.[59]

I'm not here to wag my finger and tell you that you need to quit. This is just the information on how smoking can influence pain. You can decide what to do with it. For most, quitting smoking isn't going to cure chronic pain, but it will play a part in how much, how little and the type of inflammation your body produces. And, this isn't even scratching the surface. I am just outlining some important details that you should be aware of. If you really want to overcome your pain it is something you should at least consider.

If you are thinking about quitting, seek help, speak to your GP, and get a plan together. Go online and get involved in support groups and build a supportive community around you. You can do it with the right help, and many of the effects that smoking has on your body can be reversed.

Sleep. Getting irregular sleep can increase the amount of pro-inflammatory cells that are produced. Managing sleep disturbances should be considered an important factor in the overall management of inflammation. Since individuals with irregular sleep schedules are more likely to have chronic inflammation than consistent sleepers, sleep disorders are also considered to be one of the independent risk factors for chronic inflammation. But we will speak more about this later in Chapter 7. Sleep is so important it has its own chapter.

Stress and sleep disorders. Both physical and emotional stress are associated with inflammatory cytokine release. Stress can also cause sleep disorders.[60]

Leptin and ghrelin are hormones that regulate your appetite, and when you're not getting sufficient sleep, the production of these hormones is altered in a way that creates increased cravings for sugary foods. Insufficient sleep also affects your desire or motivation to exercise, which will fall back into the energy expenditure category.

Poverty. One major problem is poverty. It's now actually cheaper to go and buy a hamburger meal than it is to cook a healthy meal at home. If you're on the breadline, this can mean having too much fast food. Almost no fast food is healthy. Most of it will be processed and high in saturated fats and sugar. I will not focus on diet and nutrition, as it is not my forte. But I will say that having a poor diet, with high sugar and saturated fat, increases the likelihood of inflammation flare-ups. This is probably not a shock to you but sometimes it has to be emphasised.

Obesity. Humans are designed to be fat. Even humans that we would consider to have a low body fat percentage have a much higher body fat percentage than most primates.[61] The average primate has approximately 5–8% body fat whereas the average skinny human has approximately 15–20% body fat. Believe it or not, humans are even fatter than elephants, whose fat percentage is approximately 8–10%.

Our capacity to have excess fat is not by accident. It's not that we are a greedy species that overindulges on food. Additional fat for the human race is a necessity. The capacity for storing extra fat is ironically one of our strengths.

A lion's survival tool is its ability to overpower its prey. If lions became hungry and then suddenly found it difficult to catch their prey, it wouldn't be long before they were replaced as the kings of the jungle. A falcon's survival tool is its eyesight. Their eyesight is up to eight times better than humans' and they can spot small prey from up to two miles away. At times of hunger, if all of a sudden, their eyesight started to diminish, they would not survive long. The point I'm making is that these animals need their strengths to be as close to optimal levels as possible to survive.

As a human, our brain is our survival tool. The human brain is much more sophisticated than those of the rest of the animal kingdom. Comparing a human brain to that of any species in the animal kingdom is like comparing the Commodore 64 to a new MacBook Pro.

The human brain is conscious, it can plan, use imagination, think ahead, navigate, speak and understand language. To run a powerful brain like this is taxing and it requires a lot of energy to do so. This is one reason why humans need this capacity for storing more energy. Running this powerful brain takes up to 20% of our energy supply. Our brains are sapping energy just to function and we need to keep them fuelled.

A drop in cognitive ability could mean we get lost, and make poor decisions that could be fatal. We need to be able to make rational and perhaps life-altering decisions in times of famine. Fat stores that energy for us to do this. Having this capacity to store excess body fat helps us not only to fuel our powerful brains, but also allows us to travel away from our food sources, explore new territory and feed our infants for longer. This ability to store energy in the form of fat has allowed us to thrive and led us to where we are today.

Our fat cells are like a backup generator. When we eat, our body stores energy in the form of fat. When we run out of food our body turns to its fat cells and converts fat to fuel to keep our energy levels up. The problem is that our ability to store energy is endless. It would be great if we could just eat and recharge our batteries up to 100% and any of the energy that was consumed after we were fully charged was discarded. But unfortunately, the human body isn't a mobile phone or a laptop, and it doesn't work like that.

The longest period for which anyone has gone without solid food is 382 days in the case of Angus Barbieri of Tayport, Fife, who lived on tea, coffee, water, soda water and vitamins in Maryfield Hospital, Dundee, from June 1965 to July 1966. His weight declined from 214 kg (33 st 10 lb) to 80.74 kg (12 st 10 lb). But after over a year without food he still survived.

This isn't something I would recommend, as it's probably highly dangerous but this story at least illustrates how good a store of energy fat is. But this ability has been misused and now we have an obesity crisis. An obese individual is classed as anybody who has a body mass index (BMI) of above 30. For the record, the BMI test should perhaps not be the gold standard test to check for obesity. It is measured by your weight divided by your height. It does not take into account muscle mass or bone density. There are more sophisticated ways to measure obesity, but these are time-consuming and expensive. Using the BMI test, people like Dwayne "The Rock" Johnson and Mike Tyson (in his prime) would be classed as obese. So, it's certainly not a flawless test. Although it's imperfect, using a BMI test gives us a general consensus on a population scale, and there is no denying that obesity levels are a real problem. Much of this stems from an imbalance of energy expenditure and food quality. There are other contributing factors but these two in particular have caused obesity levels to go through the roof.[62] [63]

There is evidence of obese humans as far back as 25,000 years ago. So, obesity is not a new phenomenon. What is new is how common it has become. There are many reasons for this but in my opinion, technology has a lot to answer for. Here's why. During our hunter-gatherer time, we would travel tens of miles every day, running, climbing, hunting, carrying firewood, carrying our young, pulling and dragging dead animals. We couldn't put on weight because we burned so much energy every day. Many of the hunter gatherers would have had bodies like our athletes do today.

Fast forward to when the agricultural revolution came along, approximately 12,000 years ago, as humans discovered how to grow their own crops. Now that food could be grown, it needed to be stored. Humans started to develop settlements and no longer had to travel for miles to search for food. Now, they could just harvest their own crops and farm their own animals. Classes developed between people within settlements: some rich, some poor. The rich could live a more sedentary lifestyle, while the poor would do most of the heavy labour. Farming was physically demanding, as they didn't have the tools we have today. Most of it was done by hand, with the help of some basic tools and animals. Around this time, the first signs of an energy expenditure imbalance were seen. The rich suddenly had an endless food source and didn't have to do any physical labour.

With the human body being designed to store energy for the next famine, weight gain became more common. However, being overweight was restricted to kings, rulers, and the wealthy back then, and the rich were few and far between while the vast majority of people were poor, with physically demanding jobs. The poor commoners had to work for their food and still expended too much energy to put on weight.

Not a lot changed for thousands of years. Up until the eighteenth century, the majority of people lived the life of a farmer. During the eighteenth century, the industrial revolution came along. With the invention of such things as the steam engine, many of the jobs that had previously been physically demanding were replaced by machines that could be mass-produced. This was the turning point. As we journeyed through the nineteenth and twentieth centuries, technology became increasingly innovative. The invention of such things as washing machines, automobiles and, more recently, the internet meant everything was becoming more and more convenient. Each generation became less dependent on physical labour as technology made life much more sedentary. Nowadays, we have the luxury of living in an era where we have running water in the house, cars to get us from A to B, and we can just go to the shop and have the option of whatever type of meat we want when we want it. We are truly living in a privileged time. For 99.9% of human existence, we didn't have these luxuries. You might say "it's great that I don't have to hunt for food, walk for miles each day to gather water or chop down firewood to build a fire in order to stay warm." And you would be right, but this convenience comes at a cost. We don't expend as much energy as we once did. Because of the huge drop in energy expenditure, we needed a way to burn off energy.

So, "exercise" was created. Exercise is something that was invented to mitigate for our loss of physical activity. Humans are the only animals who have made up an activity to burn off energy. The rest of the animal kingdom just live in their habitats. Animals have other motivations to burn off energy, whether it be playing, mating, hunting prey or evading predators. An animal isn't going to go for a run to burn off energy that could be used to fight off a predator.

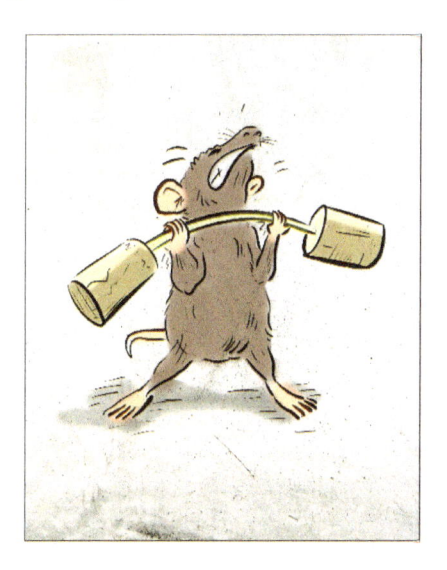

Humans have different motivations though. Because life is so convenient now, we don't expend as much energy as we once did. Exercise only became mainstream in the 1900s. Up until then it was only athletes and soldiers who exercised.

We also live in a world where there is an abundance of food sources. It is not the feast-or-famine lifestyle that we have evolved to live in. Food is available in every corner, and much of the food on our shelves is mass-produced, low quality, highly processed, high in saturated fat and high in sugar. And, although life has changed dramatically, our brain's priority is still survival. So, it will still store fat in case there is a food shortage. Your brain and body are still preparing for the next famine.

So now we overeat, with lower quality food, and we expend less energy, and with the human body being the fat storing machine it is, of course it means the rise in obesity is inevitable. Worldwide obesity has nearly tripled since the 1970s.[64] Ireland is ranked 36th in the world for obesity levels with 25% of the adult population considered obese. That is one in four people. That figure is mind-blowing to me. The UK ranks 29th, with 27% of its adult population being obese, while the United States is 14th in the world, with 36% of the population being obese. But the unwanted gold medal goes to Nauru, a small country in the north western Pacific Ocean with a staggering 61% in their adult population being classed as obese.[65]

These numbers are concerning but with further inventions like the robotic lawnmower, e-bikes and self-driving vacuum cleaners, it's only going to get worse. Additionally, ever since Covid-19 began, more and more people work from home. Today, you don't even have to leave your house to go to work. You can just roll out of bed and work in your pyjamas. Convenient for some, yes. But how much less energy do you expend during the day? If you're not getting up, commuting to work, walking around your office, heading out for lunch and then commuting home, you're left with an even larger imbalance of energy expenditure. Unless you counter that lack of energy expenditure with a lower calorie intake or more exercise, this will inevitably lead to weight gain.

Mark Zuckerberg predicts that a billion people will be working in the metaverse by 2030. If you don't know, "the metaverse" is basically a digital world where you can put on a headset at home and use an avatar version of yourself to work in a company that uses this technology. The days of sitting in a boardroom meeting may soon be a thing of the past. But it won't stop here. Soon you will be able to attend concerts, sporting events, university, and social events without even leaving the comfort of your couch. It's no wonder that half of the UK population is expected to be obese by 2030.[66]

Now don't get me wrong. I love technology, and many of those inventions are amazing; let's face it, nobody loves vacuuming. If a self-driven vacuum cleaner saves you half an hour of vacuuming and that time is used to get something more important done, I'm fine with that. But if all this convenient technology means that we just sit around all day and eat terrible food then I question if it really is a benefit to us in the long term.

The World Health Organization (WHO) now classes obesity as a disease. It's not fully clear why some people gain weight more than others. One theory is that because of adversity and famine in previous generations, the genomes have been altered to store more fat cells.

One interesting study was conducted on survivors of the Dutch winter famine. If you do not know the story it happened during World War Two when the Dutch government ordered railway workers to strike to try to halt the advance of Nazi troops through Holland in November 1944. As a result of this failed attempt, the Nazis stopped any importation of food to Holland, resulting in the deaths of more than 20,000 men, woman, and children due to starvation. The allies liberated Holland in May 1945 but many survivors of the famine suffered for decades. This was particularly true of women who had been pregnant during the famine and gave birth after it. After observing and studying thousands of the survivors, scientists discovered that among kids that were born after the famine, many were born very small and there was an increase in obesity, schizophrenia, and heart disease as they got older.

What's interesting is that there were genetic changes to survivors of the famine which were passed down to the offspring of the kids and even grandkids that were born long after the famine. This has led to some scientists hypothesising that after times of famine the human gene expression changes in order to store more fat. It is as if the body has learned from its experience and tries to better prepare for the future. The problem is that today we are not faced with famine anymore but the human body still acts as if it could be around the corner any time.

It's important to say that these are just hypotheses and there is no conclusive explanation to why some people gain weight and others don't. There are approximately 400 genes that are thought to be involved in weight gain. One thing we do know is that genes play a larger role than previously thought. Genetic changes to certain genes affect things like appetite and metabolism, which affect how well the body regulates its food intake.[67]

According to the CDC, "The brain regulates food intake by responding to signals received from fat (adipose) tissue, the pancreas, and the digestive tract. These signals are transmitted by hormones – such as leptin, insulin, and ghrelin – and other small molecules. The brain coordinates these signals with other inputs and responds with instructions to the body: either to eat more and reduce energy use, or to do the opposite, eat less and move more." Because of genetic changes, some people do not get the correct messages that they have had enough food. So, they overeat. But this happens only when there is sufficient food. Stephen O'Rahilly, professor in the field of genetic obesity at Cambridge University, explains, "You cannot get obese in a famine, but as soon as there is an adequate food supply there will be people who are susceptible to obesity." This was not as big an issue until we stopped burning as many calories as we used to.

So, you may be more likely to put on weight because of your genetics but this doesn't mean you have to. You can learn ways to know how much to eat for your lifestyle.

I don't mean to be insensitive if you are someone who has struggled with your weight. I know for some it is not as simple as reducing your calorie intake and exercising more. For some there are many emotional and psychological obstacles that need to be overcome too. Early childhood traumas, chronic stress, poor sleep habits and side effects to medication can all have an effect on our weight. And living with chronic pain can cause weight gain in itself. Frustration associated with functional limitations can lead to overeating too.

The reasons for weight gain would amount to a book in itself. I'm only here to talk about the close relationship between being overweight, inflammation and chronic pain. Chronic pain and obesity are interconnected, they're in the same circles and often share the same co-morbidities. Obesity may not directly cause pain in the way a broken leg does, but it is a risk factor to many different conditions that can cause pain. These include conditions like osteoarthritis, metabolic syndrome, fibromyalgia, cancers, depression, anxiety, hypertension (high blood pressure) sleep disorders, autoimmune diseases and heart disease. So, you could say that obesity indirectly causes pain.

One of the main ways is through inflammation. A typical inflammatory response is a defence against any infections, viruses, bacteria or injury. This type of immune response is healthy and short lived. Once the infection or injury has been resolved the immune system will stop producing inflammation, as your body has restored homeostasis. Individuals with higher fat cells have increased pro-inflammatory markers within the body. This pro-inflammatory state is present irrespective of tissue injury, virus or infection.[68]

This type of pro-inflammatory state is a low-grade inflammation that is most often present in fatty tissue, blood or visceral tissue. Why your body stays in this state is largely unknown but it doesn't seem to serve a beneficial purpose.

Leaner individuals predominantly secrete more anti-inflammatory markers.[69] Anti-inflammatory cells control pro-inflammatory cells. Individuals who are overweight have a reduction in anti-inflammatory cells, thus leaving the body in a pro-inflammatory state and more susceptible to a wide variety of pathologies or diseases as discussed above. Individuals reporting widespread pain tend to have greater total fat mass and less total lean mass than those not reporting pain,[70] and these individuals are shown to have a greater chance of developing chronic pain. Overweight people tend to have less muscle mass and lower bone density, which are also risk factors for injuries. These could lead to persistent pain due to the low-grade inflammation present within the body.

Good news

There is some good news at the end of all of this. Studies show that you do not have to lose a lot of weight to see reductions in chronic pain. By improving your metabolic health, you can start to shift the dynamic. Many dietary and lifestyle changes may be helpful in removing inflammation triggers and reducing chronic inflammation. The most effective is weight loss. For example, in patients with chronic inflammatory arthritis, weight loss alone has been shown to be independently associated with clinically significant improvement in disease activity and inflammation.[71]

Energy expenditure through exercise lowers multiple pro-inflammatory molecules and cytokines independently of weight loss. So, there are even benefits to exercise without losing weight. Any sort of resistance exercise is the basis for your body to produce a natural anti-inflammatory response which can control the low-grade inflammation.[72]

All of this tells us that you can get reductions in pain just by getting more active; some studies suggest that losing as little as 5% of body weight can reduce pain by up to one third.[73] So, you don't even have to worry about losing a lot of weight in order to start making changes. Just getting active can reduce the amount of pro-inflammatory cells and promote anti-inflammatory cell production.

This isn't a weight loss or diet book. This is just useful general information that you may or may not be familiar with. This isn't to body-shame you or to say that the pain is your fault because you have put on weight. Often when I speak to a client who is suffering with pain, they tell me they have been advised to lose weight. But often they feel that it's just a throwaway comment that is used to blame them for their pain.

Nobody wants to be told that they must lose weight to resolve their pain. It's too easy to blame weight and can leave patients feeling that their healthcare provider has invalidated them or hasn't evaluated them properly. So, if this is you, I hope this gives you more of an insight into why your healthcare professional wants you to lose weight – because it can make a difference. Being overweight plays a role in pain. It may or may not be the main driver but it will definitely contribute to it. It's not just the extra weight on your joints. To be honest, your joints are more than capable of handling excess weight, but they are not capable of living in a constant pro-inflammatory state. This is a basis for disease.

Maybe we'll get to grips with obesity and technology will fix the problem it has created with some sort of genetic therapy to stop weight gain from happening, but don't hold your breath. You have a survival body living in a world that for the most part does not have the adversity we have evolved through. Your body is trying to work for you; it's just living in the past.

Making a change to any of these risk factors can have a huge effect on how much inflammation is produced during a flare-up. By continuing to exercise at intensities that will not cause acute inflammation, tissue damage or muscle damage, you can help the suppression of chronic inflammation.

We will discuss this more in Chapter 10, but for now, make sure you take note of what is applicable to your situation. Shift the focus from weight loss to becoming healthy and you're off to a good start.

Alcohol and pain

Alcohol is used by many to help reduce the symptoms of chronic pain. In some studies, this applies to as many as 28% of pain sufferers.[75]

According to the NHS and CDC, the recommended amount of alcohol that should be consumed per day is two units for a female and four units for males (two units = one pint of beer or a medium glass of wine). But for alcohol to have an analgesic affect it takes more than this and, as with many other substances, the more you consume, the more of a tolerance you build up, until ultimately it takes more alcohol to get the same analgesic affect. This is bad news for obvious reasons, like addiction, but even for your overall health; alcohol affects sleep quality, emotions, metabolism, appetite, and motivation to exercise. Alcohol also affects your inflammatory response, which can increase the chances of autoimmune diseases. Over time alcohol misuse can cause development of peripheral neuropathy, a condition in which there is damage to nerves due to excessive drinking.

Alcohol withdrawal can be tough and can also lead to increased pain. This can motivate people to start drinking again. Everyone is entitled to have a drink. I enjoy one from time to time. At the end of the day, life is for living. But when the drink is being used to reduce the symptoms of pain, this is where you should draw the line. Alcohol is not recommended as a treatment or coping mechanism for chronic pain.

While there may be some short-term gains, over time, increased alcohol consumption makes chronic pain even worse.[76] Especially if consumed with any other codeine or opioid-based drug, it can be very dangerous. Always consult your doctor.

Our movement quality

"The body will become better at what you do or don't do"
– Ido Portal

We have just spoken about how much the world has changed in the last few decades. Not only do we not expend as much energy as we should, but also, because of our convenient world, the quality of our movement has drastically deteriorated too.

From the dawn of our existence, humans have been three-dimensional movers. We flex, extend, move laterally and rotate from left to right. Combining all of these planes of motion makes us expert functional movers. In the past we relied on movement for everything. We could climb, run, swim, carry, hunt and build with ease. All the things that were necessary for survival were made possible because of our physical ability. Today, society is set up in a way where challenging movement isn't required as much as in the past. This is great in some respects but it has gone too far the other way. Many of us we avoid challenging our body to move in new ways. We stay within the parameters of what we feel is normal for us. As life nowadays is filled with routine and schedule, most of our movements are rehearsed over and over. Nothing is new or challenging. You get up out of bed the same way, brush your teeth the same way, get into your car the same way and work the same way. Rinse and repeat.

We live in a safe zone of movement. Your safe zones are movements that you experience often. For example, a gymnast would have a broad range of safe zone movement because they experience a wide variety of movements regularly. On the opposite end of the spectrum is someone who sits down all day; their safe zones would be limited to the ranges of motion that they expose themselves to regularly. They could be experts at being in a seated position for long periods. Similar to the gymnast, their tissue will be conditioned to what they experience regularly. But they are not experts outside of those ranges and, if moved into a challenging position, they are more vulnerable to injury due to the lack of exposure or experience in that particular movement. Moving into areas that you don't have experience in are what I call "dark zone" movements. I call them this because if something is dark then you are not familiar with it. It's like walking into an unfamiliar room without the light on. Who knows what's in there?

Moving into these dark zones can put your nervous system on high alert, and rightly so. Your brain doesn't want you to get injured, so it will try to warn you before this happens. Movement in these dark zones can cause stretch receptors to fire off and tell the brain that you're in uncharted territory. Your brain will act on this and create some sort of feeling (stiffness, pain, or a feeling of strain) to get your attention. This is a normal response, and again we want this to happen as it protects us from injury.

Moving into dark zone movements aggressively or quickly can result in injury. Your tissue has little experience of these movements and is less likely to be able to adapt. Regularly moving in multiple ranges of motion gives your tissue experience in those ranges. So, by doing this, your tissue is more likely to be able to adapt, less likely to get injured and less likely to feel pain. This is why regular exposure to various movements in multiple ranges is important. It not only conditions the tissue, but it also keeps the receptors happy, and less excited when they are stimulated.

What's happening in our modern world is that more and more what we would have called familiar movements in the past are now becoming more unfamiliar. People's safe zone movements are becoming more and more limited only to what they are exposed to regularly. And again, technology is to blame.

Chairs are revolutionary inventions, there's no doubt about it. But they are overused. Today we sit for an average of eight hours per day.[77] Eight hours of sitting means eight hours of not moving, and eight hours in safe zone movements. Compare that to 200 years ago when 90% of the world worked in agriculture and sat for approximately three hours per day.[78]

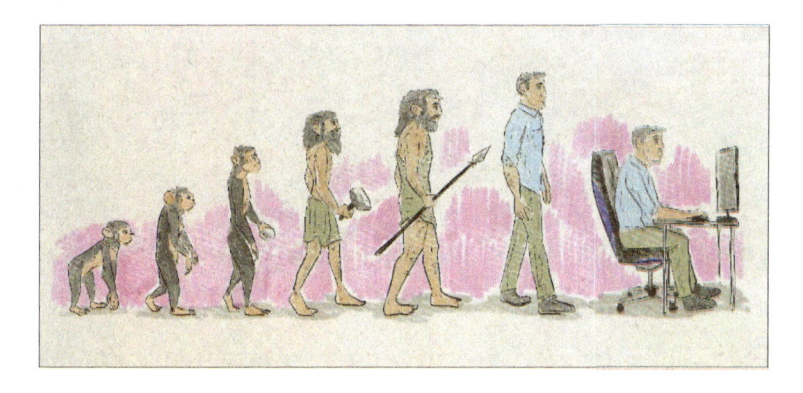

It's not just how often we sit; it's also how we sit. Sitting as we do with our hips and knees at 90-degree angles is an unnatural position as far as human movement goes. Before there was a chair in every corner of the world, humans would take the load off by hunching over in a deep squat position – basically, squatting down and getting your "ass to grass." This deep squat position is so ingrained in us that every child on the planet does it without any coaching. Even today you will see adult humans in third world countries sitting like this. But in the Western world, from the time children hit school this natural movement is discouraged because of our overuse of chairs.

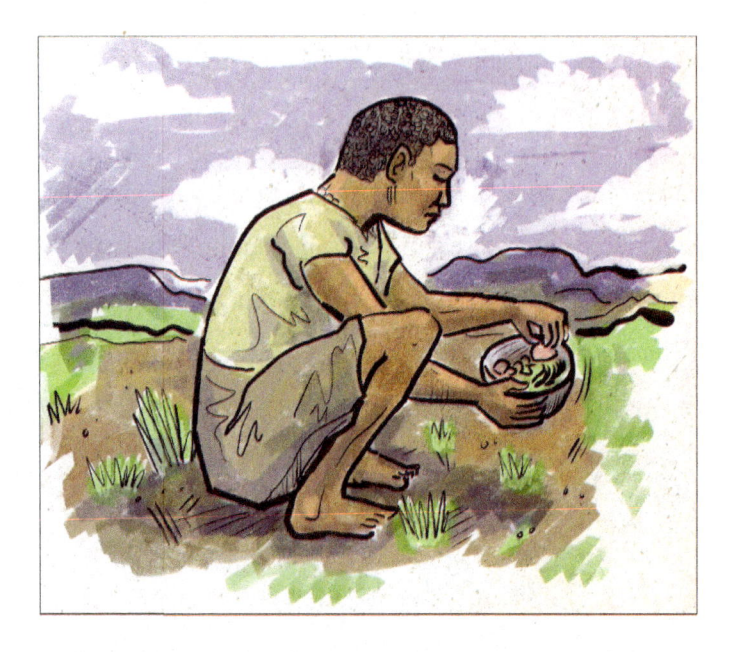

A lack of exposure to a deep squat can lead to a loss of ability to get into this position. You might wonder why that matters. I would answer that you need a similar range of motion to do all sorts of things. For instance, getting up off the ground, stepping up on a high box or climbing a ladder. Doing any of these movements proficiently requires your knee to be raised higher than your hip.

A lack of exposure to this position means a previous safe zone movement often become a dark zone movement. Or worse, you may lose the ability to do a deep squat altogether.

The brain uses a "use it or lose it" principle. It's taxing on the body to keep ranges of motion available that are not being used. The brain is always trying to conserve energy. So, if you're not using a specific movement, then your brain thinks you don't need to use it. Your brain wants to make you the most optimal version of yourself. So, it adapts to your environment. What this means is that if you spend a lot of time climbing, and you work through certain ranges of motion while you climb, then your brain will make adequate changes so that, not only can you access those ranges of motion but you also become stronger in those positions. The logic behind the brain's decision is that, because you do a lot of climbing it must be important for survival purposes. Again, the brain doesn't know if you're climbing for fun or if you're climbing to hunt. It's just adapting to the experience you're feeding it.

This goes for any activity. Regardless of whether you're Mo Farah or Michael Phelps training for the Olympics, your brain is optimising your body to be the best at your environment, purely for survival reasons. We humans have just figured out how this process works and can manipulate it so we can be better at sports. But the truth is that the human body is just adapting to the stresses we give it. I love this about the human body. I love how adaptable it is and the way we can challenge it to be able to do a wide variety of things that you may not even think are possible. But it can go the other way too; if your environment is an office or a sofa in front of the TV, it can adapt to make you better in these environments.

As the brain's priority is to adapt to make you the most efficient and capable in your environment then it should be no surprise that you see so many people develop a hunched over position with rounded shoulders.

The brain feels this position is important to you, so it adapts to allow you to be more efficient and capable in that range. The issue is that when you spend so much time in this position, you become less proficient in ranges outside of this and this is how dark zones are created.

Manual handling

Another driver of our poor-quality movement is poor knowledge of human biomechanics and pain. I believe that one contributor to this is ergonomics courses like manual handling. Manual handling courses have been brought in to help combat work-related injuries. The course itself is designed to teach the participants how to lift a load. The concept of this course is that, when faced with a heavy object, you should assess the load first, drop your hip, keep your back extended and primarily lift with your hip, while maintaining good posture while you perform the lift.

I see the argument that having an object closer to your centre of mass, then lifting with your hips, with your back in extension could be seen as a way of putting less stress on your back by involving your hips as primary lifters.

I do not necessarily agree with this principle but I don't have an issue with it being taught in the workplace. What I do have an issue with, whether it's the intention of the course instructors or not, is that many people leave with the notion that bending their back while lifting is always a bad thing. This knowledge then transfers into the real world whereby people adopt this principle of lifting everything this way, no matter how light or small the object is. I believe this causes many more problems than it prevents in the long term.

Lifting with a bent back (spinal flexion) is grossly misrepresented. Today there is a common narrative that lifting something with a bent back is bad for you. This couldn't be further from the truth. It is not only good to lift with a bent back, it is necessary to do so. Maintaining a level of conditioning in spinal flexion keeps this movement a safe zone movement. If you only ever lift the manual handling way, then you'll only be conditioned in that position and deconditioned in any other lifts.

Avoidance of spinal flexion creates unfamiliarity with a spinal flexed position thus creating a dark zone movement when you bend your back. You may feel you are "protecting" yourself in the short term by not bending your back, but in the medium to long term you are leaving yourself vulnerable to injury if you ever do lift something with a bent back. And trust me, at some point in your life you will lift something in spinal flexion.

The manual handing way to lift is not a good or a bad way to lift. It's just a way to lift. If you feel strongest lifting in that position then by all means lift heavy objects in that position. But encourage your body to lift in various other positions too.

The fact is there currently isn't much evidence to say that lifting with a bent back is bad for you. Personally, I am a big advocate for lifting with spinal flexion. It's something I do with my clients all the time. If you train yourself to lift in various ways under load then you're less susceptible to injury because your body has experience in more than one lifting position.

But just a disclaimer: if you haven't been lifting with spinal flexion don't try it for a heavy object. As with any new movement it takes time for your body to adapt and build conditioning in new movements.

To me the manual handling approach is outdated, and whoever created the model has a very simplistic understanding of how back pain occurs. In fact, manual handling courses have been shown to be ineffective in reducing back pain.[79] This is because manual handing doesn't address the many other things that might contribute to back pain.

Our whole anatomy is set up in a way to allow us to move in various ways. Your spine is articulated in a way to bend, move and lift in multiple ways. We managed to survive building the pyramids, the Colosseum and every village, town and city in history without knowing "the correct way to lift." Chronic pain is on the rise, not the decline. In summary, we don't move well anymore.

Pain as motivation

Pain is not only a great motivator of movement. It's also a motivator to not move. Movement flaws could be the result of pain and not the cause of pain. Nobody wants to feel pain and they certainly don't want to make their pain worse which is why fear/avoidant behaviour can kick in. This is fine when there is an injury and you avoid using the injured area for a short time to allow the healing process to begin. But excessive fear/avoidance is a big predictor for turning an acute pain into a chronic pain.[80]

This is where pain education comes in handy. Understanding why you're in pain can help remove that fear and help you encourage movement in ways that benefit you. Any physio, chiropractor or sports therapist worth their salt should be explaining this to you. We'll speak more about the fear/avoidance model in the next chapter.

Out of alignment

If there is ever a phrase I detest in my industry, it's that you're "out of alignment." For someone to use a phrase like means one of two things. Either they want you to believe that the human body needs to be aligned or symmetrical as a way to scare you into therapy, or they truly believe the human body needs to be aligned. Both reasons are as bad as each other. First of all, what is alignment and who gets to decide who's aligned and who's not? How is it decided? How is it measured?

There are many fake gurus out there who claim to be able assess patients' alignments through observation, and objective table tests. Unless you have sophisticated measuring tools such as force plates, these are not much use. Table tests using things like leg-length discrepancies have been shown to be unreliable, while visual assessments from practitioners have shown that therapists cannot agree on posture through visual assessments alone.[81]

Why are humans so dead set on symmetries? We don't apply this idea of alignment to any other animal. A vet would never say that your dog is in pain because he has an anterior tilted pelvis or your cat has one shoulder lower than the other. These conversations would never crop up because they are ridiculous. But not in human terms. Apparently, we're the species that needs to have alignment.

We focus our attention on trying to maintain good alignment by keeping our back straight, shoulders level and pelvis in the correct position, in activities from sitting to lifting to walking and even sleeping. And this alignment ideology is commonly used to diagnose pain.

The relationship between asymmetries, posture and pain has long been debunked but it doesn't stop most therapists looking at pain from this point of view.[82] People who have awful widespread pain often have "perfect posture" while other people who have what would be considered to have a poor posture have no pain.

People come in all shapes and sizes. Some of us have flat feet, some have high arches, and some have more or less of an anterior or posterior tilted pelvis. We are all different, we all look different, and we all have different shaped joints and features.

Much of how we align is genetic but some of it is influenced by our environment and lifestyle. It's not so easy to change posture. You cannot just get realigned by adjustments or massages. Joints don't just move in and out of place. Humans are not machines.

This is living, breathing tissue and the position it's in is due to a mixture of genetics, tissue health, exposure to loads and experiences of ranges of motion.

The human body is not a car. A car doesn't have consciousness, a personality, fears or worries. A car doesn't need eight hours of sleep a night, good nutrition or good mental health.

Cars don't adapt to their environment. A car has mechanical parts that move to create a vehicle that moves from A to B. In some ways it would be great to be able to just plug yourself into a computer to find out which part was faulty, get a new one and move on with your life but that's not reality.

The current obsession that everything in the human body should be aligned and symmetrical is not just wrong; it's malignant.

In my opinion movement trumps posture all day long. In my opinion poor quality movement is a far better predictor of pain than posture.

The cerebellum is an area of the brain that is dedicated to motor control, muscle tone, movement, balance and coordination. Cerebellum means "little brain" in Latin: it sits at the underside of the brain just above the brain stem. The cerebellum makes up 1/10 of the brain but contains over 50% of its cells. This is how important movement is to the brain: it has dedicated more than half of its brain cells to this small structure. Movement is part of us and we are starting to lose sight of this.

Sitting for eight hours a day cannot be compensated for by one hour of exercise three days a week. It doesn't matter how perfect your posture is, or how aligned you are. If you don't move well and often then you can land yourself in trouble. There is no ergonomic chair, desk, mattress or perfect posture that will reverse the effects of poor-quality daily movement. As a species we need to start moving better more often.

Genetics

When we think about traits, we often refer to them in the form of personality. In terms of genetics, a trait is something that can be measured physically or behaviourally. We see this when kids resemble their parents in behaviour or appearance. Ancient civilisations always presumed that there had to be some sort of biological mechanism to the passing on of traits. There just wasn't the technology to explain it. Today we have the ability to explain this. Now we know that we inherit genes from our parents and these genes set the stage for who you are as a person.

Your genes contain a set of instructions that your body reads like a recipe and builds proteins based on the genetic instructions. These genes are modified with each generation. You get 50% of your genetic code from your mother and 50% from your father. This has happened from the dawn of time. This is how we can trace our genes back to long before we were apes.

Just like baking a cake, when you have a recipe, it's easy for you to read the instructions to determine what to do. You could have flour, eggs, sugar, butter, chocolate, milk and icing. You know what temperature to preheat the oven at and how long to bake the cake for. The instructions tell you what order to put the ingredients in, and how long to have the cake in the oven for. Whatever the recipe says, just follow the instructions and you'll have yourself a lovely cake. Your genes contain instructions that tell your cells to make molecules called proteins. Because of these instructions, your body knows what to make, how much to make and when to make them. Because of these instructions your body knows how tall you should be, what colour skin you have, how many teeth you have, where to have hair, how much of it to have and so on.

We share many genes with all animals around the world. We share 96% of our genetics with a chimpanzee, 61% with chickens and, oddly, over 50% of our genes with a banana.[83]

Every human is different but in regards to genetics we are 99.9% the same. If an alien was to look down on our planet and look at our species, they might say we all look the same and they would be right to a certain degree. We are only 0.1% different genetically. You are almost identical to everybody you love or hate. Every hero or villain has almost the same genetic code as you or me. But that 0.1% is enough to make a huge difference. That 0.1% is the reason why we all have different features in terms of sex, height, eye colour, hair colour, bone structures and temperament. Genes also affect pain sensitivity and pain susceptibility. They play a role in weight, how inflammatory your immune system is, your tissue tolerance level and how prone you are to stress and anxiety.

Every facet of pain is intertwined with genetics. Certain genes predispose individuals to chronic pain, while others mitigate its likelihood. In the past, it was believed that, once your genetic code was set, there was no room for change. However, scientists have shown that while the genetic code remains immutable, gene expression can be altered. Gene expression refers to the activation or deactivation of genes.

Some genes might exist without being expressed. Possessing a gene doesn't guarantee that its associated traits will manifest. Genes linked to cancer, inflammation, chronic pain, heart disease, obesity, and diabetes can be turned on or off by our experiences, diet, stress levels, alcohol consumption, nutrition, smoking, and sleep patterns. Conversely, certain genes with anti-inflammatory, anti-cancer, and pain-relieving properties can be silenced. Genes that amplify or suppress characteristics are equally malleable.

Our lives exert a profound impact on gene expression. Take height, for instance – this is a trait influenced by genetics but also moulded by environment. Even identical twins raised in disparate settings show that a deprived environment can stifle their potential height. In a rat study, pups nurtured by a more caring mother exhibited enhanced resilience to stress due to changes in specific genes. Conversely, rats given less nurturing displayed poorer stress management due to a lack of genetic modifications. Remarkably, these genetic changes were transmitted to the second and third generations of pups.[84]

As identical twins age, they grow apart genetically. Even twins leading relatively similar lives manifest distinct gene expressions. Your environment is an ongoing sculptor of your genetic profile. This process of gene expression is called epigenetics. In essence, tending to your health, both physical and mental, directly influences your gene expression. You won't know if you have genes that specifically relate to your pain. So, it's not something that I expect you to write down at the end of this chapter. But it's useful to know that genetics play a role in pain and environment plays a role in gene expression.

Pain medication

Chronic pain sufferers are no strangers to pain medications, which play a central role in managing their discomfort. They're often the first thing that comes to mind when pain occurs and sadly can be the only treatment provided for a chronic pain. The use of pain medication is a booming industry, valued at $75 billion annually in the United States; this is projected to increase to $94 billion by 2028. However, this rising trend comes with concerning consequences; an increasing number of individuals are becoming dependent on these medications.

There is a diverse array of pain medications, with each having their distinct mechanisms. One of the most commonly used pain relievers is acetaminophen, also known as paracetamol. It is the mildest in terms of potency, and is frequently employed to alleviate mild to moderate pain. Surprisingly, the precise mechanisms through which paracetamol operates remain somewhat unknown even to this day. Nonetheless, it appears to obstruct the synthesis of prostaglandin, a hormone-like substance generated at injury or infection sites, ultimately reducing pain.

Non-steroidal anti-inflammatory drugs (NSAIDs) represent another widely available over-the-counter option for pain relief. An example of these would be Ibuprofen. They function similarly to paracetamol but offer the added benefit of reducing inflammation. A characteristic not shared by paracetamol.

It is important to note that neither of these types of medication significantly affects tolerance or physical dependence. However, some individuals may develop psychological dependence, manifesting as an emotional or cognitive inclination to take pain medication. This is the case with many of my clients. For instance, one might feel the need to take medication before engaging in physical activities like golf, long journeys in the car or even work, in anticipation of potential pain. This repetitive behaviour can lead to psychological dependence.

Certain antidepressants are also utilised in pain management even when depression isn't a factor. These antidepressants are prescribed by doctors in an off-label capacity as they were not originally designed for pain management. They just have an analgesic affect. However, according to the Mayo Clinic, they don't work immediately. "You may feel some relief from an antidepressant after a week or so, but maximum relief may take several weeks. Antidepressants may increase neurotransmitters in the spinal cord that reduce pain signals." The painkilling mechanism of these drugs still isn't fully understood.

This brings us to opioids, possibly the most famous type of drug out of all painkillers. But before we talk about opioids, I want to set the stage by discussing the brain's motivation and reward system. In the brain we have a reward mechanism that is designed to reinforce behaviours that are important for survival. These include eating, drinking, having sex and socialising. The brain needs ways to learn what is important for us. So, it uses this mechanism of reward.

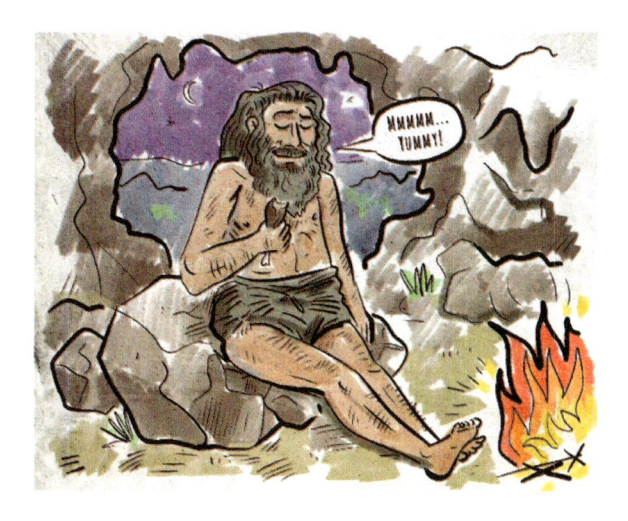

Let's take eating for example, and go back to the Stone Age to your distant relatives. Imagine your ancestor is sitting in his cave and he's hungry. Back then, you couldn't just open the fridge and make a sandwich. When your ancestor has decided he wants some food, a neurotransmitter called dopamine that is involved in motivating seeking behaviour is released. It's dopamine that helps motivate him to leave his cave, grab his spear and seek out his dinner. When the caveman finally catches and eats his dinner there is a release of neurotransmitters such as serotonin, oxytocin and endorphins which give him a feeling of pleasure. This feeling of pleasure makes your ancestor feel good. There is also a release of dopamine which helps reinforce the likelihood of the behaviour being repeated.

The feeling of pleasure is the reward for all his hard work hunting for his food. The fattier and higher in calories it is, the better. It's one reason why high carb foods are still so appealing to us today. The problem today is that high calorie foods are available in abundance. I'll touch more on this a little later. Anyway, the pleasurable feeling with the surge of dopamine helps the brain learn that this behaviour is good, which increases the likelihood of the behaviour being repeated. Just as pain and learning are tied together, pleasure and learning are too. The brain needs ways to learn what is good and what is bad for survival. If the feeling wasn't pleasurable, you wouldn't repeat it. As a result, the neurocircuitry in the brain changes to increase the odds of the behaviour being repeated. This is why we seek out food again. The same principle applies to drinking, sex and socialising.

Opioids are a class of drugs derived from or designed to mimic natural substances found in the opium poppy plant. These substances operate by binding to opiate receptors in the brain. Chemicals from opioids mimic the brain's own neurotransmitters such as enkephalins and endorphins, and bind to the opiate receptors, providing temporary pain relief, pleasure and even euphoria.

Marcia Meldrum, an associate researcher in the department of psychiatry and biobehavioural sciences at the University of California, Los Angeles, states that "The thing about opioids is they are very effective in interrupting and shutting off pain signals in the brain. They are very, very effective. But they are also very dangerous."[85]

This is because that's not all they do. In the brain's reward system, there are also opiate receptors. When opioid medication is taken, these chemicals also bind to the opiate receptors in the reward system, releasing dopamine. The artificial spike of dopamine is much larger than natural spikes that you would get from exercising or eating dinner. So, the brain thinks that this behaviour is extremely important.

Opioids are also very good at covering up emotional pain and trauma, giving a sense of calmness, relaxation and wellbeing. This can be particularly appealing for people who suffer with depression or anxiety. The calmness and sense of wellbeing offer an escape from the emotional challenges that are faced on a daily basis. For this reason, it's probably not a shock that people with mental health issues are at a higher risk factor for opioid addiction.

This can all be helpful in the short term. However, long-term consumption of opioids can have catastrophic consequences. You see, the brain is clever. When there is an unnatural spike of dopamine after taking opioid medication, the brain realises that something isn't right. The brain is always trying to maintain its homeostasis levels so it seeks balance. It recognises the unnaturally high dopamine levels caused by opioids and reacts in two ways: by reducing natural dopamine release and by reducing the number of receptors available to absorb dopamine. This lowers the natural dopamine baseline, creating a need for increased opioids just to feel normal. This phenomenon is called "tolerance" and it means the brain requires higher doses for the same analgesic effect.

Because dopamine doesn't work exclusively in the reward system and is also involved in memory, decision making and judgement, when tolerance levels are affected, these areas are affected too.

Additionally, pain shares many of the same brain regions as emotion. When pain medication changes areas of the brain that are involved in pain, areas involved in emotion also change. This can lead to a need for opioid consumption to keep emotions in check. Without them, anxiety and depression can be exacerbated. Increased tolerance levels can get out of control over time.

Opioids are the most common group of drugs misused worldwide. The United States has faced an opioid epidemic, primarily stemming from the over-prescription of these medications. OxyContin, a widely used painkiller, in particular, has been extensively documented as a key contributor to this crisis. But there are many more of them. They all have different potency levels but basically work on the same reward mechanism. Other examples of opioids include morphine, heroin, codeine, oxycodone, hydrocodone, and fentanyl.

Over time, repeated consumption of these drugs and the huge spikes of dopamine mean that the brain learns that this behaviour is important. When it does this it's very hard to change it. Remember the one reason the reward system has developed is to reinforce behaviours that are important for survival. "Large surges of dopamine 'teach' the brain to seek drugs at the expense of other, healthier goals and activities."[86] Normal pleasurable things become less pleasurable. I want you to bear this information in mind when we are setting goals in the final chapter, as motivation will be a key component to overcoming pain.

Reducing opioids

One big challenge for people tapering off opioids is that when they reduce consumption there can be an increase of pain. As the brain is always trying to regain its balance, one thing it does is increase the intensity of pain in order to encourage the pain sufferer to take more opioids. It's almost as if it is saying, "Oi, where are my pain meds?" This makes it very difficult for long-term users of opioids to quit, because of the increased intensity of pain when initially cutting down.

What's important to note at the end of all of this is that the brain isn't seeking opioids; it's seeking balance and it will do what it can to restore it. And if your natural dopamine levels are depleted then it will do what it can to get them back. This can include symptoms such as increased anxiety, depressive moods, withdrawal symptoms and intense pain.

There is no question that opioid medications are the most effective type of pain relief. But the jury is out on the benefits of their long-term use. The recommendations for the use of opioids long-term swings like a pendulum. Currently, as of 2023, the International Association for the Study of Pain (IASP) strongly advocates for access to opioids for the humane treatment of severe short-lived pain, using reasonable precautions to avoid misuse, diversion, and other adverse outcomes. At the same time, it recommends caution when prescribing opioids for chronic pain. There may be a role for medium-term, low-dose opioid therapy in carefully selected patients with chronic pain who can be managed in a monitored setting. "However, with continuous longer-term use, tolerance, dependence, and other neuroadaptations compromise both efficacy and safety." In other words, the negatives outweigh the benefits.

We know that there are many risks and side effects to taking opioids long-term. These include cognitive changes, gastrointestinal issues, poorer immune function, addiction, overdose and death, to name a few. In 2019, approximately 480,000 people died worldwide from opioids (WHO data). These figures are still rising. As genetics and your environment (current and that of your upbringing) are major risk factors for addiction, proper screening of these can reduce the chances of this addiction occurring in individuals.

Opioid-induced hyperalgesia

Opioid-induced hyperalgesia (OIH) occurs when opioids paradoxically enhance pain. It's like the medicine is making the pain worse instead of better. This kind of pain can be the same as your original pain or it can spread to different parts of the body. It's not clear how common OIH is and the precise mechanism is not fully understood. OIH is likely to result from multifactorial changes that occur with opioid exposure.[87]

OIH should be suspected when increased doses of opioids exacerbate pain or the subject's pain changes in terms of characterisation (e.g. burning) or location without evidence of a new pain source or injury.[88]

As the mechanisms for this phenomenon are not fully understood, prevention may serve as the best treatment. Recent studies suggest that OIH may be preventable with screening and delaying elective surgery when needed. Treatment of OIH requires tapering opioids and use of alternative pain management techniques. It's an extremely complex issue that usually needs a pain expert to diagnose and treat. Reducing opioids can initially increase pain which can really frustrate the pain sufferer and tapering takes time, which can also be a huge burden on the sufferer. But when the tapering gets to a certain point, the pain intensity starts to shift and the pain reduces.

At this point, I would just like to remind you that I am not a medical doctor MD and you shouldn't take this as medical advice. This information is purely for educational purposes. Always consult your own doctor when using or tapering off medication.

NOTES

Chapter 5

Psychological

"So, you're saying the pain is in my head." These are usually the first words someone says when their healthcare provider mentions pain and psychology in the same sentence. Immediately they switch off, stop listening and lose trust in the healthcare provider. And why wouldn't they? Someone has just suggested that their pain is not real, just imagined.

Straying away from the conventional approach of pain being solely a physical sensation is a delicate subject. But this is because of the fundamental misconceptions about why we have pain. The consensus is that pain is due to tissue damage or the threat of tissue damage, and psychology is something to do with your mind. 2+2=5 and that means that you said that the pain is in my head and I am imagining it.

Chronic pain sufferers have been through the wringer. In their life, they have been exposed to all kinds of people who don't believe they are in pain. When you're suffering with pain, someone suggesting that it's imagined is as insulting as it gets. But welcome to a pain sufferer's life. So, if the healthcare provider mentions "psychology" or "psychological" this can be taken to mean your healthcare provider doesn't believe you.

So, it's a delicate topic to approach. Trust must remain or the relationship is broken. A broken relationship between healthcare provider and patient will most certainly affect recovery. I'll speak a bit more about this in the next chapter. When you're in healthcare, it's important to know your audience. I have learned to know my audience – probably the hard way. Certainly, I have made mistakes in the ways I have approached difficult topics with past clients but I think that I have learned from them.

You should never be made to feel that the pain you are experiencing is imagined or in your head. Never! If you have left a treatment room feeling like this, it is a failure on the part of the healthcare provider and nothing to do with you. Psychological aspects of pain can be approached more directly with some people, while with others it has be a little more subtle or gentle. As you will learn in this chapter, the psychological aspect of pain is certainly not "imagined pain." However, there are many ways your psychology can influence your pain. The psychological aspect of pain is just as important as the biological aspect of pain. And, in my opinion, it is much more interesting. Psychology is more than just your thoughts. Psychology is the study of human behaviour and emotions. Pain psychology is the same thing. It is the study of human behaviour and emotions in the context of pain.

But remember these are just influencers; when there is chronic pain there are many influencers that are involved in the overall experience of pain.

Personality and pain

You may have heard the term "nature or nurture." Scientists debating which influences your personality more goes as far back as the chicken or the egg debate. The nature argument is implying that you're born with a personality; it's just your genetics and there's nothing anyone can do about it. By contrast, the nurture argument suggests that you are born as a blank slate and you develop your personality through your upbringing – everything from your parenting and education to social environment, culture and religion. Today it is widely accepted that personality is created by both genetic and environmental factors. But there is still no consensus on which one plays a larger role.

Understanding personality traits is useful because it helps us understand human behaviour. If you understand your own traits, it's easier to understand why you are the way you are. The "five-factor model of personality" is one of the most widely used and arguably the most accurate personality trait test. This model breaks down personality into five areas (Openness to experience, Conscientiousness, Extroversion, Agreeableness and Neuroticism). Each of these traits would be scored on a scale of 1–100 to give a person a reasonable evaluation of their personality.

When dealing with pain I really want to focus on the trait of neuroticism, and specifically the people that score above average to high on this chart. This personality trait is most associated with negative emotion. People who score high on this chart respond poorly to environmental stress, interpret ordinary situations as more threatening, and can experience small frustrations as overwhelming. However, if you score low on this trait, it doesn't mean you feel more positive emotions; it just means feeling fewer negative emotions. Feeling more emotionally positive is most associated with the trait of extroversion. It's useful to take the test to see how well you score on this particular trait but it's not necessary. Usually, people who score high in the trait of neuroticism are well aware how they think and behave. Someone who scores high on this trait would respond more negatively to irritability, anger, sadness, anxiety, worry, hostility, self-consciousness, and vulnerability than somebody who would score low in this trait.[89]

There are multiple facets to neuroticism.[90] Anxiety and depression are two facets that are commonly co-morbid with persistent pain so we will pay particular attention to these.

Anxiety

Anxiety is closely related to fear, with both sharing the same physiological response. Fear is an emotion that helps us deal with an identifiable threat, such as being confronted by a bear or being at a cliff-edge. It relates to a real, known, external or subjective danger. Anxiety on the other hand is an internal, often unidentifiable anticipation of threat. A key aspect of anxiety is uncertainty. It's like walking down a dark unfamiliar road. You don't know what you're afraid of. You're just afraid. Anxiety stems from your mind's interpretation of the possible dangers. It's persistent worry and fear, not just about stressful events but about everyday situations. *Roughly speaking, fear is about something outside the mind and anxiety is inside the mind.* People with anxiety have a low threshold for fight-or-flight, meaning it can get triggered easily.

Whether it's fear or anxiety, the fight-or-flight response is still being triggered. We have discussed earlier what happens during this response, but just to recap, when the fight-or-flight response is activated, the heart rate is elevated, breathing increases, pupils dilate, stress hormones are secreted into the bloodstream, muscle tone is engaged and all unnecessary systems are downgraded, including the immune, digestive and reproductive systems, to make more resources available to help deal with the threat at hand.

Being anxious can have advantages; you are more self-aware, and you can anticipate obstacles, remain cautious and take fewer risks. People with higher levels of anxiety are usually better at reading situations, interpreting data and being more realistic, or even cynical. Anxiety can help you prepare for something important, whether it's an exam, a presentation, or an important meeting. Fearing the unknown and being uncomfortable with uncertainty can motivate you to study harder or prepare for the unexpected. This preparation helps you deal with any curveballs that may come your way. This can lead in turn to better performance. So, there are advantages to being fearful or anxious, even in this modern world. But these same characteristics can become disadvantages when dealing with personal issues such as an injury and pain. A great predictor of chronic pain is someone who overanalyses their own pain. We call this catastrophising.

Catastrophising

Catastrophising takes this level of analysis and prediction to the extreme. It's where you worry or think about future situations as a potential catastrophe. It's a way of overanalysing, interpreting information and coming up with a conclusion that is usually the worst-case scenario, and then ruminating over this conclusion. For example, if you're studying for an exam, you may conclude that you are going to fail the test because you always fail tests. Because of this failure, you won't ever be able to get a job, therefore you won't be able to pay rent or support yourself. Once the conclusion is reached, you may accept your faith and give up. What's the point in studying when you're going to fail anyway? Instead of working hard to prevent the consequences of failure, giving up is the best option. In a way, you're saving yourself from the feeling of actually failing. It's literally taking Homer Simpson's advice: "Son, you've tried and you've failed. The lesson is, never try."

A person who often thinks this way is called a catastrophiser. They may not even know that this is how they think or speak. They may have grown up in an environment where thinking this way was normal. In situations like this, it can be hard for them to see that this thinking is irregular; it could take a friend or therapist to explain this to them. People can catastrophise when it comes to pain too. In the context of pain, it's called pain catastrophising. This is a tendency to magnify the threat level of pain. A common example of this is that someone with a headache thinks it must be a brain tumour.

Pain catastrophisers take more opioid medication, are associated with longer stays in hospital and more often develop chronic pain post-surgery.[91] It's common practice for surgical consultants to explain the possible negative outcomes post-surgery. This can result in the nocebo effect (a negative result based on negative expectations). There is no easy way around this because it's not only ethical to explain possible negative outcomes to a patient, but it's also illegal not to explain them.

This is where the language used between healthcare provider and patient is imperative. If the choice of words used to a patient who is a catastrophiser is not perfect, it can result in the nocebo effect, (more on this in a minute), regardless of how successful the surgery was. It's a great example of how our thoughts and beliefs affect pain. We all catastrophise in some form or other, especially during times of stress. It's a way we prepare ourselves for whatever disaster is about to come. Generally, it's irrational thinking based on limited knowledge. You may conclude a headache is a brain tumour or that turbulence on a plane means the plane is about to crash. But if this catastrophic thinking is a common occurrence, then it can be a sign of an anxiety disorder or depression.[92]

If you are always worrying or anticipating danger then you will strengthen these neuropathways. The brain changes to be better at what you are doing, even if it's just thinking negatively. There are few if any benefits to this way of thinking. The only purpose it may serve is to somehow help you prepare for possible outcomes, but even then, the prediction is likely to be out of proportion to the problem. Cognitive behavioural therapy (CBT) can help with reframing these negative thoughts and help you learn to think in a more helpful way. With practice, the brain can reorganise and form new pathways and connections that ameliorate this negative way of thinking.

Neuroticism isn't the most desirable trait to have but it's not totally useless. It has served a purpose, more so in history. Out of the five personality traits it's the one that's most influenced by environment, particularly in childhood. Children who have grown up with insecurity may develop a brain that is more sensitive to threat. You can understand this, because if a child's brain is developing in an insecure environment, then it's only logical that the brain would develop to be more sensitive to that world.[23]

On average, females score higher than males in neuroticism. This makes sense; throughout most of our existence on this planet, women were the primary caregivers who had to nurse our young. Being sensitive to threat was thus paramount. On average, females are also at a physical disadvantage to men which means they face a greater risk of aggression or sexual assault, especially during times when societies weren't set up to protect women. Males on the other hand needed to be less anxious or fearful because their primary focus was to provide for their families. Being too anxious or fearful would not be favourable during times of hunting or defending your family. This is also a reason why, when females are choosing a partner, they tend to look for males who display low levels of neuroticism.[94]

Knowing what your personality traits are is not a necessity when it comes to resolving your pain, but it can be beneficial to know why you react to things in certain ways. If you become aware of this then it may be easier to control fear, worry and anxieties. Later in the book we will concentrate on ways to control these feelings. Becoming aware of when you're feeling this way, particularly when you are in pain, will help you learn how to counteract this. Moderating the negative emotions can lessen the perceived threat, and this can lessen your pain.

Depression

Depression is the most commonly diagnosed mental health condition. It comes in many forms and affects each person in different ways. According to the WHO, up to 4% of the world's population suffer with some form of it at any one time. Major depressive disorder (MDD) or clinical depression is the most common of type of depression. It is characterised by persistent low moods, loss of interest in your favourite activities and a lack of motivation for a period of two weeks or more. If someone says they have been diagnosed with depression, they are probably talking about this condition.

Depression isn't a new phenomenon. In fact, there are documented examples of depression dating as far back as the second millennium B.C. Back then depression was seen as more of a spiritual issue than a physical condition. It was believed that sufferers had demonic influences and, because of this, exorcisms, starvation or trepanations were performed to rid the person of evil spirits. Treatment for it was performed by priests rather than doctors.[95]

In the fifth century A.D., the Greek physician Hippocrates claimed that depression (or "melancholia") was due to an imbalance of fluid within the body – specifically, an increase of black bile in the spleen. The proposed treatment was to restore balance between the four fluids (blood, yellow bile, black bile, phlegm). He did this through bloodletting, exercise, diet and baths. Elsewhere, medieval Europeans believed depression was contagious; as a result, sufferers were to be killed or locked up in prisons away from society.

It's no surprise that the spiritual and demonic influence was still very much ingrained in European society as European thinking was dominated by Christianity.

Around the nineteenth century, the thought process started to shift away from the spiritual towards a more biological explanation. People who were desperate for help would turn to experimental lobotomies to ease their symptoms. Lobotomy had been shown to alter behaviour, and some patients seemed to improve after the procedure. But many also suffered severe and irreparable brain damage.

Today lobotomies are considered barbaric and unnecessary.

Eventually psycho-analyst Sigmund Freud proposed his theory that depression was due to an inner conflict and suggested a less invasive talk therapy. Variations on this are still used today and can be extremely effective in helping people.

Nowadays, the mainstream narrative is that depression is due to a chemical imbalance in the brain, although the evidence to support this theory isn't solid.[96] Treatment using antidepressants is widely used to correct the brain's so-called chemical imbalance but this approach is disputed, with many claiming that antidepressants are not much more effective than a placebo.[7]

How depression develops is still somewhat of a mystery. Much like anything that happens within the human body, depression is very complex, usually multifactorial and not as simple as one chemical being too low or another being too high. Some people seem to be genetically predisposed to having depression. How much influence this has is unclear. If a parent had depression, studies have shown that you are three to four times more likely to have it,[97] but it doesn't mean you will definitely have it. How you were raised, especially in the early years, can be a risk factor in the development of depression. Severe childhood physical or sexual abuse, and childhood emotional and physical neglect can be factors. Losing a parent early in life also increases the risk to some extent. Other psychosocial factors that greatly affect depression include prolonged life stresses, including financial problems or bereavement;

chronic pain or illness; and taking drugs, including cannabis, ecstasy and heroin.[98] Social isolation and loneliness are also thought to be big contributors that played a significant role in how depression rates sky-rocketed during the Covid-19 pandemic. More on that later.

Most modern-day approaches will involve a combination of exercise, dietary changes, psychotherapy, other forms of therapy, and the use of antidepressants.

Why we can get depressed

You may wonder why we have the capability to have low moods in the first place? What's the advantage to this? If evolution is the survival of the fittest, what purpose does low mood serve? It's difficult to imagine that depression or depressive behaviour has or at least had an advantage. But in her infinite wisdom, Mother Nature doesn't do things for the sake of it. There will always be method to her madness, or at least some sort of underlying purpose. In one study, it was found that low mood and depression is a useful adaptation to prompt an animal to withdraw after losing social rank. The argument is made that withdrawing and being more submissive allows it to live to fight another day. By contrast, animals who don't withdraw could be killed or ostracised from the group or tribe.[99]

Low mood also makes you more sceptical and improves your ability to detect deception, both of which can improve survival chances. It can increase concentration levels and be beneficial to motivation.

Withdrawing from society also gives someone an opportunity for deep thought and reflection.

Depression and inflammation

Another intriguing theory, put forward by internationally recognised psychiatrist Dr Charles Raison, is that depression could have served a vital survival function in the protection against infection. We all experience this nowadays. If you get the flu, you feel drained, tired and fatigued. All you want to do is go to bed and avoid going outside. The last thing you want to do is go to work or meet up with friends. Back before the discovery of penicillin, infection was the biggest killer among humans. If you were a hunter gatherer who had been infected, whether from a small wound or a flu virus, it could be life-threatening. When the immune system is activated to fend off infection, depressive moods inflict a lack of motivation. This can be seen as a useful strategy so the infected person will rest and conserve their energy to help fight off the infection. Social withdrawal could also be explained as a way to help contain the virus and stop its spread. Child mortality was as high as 40% as recently as the early twentieth century, so for the survival of the species, a motivation to socially withdraw until the infection was fought off is a useful method for the overall survival of the human race.[100]

Social withdrawal would also protect you from being attacked by other tribes or predators when you're at your weakest or most vulnerable. This theory is supported by research showing that healthy volunteers who are given a flu virus can develop depressive symptoms. Furthermore, people who are suffering with inflammatory conditions such as rheumatoid arthritis and cancer and are given anti-inflammatories show an improvement in mood.

Dr Raison stresses that this is not to say that depression is an inflammatory condition. But this relationship does appear in approximately 30% of patients. And the theory does help explain why pain and depression so often co-exist.[101] Many people who suffer with a chronic pain condition are co-morbid with inflammatory conditions such as obesity, cancer, diabetes, osteo-arthritis and rheumatoid arthritis. Additionally, many of our modern lifestyle choices contribute to a pro-inflammatory state. Prolonged stress, lack of sunlight, poor physical fitness, poor sleep quality and a sedentary lifestyle are all well-documented risk factors for an overactive immune system. If this connection between inflammation and depression is real, then it's plausible that many modern lifestyle choices could contribute to the body's natural survival response by inducing depression or a depressive state.

Pain and depression

So, chronic pain and depression often co-exist and both exacerbate each other. Pain makes depression worse and depression makes pain worse.

The most common form it takes is "pain-induced depression." This is depression that develops after the onset of pain. It's been shown that up to 85% of people who suffer with chronic pain develop depression. People who have both chronic pain and depression have a worse response to medication, and treatment outcomes are worse than for people with either pain or depression on their own.[102] While the exact mechanisms underlying the relationship between pain and depression remain subjects of ongoing research, there are several theories and observations worth considering. One explanation is that living with chronic pain can naturally lead to depression as a psychological consequence. The significant impact on an individual's daily life and functioning, coupled with the distressing nature of persistent pain, can understandably lead to the development of depressive moods. On the surface, this would seem like the most logical explanation. The sufferer's life has been greatly affected, so depressive moods are inevitable. This has been the mainstream thought process up until recently and although there is definitely merit to this explanation there are other factors to consider.

For instance, pain and depression occupy similar brain regions, and their neural pathways intertwine (in the insular cortex, prefrontal cortex, anterior cingulate, thalamus, hippocampus, and amygdala).[103] The emotional aspect of pain, combined with the physical sensation, plays a critical role in motivating appropriate behavioural responses. If you were not concerned or worried about a broken ankle, for example, you might not take appropriate action to address the injury. So, the intertwining of pain and emotion is essential for motivating appropriate responses to protect and care for our bodies.

When pain persists and becomes chronic, the plasticity of the brain changes. Old pathways loosen and new pathways form and strengthen.

Because pain and emotion are so deeply intertwined neurologically, areas involved in mood management and emotional regulation change too, and not for the better. This also appears to be a solid explanation why depression so commonly develops after chronic pain conditions.

Opioids, pain and depression

Another explanation is the long-term effect of opioid medication. It's well known that side effects from opioids include sedation, lack of motivation, anxiety and depression. This can be a catch-22 for some people who take opioids because the only thing that helps with their pain is the medication, but because of the side effects, they lack the energy and motivation to do things that would help reduce or resolve their pain in the longer term. We know now that taking opioids over long periods negatively affects the way that pain is influenced (as discussed elsewhere) and can affect other things such as sleep quality and appetite, all of which can combine to result in depression as a side effect.

Grief

"Grief is the price you pay for love" – Queen Elizabeth II

Grief is the natural response to loss. It's the emotional suffering that is often associated with the loss of a loved one. But any important loss can trigger the same grief reaction. When persistent pain kicks in and starts to take over, in an effort to try to alleviate symptoms, the first strategy can be a reduction in activities. Hobbies, exercising, and social roles are usually the first to be minimised, followed by career and finally responsibilities at home. What tends to happen with chronic pain is that, most of the time you lose things gradually. Of course, this isn't always the case. If the pain is induced by a trauma or an accident then the loss can be abrupt. But in my experience, most of the time these losses creep in and develop from there. And like any loss, this leads to grief.

Mark Twain famously said that "Nothing that grieves us can be called little; by the external laws of proportion a child's loss of a doll and a king's loss of a crown are events of the same size."

Grief is a subjective feeling. It's about your own experience and relationship with the person or thing you have lost. It's about how much you are craving or longing to be reunited with what you have lost.

It may be difficult to distinguish between grief and depression because they share similar symptoms. But they are distinctly different. They both lead to intense sadness, loss of appetite and insomnia. Grief comes in waves and is triggered by thoughts, memories or reminders.

Grief is a motivational process. There can be a difficulty accepting the loss, causing the grief. Grief is usually less intense in situations where friends or family rally around for support and tends to get better over time. Antidepressants rarely work for grief.[104]

Depression is present regardless of who is around. It can be described as a deep emptiness or sadness. Depression differs from grief, as it's not a motivational process. You're not actively seeking or craving something.

In fact, the opposite is true. You would prefer to be alone and withdraw from the world.

Because grief and depression share so many symptoms, it can be difficult to distinguish between the two unless you are a trained professional, especially if the grief isn't related to a death. If a loved one dies, it's expected that you will need time to grieve. Family and friends will usually give you the love, empathy and compassion that you need. The same can't be said for the loss of other things in your life. In fact, people may not even know that you're grieving. You may not even know you are grieving yourself.

The psychiatrist's Diagnostic and Statistical Manual of Mental Disorders (DSM) IV specifically lists grief as an exception to the diagnosis of clinical depression. So, if you're feeling low after the loss of a loved one, there will be hesitancy to diagnose depression rather than allowing for a natural grieving period. This has changed in the latest edition, the DSM V, because grief can often trigger episodes of depression.

We know one role of the brain is to make predictions. It does this through learning from lived experiences. It forms a neural map of the environment and everything around it. This makes it easier for the brain to comprehend and navigate the environment without needing to process things. For example, when you see the sensor light come on outside the house at 6 p.m. you know it's your partner. You anticipate that any minute they are going to walk in the door, complain about someone at work or ask what time dinner will be ready. Having created this neural map, the brain makes predictions. This means that you don't need to assess or process every incident with the same level of scrutiny. Without this process you would spend all of your time processing every bit of information you receive every day. This prediction process is more efficient and less energy-sapping.

When someone or something that is important to you is taken away, there is a neurological change. The brain tries to make sense of and navigate this new world. But the brain won't change overnight. It's been wired and conditioned over time. If you lost your partner and around 6 p.m. you saw the sensor light coming on outside, there would be the expectation that your partner is going to walk through the door. When this doesn't happen but the reminder is there because the brain is trying to make that connection and can't, grief is the result.[105]

Over time the brain reorganises itself and forms a new map. This doesn't happen overnight. It takes weeks or months for the brain to reorganise itself. When it's the loss of something or someone that you love, there is a high-level emotion attached to each experience, which is the reason why grief is such an emotional challenge.

Finally, depression can often have no identifiable cause. Grief always does. These are the main differences between depression and grief.

Chronic prolonged grief

If you have lost a loved one, yes, it is hard, but time is a healer; in most cases, life goes on and, in most cases, the brain reorganises itself and you'll eventually get back to yourself.

When it comes to chronic pain and you have mourned the loss of your identity, career, and hobbies, you are left with debilitating pain, no career to drive you on, no hobbies or social life to keep you happy, financially under pressure and without purpose or meaning in your life.

And I believe this is a big contributory factor in pain-induced depression that is not spoken about. In this scenario, many of the things that you love about your life have been affected or taken away. You are left with no goals, no purpose, no drive and no hope: an emptiness that cannot be filled because pain has taken it all away. A human being without a goal, without something to aim for, without meaning or purpose, has nothing. Humans are goal-orientated animals. We need motivation to drive behaviour. Hunger gives us a desire or a motivation to find something to eat. Thirst gives us motivation to drink. When a human loses their purpose and has no goal anymore, what will motivate them to get up in the morning?

The natural and most primal thing to do is to withdraw from the world, reflect and think deeply. However, where there is no hope or light at the end of the tunnel, the reflection can just lead to ruminating on how bad your life is. It doesn't help that, with social media, everyone else's life seems so perfect. Pictures of new cars, holidays, promotions at work and personal bests in the gym are all posted online. None of this makes you feel good about yourself or your life and can further spiral you downwards.

Depression is a complex problem and pain-induced depression is even more complex. It can be one or all of those examples that causes it. In any case, the first and most important way to overcome these feelings is to find motivation again. Renew the hunger inside of you. Goal-setting is crucial for this. More importantly, the goals must be realistic. Focus on the things you can do, not what you can't do. This will be the first thing we do in the final chapter and will be one of the building blocks to your recovery.

Your belief system

"We see the world, not how it is, but as we are" – Stephen Covey

I would argue that beliefs are probably one of the main influencers of chronic pain.

Our beliefs come from information we consider to be true. I emphasise the words "we consider." Just because you consider it to be true doesn't mean it is. A belief is essentially a conclusion that we have accepted as the truth. But a conclusion is the product of a starting point. So, a belief must start from somewhere. Beliefs are generally formed in two ways: by experience (in education, events, and influences from our environment), or by accepting what others tell us to be true.[106]

When I speak about beliefs, I am not just talking about religious beliefs. Although there is not really anything different between a religious belief and a regular belief. Beliefs (religious or not) give you direction. Having a belief helps gives meaning and significance to things. How you think and how you behave will correspond to what you believe. You may believe in God and think that being a good Christian in the eyes of the Lord means you should be a good person. This might mean going to church every Sunday, always being friendly and respectful to others and donating to charity.

You may believe that to be a good employee you need to be hard-working, punctual and reliable. As a result of this belief, you get up every day, show up for work on time and put in a good shift. You may also believe that to be a good parent you must never have your child wanting. So you give them what they ask for. Other parents may have the belief that it's important for their children to learn the value of money, so they make their kids do chores in order to give them what they want. Beliefs are like an inner guide. They orientate us and help us navigate our complex world.

Forming beliefs serves many purposes. A belief helps in decision-making, dictates behaviour and helps us come to conclusions quicker. Without a preconceived belief, we would have to register and try to process all new information all the time.

We start to form our beliefs by taking in sensory information from our experiences. This sensory input travels up to the frontal lobe of the brain and where it is made conscious.[107] This is when the brain registers the sensory information and it may become a thought. If the information is then accepted as the truth, a belief is formed.

So, the brain takes a representation of how the world should be in the form of your beliefs. This gives your brain a template to work from and you fit your experiences into the template to make sense of the world right now. Critically analysing everything in your environment would be too time-consuming and taxing for the brain. For survival purposes time is of the essence, the brain connects the dots and fills in gaps in order to construct an explanation for the world around it. By filling in gaps and jumping to conclusions, the brain saves time by constructing its own explanation in real time rather than trying to evaluate or analyse the whole situation critically. This means fitting a story around a belief.

This is not a flawless system by any means. But the brain needs to compromise on accuracy for the sake of efficiency. Our lazy brain is always trying to conserve as much energy as possible for when it may need it for survival purposes.

You may think this is a bad system, but it has served our species very well over the course of time. Let's imagine that 20,000 years ago one of your ancestors was out hunting in an unfamiliar forest and heard a rustling in the bushes. Their brain would have to take whatever information was available and reach a conclusion very quickly. Even if it's just the wind blowing the bushes, their brain would skip the process of trying to construct an explanation for why the bushes could be rustling. They may have had past experiences of predators jumping from bushes. Or, they could have been taught by parents or members of their tribe that if you hear a bush rustling then it could be a predator. So, the gaps are filled and a conclusion is reached in order for them to make a decision.

Another example is the context of pain; people administered a painful stimulus with a red laser will feel more pain than if it is administrated with a blue laser. Red signifies danger so our perception of the stimulus is altered because of this.[108]

Confirmation bias

Once the information is accepted as the truth, the belief is formed. Dr Michael Shermer's *New York Times* bestseller *Why People Believe Weird Things* explains that once we form a belief, our brains immediately look for information to support it. This means seeking out information that backs up and reinforces this belief, thus making the belief stronger. But here is where the interesting part happens. Once the belief is formed, you will also filter out or disregard information that challenges or contradicts the belief. This phenomenon is called confirmation bias and it happens to everybody all the time. Conformation bias is the tendency to selectively gather evidence that confirms our preconceived beliefs and assumptions.

There are a few theories as to why we do this. Firstly, reaffirming beliefs makes you feel good about yourself. By contrast, challenging your beliefs is emotionally distressing and can make you feel bad about yourself. Therefore, when their beliefs are challenged, people can get defensive.

We spoke before about the way the body is always trying to maintain homeostasis. Someone challenging your beliefs or contradicting them can be perceived as a threat. Often this can result in you feeling uncomfortable, getting into a heated argument or all out physical aggression. This is your body moving away from homeostasis and into a fight-or-flight response. Humans use confirmation bias to restore homeostasis. By doubling down on your beliefs and searching for information that affirms what you believe to be true, you reduce the distress and restore balance within the system. In a way, confirmation bias is a way for people to emotionally protect themselves.

Changing your beliefs, especially highly valued ones such as religious, political, or deep core beliefs can be time-consuming or energy-sapping as you will be using areas of the brain that are involved in higher reasoning processing. It's emotionally more satisfying to critically analyse information that we disagree with rather than changing our own beliefs.

Secondly, confirmation bias also helps strengthen connections between humans. Again, we can look to our ancestors to help you understand why this process happens. Humans are social animals and we want our tribe to be the strongest. The stronger your tribe is, the safer it is from predators and other tribes. To go against your tribe would mean jeopardising relationships between tribe members, which could weaken your tribe. So, your tribe sticks together and you will defend their decisions and actions.

We still use this system today. Your tribe could be your favourite political party. We will favour our political party and defend their policies regardless of whether they are bad policies or not. We feel safer if our tribe is in charge i.e., in government. Anything positive our political party does will be remembered and will strengthen the feeling that we have the best party. On the other hand, anything that looks dodgy or suspect will easily be forgotten about or disregarded.

So why is confirmation bias important when it comes to pain? Whenever we encounter new information, we see this information through the lens of our own beliefs. This is an unconscious process but we will look to affirm what we believe to be true.

"Claire" was a client of mine. She had suffered with back pain on and off for five years or so. Claire believed that the reason that she had the pain was because of an old injury that had not healed properly. This bothered her for some time, until she finally decided to get something done about it. She decided to go to her local GP to find out once and for all what was going on with her back. He told her by observation only that she had a prolapsed disk in her back. She just accepted this without analysing how her GP knew this by just looking at her for two minutes. The fact that he had no evidence to this diagnosis such as an MRI or X-ray was irrelevant. In fact, his diagnosis was merely an opinion. But this did not concern Claire because it confirmed something that she already believed.

There was plenty of evidence against the GP's diagnosis, for instance, why would the pain be on and off if there was a prolapsed disc sitting on a nerve? However, she didn't consider this.

The thing about beliefs is that one belief can trigger a cascade of other beliefs too. Claire decided to avoid bending or ever sitting or kneeling on the ground because of this belief. One day she had got on the ground and been unable to get up. This only strengthened her belief that it was not safe for her to be on the ground because of her injury. Over time, she lost the ability to get down on the ground.

Whether or not Claire's belief was right her or wrong doesn't matter. *As humans we respond to the perceptions of our reality and not reality in itself.*[109] It's up to the healthcare practitioner to understand this and look out for these negative beliefs as these negative beliefs with likely be dictating her behaviour. And certainly, make sure they are not instilling new negative beliefs themselves.

In Claire's situation when she came to my clinic and after hearing her story, I felt the best option for her was to get an MRI to see what was actually going on. If she came to me before her visit to her GP, I wouldn't have sent her for the MRI because I wouldn't have suspected a prolapsed disc. But because her belief was so ingrained and reinforced by a person who she trusted I felt this was the best option. The MRI result showed no prolapsed, just some general degeneration and a disc bulge. All normal for someone her age. This allowed me to help her change her negative belief, remove the fear, take the shackles off the recovery and allowed her to start moving again.

Words matter

I was told by a physiotherapist when I was a teenager that I had "athletic groin syndrome" after I got injured during a football match. I was given no more information on this. I'll never forget it because all I could remember was the word "syndrome" without any context or meaning behind it. I was left frightened and at my next appointment with him, I asked him again to explain what "athletic groin syndrome" was to me. He basically explained that the muscle in my groin was weak and it needed to be strengthened. I thought to myself, *why didn't he just say that in the first place?*

If you have been suffering with any sort of pain for long periods, you have almost certainly been subjected to multiple diagnoses from doctors, surgeons, physios, chiropractors, or sports therapists. Time and time again the wrong language is being used by healthcare practitioners. Multiple diagnoses using very scary words and little to no explanations to accompany them.

It's unfortunate that at this stage there is so little consideration given to the words that are being spewed from people in lab coats right down to the physio giving a sports massage. On a daily basis clients inform me what their healthcare providers have said to them. Things like "You have the back of a seventy-year-old" or "I think you've slipped a disc." Is it ignorance, a lack of consideration or compassion for the patient's feelings? If you are someone in a high position of authority you better understand that what you say is gospel. Your patient will hang on to every word you say. If you tell them that they have a back like a seventy-year-old they will act like it. If you say that you've never seen a back as bad as this one, well then, you have potentially ruined that person's life. This may sound exaggerated but I have seen this on a daily basis: when someone in high authority tells a patient a phrase like that, the patient's whole life is turned upside down, especially if they are someone who is receptive to this type of information.

What if their back pain was driven by stress and lifestyle choices and now this person has been told they have the back of a seventy-year-old? You may get some people who can brush these negative statements off, but many people will catastrophise and their behaviours will change with this information. You might argue "Well, healthcare providers need to put a label on the problem and athletic groin syndrome is a universal language that every healthcare provider can relate to." If this is your argument that's fine, it's a valid one, but at least explain what athletic groin syndrome actually means.

When people come to my clinic, I will just use terms like "cranky nerves" to explain nerve pain, "sensitised joint" to explain joint injuries or "a muscle injury" to explain, you guessed it, a muscle injury.

I don't focus so much on the pathology or previous diagnoses. Obviously, they are important and taken into consideration, but I prefer to focus on the person and try to build a better and more resilient version of themselves. This starts with clear understanding through simplified education and reassurance. Changing up the language can be enough to take on the potency of the problem. Sometimes the language that is used can be more pathological than the pathology itself. Claire's case was a prime example of this. Once there is a clear understanding then we can focus on building strength and confidence, and, ultimately reducing the symptoms.

Our words matter and can be the difference between a treatment failing or being successful. In my opinion there needs to be more focus on communication skills at university level because if the health provider doesn't have good communication skills, then I would argue they are not prepared to deal with their patients regardless of how academically competent they are.

I question why at this stage with so much knowledge as to how the body works we don't realise how important language is. And the higher up the medical hierarchy the healthcare provider is, the more weight their words hold.

What benefit does information such as "You're going to need a hip replacement in ten years" have to a patient? Or "You have the back of a seventy-year-old" to a young adult? But this language is used on a daily basis. It will only serve to frighten a person and can greatly affect their life. I'm not suggesting that a healthcare provider should lie to a patient but they have to ask themselves how helpful their information is to those they're giving it to. As well as that, reassuring information often isn't provided. Words can be damaging, and we in healthcare need to recognise this and do better.

Limiting beliefs

A positive belief can make you feel like you can do anything. Very few people achieve anything great without believing it's possible. This is not a cliché. Humans have unconscious processes that follow their beliefs. If you look at any top athlete in the world, they have got to where they are by believing it was possible. Without that inner belief, the drive or motivation just wouldn't be there. Why would you get up every day and grind through the training if you didn't genuinely believe that your goal would be achievable? This goes for business, education, and most other spheres of life.

By contrast, limiting beliefs are negative beliefs that we hold to be true about ourselves. These limiting beliefs can hold you back from achieving your goals. Pain forms limiting beliefs. Actually, I'll rephrase that: a poor understanding of pain forms limiting beliefs. One of the most common limiting beliefs is "I can't." This could be because of the belief that you are broken, injured or that you are wearing yourself away. Or there may have been many failed treatments and you believe that you cannot be "fixed."

Limiting beliefs set a ceiling. These ceilings are very low. Often much lower than they should be. Imagine a big house with a low ceiling and this is what a limiting belief looks like. There is so much more potential beyond the ceiling that has been constructed by your thoughts and experiences.

Tony Robbins says, "beliefs create, and beliefs destroy. The problem is that most of us are not conscious of our beliefs. A belief is nothing more than you being absolutely certain of what something means." When you are certain about your beliefs, your behaviours will align to them.

Beliefs dictate your behaviour

Imagine you are walking through an old house and suddenly you come across a nest of tarantulas. If you are anything like me, you'd run as far away as you could. This is because of the meaning I have attached to spiders. Humans attach meaning to everything around us. Effectively we put labels on things and assume they are correct.

Attaching meaning helps the brain interpret information and make predictions. We assign meaning to something through the lens of what we believe to be true. Many of us believe spiders to be a threat, so we get grossed out by them, or become fearful as a result. So, most of us will attach a sense of danger to spiders. As a result, when we see a spider's nest it results in a fight-or-flight response. I may freeze, tense up or run away. I cannot remember why I don't like spiders, I just don't. But if I see one, especially if it's a big one, I will avoid it like the plague. My behaviour changes to avoid something that I fear. Spiders are scary to me, but not to an arachnologist. An arachnologist is just going to find them interesting. This is because of the personal meaning they have attached to spiders. Because of the meaning the arachnologist has attached to the spiders their behaviour is to become interested and investigate the nest.

Fear and anxiety are emotions designed to keep you alive. They are uncomfortable feelings for a reason. Nobody wants to feel fearful or anxious, which is why your behaviour changes to help you avoid these uncomfortable feelings. "Avoid" is the key word. Afraid to speak in public? Why? Generally, there is a belief that you will mess up or people won't take you seriously. Often this is a result of an experience from the past. Your brain stores the memory of an experience and has attached a sense of danger to it. So now your body is set up to avoid situations that involve public speaking. As a result, any time you are asked to do some public speaking your brain kicks into gear and tries to get you out of that situation by moving you into a fight-or-flight response.

Similarly, you could attach danger to bending because your belief is that you have a slipped disc or have arthritis and bending is going to wear away your back. Bending may have caused pain in the past so that seems a good enough reason to attach danger to bending, just as Claire did. So now your behaviour is to avoid bending. You can associate danger with anything, such as walking, running, lifting, sitting or slouching in a chair. Pain is a protective mechanism just like anxiety is. Its job is to keep you safe and avoid any real or perceived danger.

So, if your belief is that bending is going to wear away your back or cause a disc to "slip out" then of course that is a good enough reason for your nervous system to feel threatened by that movement. And any time you bend, your nervous system can quite rightly generate pain to get you to avoid bending. This isn't to say that your perceptions are wrong. You could be totally justified in believing that a movement is harmful to you.

This is where the conundrum is. If your nervous system's job is to keep you safe and it's painful to move, then surely, it's not safe to move. So, you should be justified in this belief.

Yes, this is true. But sometimes the nervous system can become over-sensitised and over-protective. The nervous system responds to the information it's being given so its response is influenced by your experiences, actions, behaviours, and thoughts. You may have injured yourself months or years ago and since then the tissue has healed, but because of the way you behave, move, and think, and your fears, worries, and stress since the initial injury, the nervous system has more to consider than just tissue injury.

Your nervous system is doing its job to keep you safe but it's basing this on what you believe to be true. Your thoughts, movements, behaviours, fears, worries, stress will all be driven through this belief system.

Placebos

The placebo effect works through the power of belief. Placebo pain relief makes individuals experience pain relief simply by virtue of the anticipation of a benefit.[110] A placebo doesn't cure a problem; it just modulates that area of the brain that is creating the symptom, as the brain believes it is going to work. When a new medication is being trialled, many of them get tested against a placebo. If the results are not better than the placebo, then the medication isn't fit to be brought to market. A placebo is essentially "medication" without any active ingredients. They are often referred to as "sugar pills."

Placebos won't cure tumours or heal a broken limb. The power of positive belief only modulates areas of the brain that influence the symptoms, such as pain, anxiety, or nausea.

One study was conducted in Stanford University on a college student who was suffering with chronic pain following a safari accident. The student had suffered a crush injury to his arm the previous summer. Doctors stroked the area of his arm where the student's injury was and he experienced terrible burning pain rated at 7 out of 10 in his arm where the old injury was. This was confirmed by increased activity in many areas of the brain that are involved in a pain experience. Doctors then put an IV in his arm and told the student that they were going to start putting in a powerful pain medication. Little did the subject know that there were no pain relief ingredients in the IV. Despite the lack of active pain relief, what they found was the subject's pain went down dramatically to a 3/10 with the same stroking stimulus to his arm. This was also confirmed by a decrease in activity in the areas of the brain involved in the subject's pain experience.[111]

Similarly, "sham surgeries", which are surgeries without any physical interventions, were conducted on patients with knee osteoarthritis. There were two groups, the controlled group and the placebo group.

The control group were given real arthroscopic lavage or arthroscopic knee surgeries whereas the placebo group were given skin incisions which were immediately sewn back up to give this group the illusion that they undergone surgery. The results after a 24-month period were no different between the placebo group and the control group.[112]

If the expectation is that the treatment is going to work it can make immediate changes and take the handcuffs off recovery, remove the fear, worry and despair and replace it with positivity and hope which can be enough to kick-start the recovery. Having a positive belief can be powerful. But you have to believe it is going to work. It cannot be fake or pretend belief.

Don't worry. I'm not here trying to get you to pretend that things are going to be okay. That would just be wishful thinking. But you will probably have formed some limiting beliefs along your pain journey. On an individual basis it's impossible for me to be able to go through what negative beliefs you could have formed yourself. This takes a good therapist with knowledge of the way beliefs affect behaviour and pain.

What I am trying to give you is hope that, through education and understanding, you may come to see that things are not how they seem. As a by-product of this process, your beliefs should change.

The nocebo effect

Having a positive belief about a treatment can be powerful, but equally having a negative belief can leave you powerless, especially when you are in pain. One of the most common beliefs people have when they are in pain is that they are damaged, broken or that the more they move, the more they are wearing away their body. This is certainly not a useful belief. Especially if it is not true. Such beliefs can put the shackles on your recovery. You will only be able to recover as well as you believe you can.

So now we move on to the nocebo effect, which is the result of a person having a negative outcome to a treatment due to a negative expectation. The nocebo effect is lesser known than its counterpart, the placebo effect, but, ironically, it is more common and has greater effect on negative outcomes compared to positive outcomes of the placebo effect.[113]

The nocebo effect is prevalent in interactions between patients and healthcare workers. Many treatments do not work because patients have a negative attitude to the physician or the treatment given. If there is a lack of trust in the person or treatment, or if you just believe that the intervention won't work, then you're more likely to get a negative result. This goes for any treatment, whether it's medication, surgery, exercise or manual therapy. Perhaps you've experienced this when initiating treatment with a healthcare provider you didn't trust, resulting in a negative outcome. Many patients that feel their healthcare provider invalidated them can have negative outcomes due to the nocebo effect.

In one study, participants who embraced a biomedical perspective regarding the cause of chronic low back pain (CLBP) believed that the pain stemmed from the structural vulnerability of their spine. This belief was influenced by advice from healthcare practitioners and findings from MRI scans.

Interestingly, those who experienced greater disability were the ones who maintained a more pessimistic view of their back pain. Conversely, individuals with less disability tended to hold more positive beliefs about their condition that weren't shaped by interactions with healthcare practitioners.[114]

Stay off the internet

Beliefs can take root anywhere, not just in a doctor's office. In today's digital age, information is at our fingertips, and Dr Google is always ready to reinforce what you already think is true. Due to something called confirmation bias, the more you search, the more convinced you become of your beliefs.

When it comes to dealing with pain, Dr Google can sometimes make things worse, especially if you believe you're somehow damaged or broken. If that's your belief, you'll almost certainly find ways to strengthen it online.

Here's a crucial piece of advice for anyone dealing with pain: Stay away from the internet. There are generally two scenarios where people go online in this situation. First, if you've recently been injured or if your doctor or physio used confusing terms during your appointment, you might turn to Google for clarity.

When you've just been hurt, you may be looking for reassurance or trying to save money on treatment. Alternatively, you might simply be a curious person who wants to better understand your condition.

Regardless of your reasons, I wouldn't recommend it. All you'll find online are numerous diagnoses, and the prevailing trend is to self-diagnose with the help of Google. Trust me, you'll find a diagnosis, but more often than not, it won't be the right one. I understand the human desire for a diagnosis because it seems like having one would lead to a cure. However, as you've seen, dealing with chronic pain is not as straightforward as a Google search.

When you self-diagnose, confirmation bias kicks in, and you unconsciously start confirming what you already suspect. The result is often confusion and fear. It's easy to get lost in the search for a diagnosis that brings you comfort, but ironically, this can make matters worse. A simple sore toe could end up linked to a serious condition if you dig deep enough. Imagine the anxiety of diagnosing yourself with a severe ailment, only to wait days to see your GP.

The nosy neighbour

We all have a nosy neighbour in our life. These are the people who think they know it all; they are people who love to voice their opinion and diagnose your pain, even though they have no qualifications to do so. They may have had pain in a similar area or have a friend or loved one that had pain so that makes them an expert. These people are as common as the cold. They can also be very dangerous. Their words shouldn't hold as much weight but depending on how convincing the nosy neighbour is and how receptive you are, their words may have a negative impact on your life.

I have a friend who was watching a football match with me; a player that we both knew walked past limping from an injury a week earlier. My friend told him he might not play again because of the knee injury. I challenged him and asked how he could say this; his reply was "I know knees." I found this hilarious at the time, but the more I thought about how often this happens on a daily basis, the more I realised the downside of putting negative thoughts into somebody's head. Different people will take this information differently. Some are receptive and will take it on board and others will just brush it off and not take any notice. It's the people that are receptive to this type of information that I worry about. These are the type of people that hear something and then go onto Dr Google to confirm the diagnosis. They will search the symptoms until they can find one because this is what they are after. Think about confirmation bias. It doesn't have to be a person in a lab coat or a physio who gives out this information.

This can start from anywhere. Having an answer and a diagnosis, then it's easier to find a cure, isn't it? Some people are more receptive to a diagnosis that involves a quick fix, which is why they jump from practitioner to practitioner.

I'm realistic and I know that this will happen and will never change. People in most cases genuinely want to help and they don't mean to inflict negative thoughts on your psychology. You're the one left thinking about what they say. The nosy neighbour will go about their day and not give a second's thought to what was just said.

Fear avoidance model

After an injury, it's perfectly normal to feel some fear, worry, or anxiety towards movement. This reaction is your brain's way of being cautious, reminding you of the past injury, and trying to prevent it from happening again. Remember the brain's goal is survival and if you keep getting injured your chance of survival decreases. Injury will affect your ability to hunt, evade predators, find shelter and even searching for a mate. It's imperative that your brain does its best to protect you. So, in this regard, it's important for the brain to attach fear, worry and uncertainty to something that was previously harmful.

Now, the Fear Avoidance Model is an essential concept to understand. It starts with an injury. Following that, you might decide to avoid certain movements associated with the injury, such as bending your back after a back injury or reaching overhead after a shoulder injury.

While withdrawing from the activity results in decreased pain, there can be some positive reinforcement within the brain. This can keep you repeating the avoidance behaviour, which in turn over time can increase the fear.

This happens all the time with clients of mine. Pain is such a great motivator to avoid certain behaviours. The repeated avoidance of such behaviours can actually increase fear and disability and ultimately reinforce pain, as shown in the figure below.

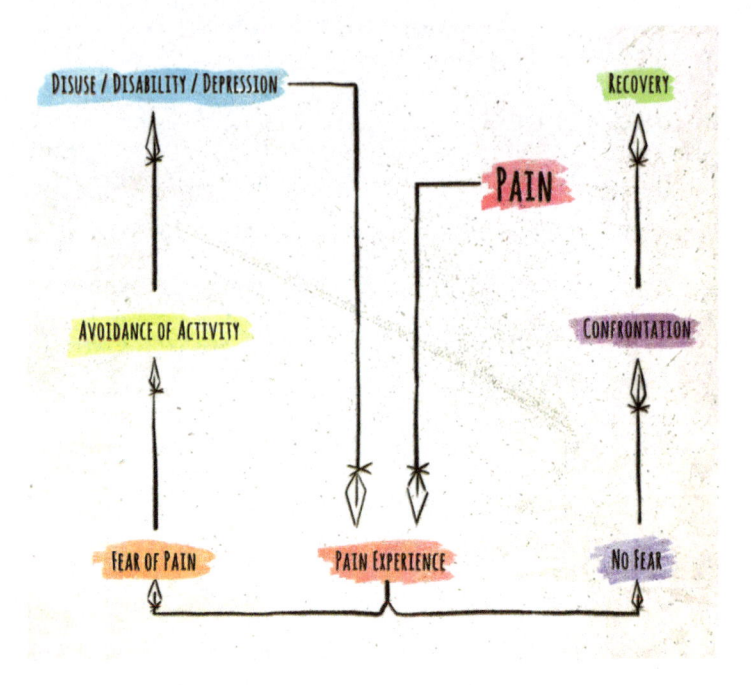

Long term avoidance of activity contributes to greater levels of disability due to physical deconditioning and increased fear.

It has been shown that greater pain-related fear has been associated with lower levels of physical activity among persons with low-back pain and that people with low-back pain who remain sedentary experience greater levels of disability over time.[115]

Sometimes, negative beliefs about what to avoid can be from your own interpretation of why the pain is there. Or they can be influenced by others, like nosy neighbours, healthcare professionals or results on images (MRIs and X-rays).

However, it's important to understand that avoiding these actions doesn't actually solve anything. Avoiding the problem only weakens you and makes you more vulnerable. Sooner or later, you'll have to confront these challenges, and avoidance won't help when that time comes. Avoidance strategies may help in the short term but over the long-term cause bigger issues.

How do you identify and change beliefs

Beliefs are what you have accepted as the truth. They could be a long-term core belief, a religious belief or just something that you are passionately in favour of. Some of them are easier to change than others. You may be willing to change them or not.

You cannot wake up one day and decide you won't think this way anymore. Remember these beliefs are ingrained into your unconscious and most of your feelings and decisions are based around the belief.

One remarkable study involved a schizophrenic. This woman was observed to have a split personality. Under normal conditions, her blood glucose levels were normal. However, the moment she believed she was a diabetic, her entire physiology changed to become that of a diabetic, including elevated blood glucose levels.[116] So, your beliefs are so powerful they can even affect your physiology to a certain extent.

You could have a lot invested in your belief. Many people base their reputation on a belief, so they have a lot more to give up.[117] So, changing them isn't straightforward. First, you need to be willing to challenge your belief. If you are not willing to change your beliefs, throw in the towel. Put the book in the bin. Actually, don't put it in the bin; I have spent a lot of time writing it.

Some people are so invested in their belief it's almost impossible for them to accept information that's contrary to their beliefs. Have a look at "Flat Earthers" for instance. This is a prime example of confirmation bias. There is so much evidence that challenges and outright debunks the flat earth theory, but to someone who is heavily invested in a belief, all that evidence is disregarded. You may wonder why somebody would just disregard such compelling evidence that the earth is round. To understand this, you need to look at the motivations of the person in question. To be a flat earther means you are part of an exclusive club. You may have built a community around you, made friends, and have social benefits based on this belief. To challenge the belief and accept that it is in fact a sphere is not in your best interests because it would mean giving up the flat earth club membership. So even the most compelling evidence is disregarded.

If you are receptive to changing your mind then we are off to a great start.

"An opportunity for changing the way someone thinks magnifies when his or her thinking is muddled, turbulent, confused, uncertain or anxious."[118] In other words, if someone is unsure what is going on with their pain or injury, their ability to alter their belief about their pain is greatly increased.

Next, we need good quality concise education, with logical explanation. This is what I hope I am providing here. In the context of pain so many people's beliefs can be swayed with good communication and the reasoning behind it.

Finally, the only true way to change your beliefs with regard to pain is through experience. This means experiencing new things that you previously avoided or even believed were bad for you. (But on a scaled down version of the movements to allow you to build up tolerance and confidence again. This is what I will help you with in the final chapter.)

When we choose to change our thoughts, we become open and receptive to pieces of sensory information previously blocked by our beliefs, there are bursts of neurochemicals in the brain, new synapses are formed and things begin to change.[119] It's like the brain has taken away the filter and is ready for change. When we change our thinking, we change our beliefs, and we change our behaviour.[120]

Your identity/self-image

Your personal identity, often referred to as your self-image, is essentially the way you perceive yourself. When you gaze into a mirror, you witness a reflection of your physical appearance, but this doesn't capture the full essence of who you are. You see the real you in your mind.

Your self-image takes shape through a combination of intrinsic factors such as height, weight, eye colour, hair colour, race, gender, sexual orientation, as well as psychosocial elements like culture, religious beliefs, personality traits, education, upbringing, and life experiences. It begins to form in childhood and evolves over time. The person you are today is not the same as you were five years ago. Life is a journey, and both internal and external factors lead to change. You may have completed your education, started a family, advanced in your career, retired, discovered new passions, or faced challenges such as injuries that altered your life in various ways.

Internally, you might have grown emotionally stronger or encountered situations that affected your confidence. As life unfolds, our interests, responsibilities, and lifestyle adapt, but fundamentally, we remain the same at our core.

Within your identity, there are various roles you take on. Each of these roles comes with internal expectations and personal meanings about how to embody them. Your self-image and beliefs guide your actions and behaviours in these roles, defining how you think they should be enacted.

For instance, consider two parents: one may be strict, while the other is easy-going. Both are parents, but they interpret and play this role differently. Neither approach is inherently right or wrong; they are merely distinct individuals who view the parental role through the lens of their own beliefs and self-image.

This perception is rooted in your core beliefs about what it means to be a parent, influenced by your values and your experiences, including your upbringing and the influence of others. Attempting to act in a manner that contradicts your core identity can feel alien because it goes against your internal understanding of yourself.

Even people who know you well will form expectations based on their understanding of your self-image, as they recognise the unique qualities that define you.

We all have an identity; we are all unique. Most people will float through life and never have to think about who they are, until it's gone.

Loss of identity

What would happen if all of a sudden you weren't able to be the "you" that you know so well anymore? What if you were in too much pain to be the boss, colleague, friend, or parent? If you couldn't play the role the way you would like to play it, would you be the person you want to be?

You can start to lose your identity abruptly, from a trauma, or after an accident, or it can be a gradual process starting from a small acute pain that starts and doesn't go away. You can lose your identity from being forced to adapt to your current circumstances because of your pain. It may not be possible to be as sociable as you once were or you may not be able to fulfil your self-imposed roles at home, work or in the community.

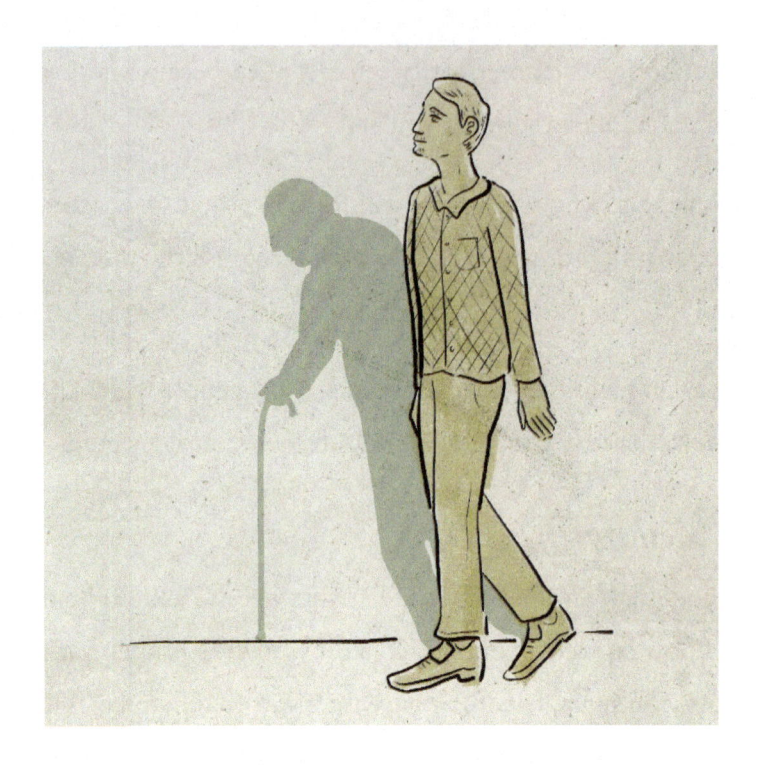

When you cannot fulfil these roles, you may feel like you are losing a sense of who you are. Many new mothers go through this loss of identity because, in most cases, careers and social life can take a back seat when there is a new priority in life. Although this can be tough on mothers, it's easier to accept as, in most cases, it was their decision to have a child. Moreover, there's always the added bonus of having a new baby to look after. When it comes to pain, it's never the person's choice to be in pain. So, when your life has been interrupted for a long period of time it isn't as easy to accept.

Maintaining your true identity when living with pain is incredibly hard. Eventually pain forces you to accept the new you. You can try to resist your pain and continue through life, but eventually pain will grind you down.

Let's not forget that pain's role is to draw your attention to perceived or actual danger. So, if what you are addressing isn't what needs to be addressed, then the pain is going to persist until you do address that. It's as simple as that.

When a shift of identity is forced upon you, pain starts to reorganise your identity. Your thoughts, behaviours, habits and actions change. A different identity or self-image arises, usually not for the better. Identity changes are not something that happen overnight. It's a gradual process that is modified by failed treatments, poor education, poor advice and disability. It can creep up on you until you can't believe how much you have changed.

New identities come with new labels. These labels can come from healthcare professionals, friends, family or your own research. All of a sudden, they are part of your everyday conversations. "Hi, I'm Sharon, I have fibromyalgia." "Hi, I'm Kevin, I have chronic low back pain." Unfortunately, in my experience because pain has such a profound effect on people's lives, it becomes who they are and almost engulfs their identity, making it the primary part of their life. When someone's identity or self-image is that they are in debilitating pain and can't do anything, then their actions and behaviours will align with this.

How you see yourself will affect how you act in the world. If you see yourself as a fearful, broken, injured person who has never healed right, your behaviours and actions will reflect this. You will be more protective and guarded in fear of "damaging" yourself further. The language you use in relation to yourself will be of a more cautious or protective nature. You can develop protective postures, make groans and grunting sounds when moving but all of this is playing out the role of your new identity.

In his book, *Psycho Cybernetics*, Maxwell Maltz compares our identity to a thermostat in a room. Imagine that your thermostat is set at 20 degrees Celsius. Somebody opens a window and the room temperature drops to 18 degrees. The room temperature is a little uncomfortable because you are used to the room being 20 degrees. The thermostat kicks in and the heat comes on until the temperature in the room increases to the familiar 20 degrees again.

Our identity or self-image is like this. If you come to see yourself as a person in pain, your behaviours and actions will align to your identity and keep you on track with how you see yourself. If there is any attempt to veer away from this self-image, you will quickly recalibrate and bring yourself back to where you feel comfortable, ironically making you uncomfortable again. The brain loves familiarity because it means it can predict things better. Even if the prediction is pain and disability.

Let's go back to the story of our ancestor in the strange forest looking for food. He heard a rustling in the bushes. Because he wasn't in the comfort of his own forest it made it more difficult to be able to predict what was in the bushes. His brain immediately went into a fight-or-flight response and evoked fear and anxiety even though it was only a rabbit in the bushes. When your identity is of someone in pain, moving away from that means moving away from the familiar. The brain sees familiarity as safety, even though this safety means you're in pain. Moving into the unfamiliar means the brain cannot predict what's going to happen and the brain doesn't like this.

In a way it's self-sabotage. This is common for overweight people who lose weight. Many don't see themselves as a skinny person even though they have lost so much weight. As a result, their actions and self-sabotaging behaviours often mean that their weight loss gains are short lived. Like the thermostat, they want to restore equilibrium, which for them means putting weight back on.

If you are in pain for so long that you only see yourself as a person in pain then that is where your internal thermostat is set. An identity shift will be required to achieve long-term pain-free results or, at the very least, less debilitating pain. Otherwise, your self-sabotaging behaviours and actions will steer you back towards your identity, which is "the person in pain."

If you're not sure if this is you, take a minute and think to yourself who you see yourself as now. Do you see yourself as a person who is in pain? A person who is broken? Can you imagine yourself being pain-free at some point in the future?

After reading this paragraph I want you to close your eyes for a minute to visualise yourself being someone who is pain-free, doing all the things that you would do if you had no pain. How does that feel? Does it feel natural and normal? Or does imagining your life being pain-free feel alien to you? Can you imagine this or is it a struggle? How do you feel inside? Does this elevate your heart rate? Do you feel a bit uneasy or does this feel okay? Or can you not imagine yourself being in pain at all?

If you can only see yourself as being a person in debilitating pain, then there is an identity issue. The self-image you have of yourself is of a person in debilitating pain. The unconscious thermostat is set to this which may be making it more difficult to change external issues, as internal issues drive external changes.

We will speak more about how we are going to put this way of thinking into practice later in the book. For now, take note of this and we'll come back to it.

NOTES

_____
_____
_____
_____
_____
_____
_____
_____
_____
_____
_____
_____
_____
_____
_____
_____
_____
_____
_____
_____
_____
_____

Chapter 6

Social

The least researched area of the biopsychosocial model of pain is the social aspect, even though everything we do in life is partly due to some sort of social or environmental motivation. There is endless biological and psychological research in relation to pain but, when it comes to the social side, the research falls short.

Can your social life really influence pain? Your social life is a pretty broad term so I have broken it down into two categories to make this easier to talk about. There are outer social circles which include a broader social context, religion, politics, culture, and society as a whole. These areas can certainly influence chronic pain, especially with the politics of our turbulent times. This can lead to stress that certainly affects the sensitivity of our nervous system. Although there is merit in talking about the outer social circle, I would like to focus on the social aspect that is in our control.

This leads us to our inner social circles, which will include your close social contacts such as family, friends, neighbours, and those related to hobbies, work and healthcare. These are our everyday social interactions. Pain can have a detrimental effect on your social life but your social life can also have an impact on your pain; this is another reciprocal relationship.

This is a relatively unexplored area – most healthcare professionals would not even think to explore it. And let's face it; when you are suffering with pain, would you think it's due to, or at least influenced by, something that's going on in your social life? People don't usually consider their psychosocial environment because it's easier to assume that their pain is due to tissue health. There is a stigma that suggests that, if the pain isn't something physical, then it must be all in your head. Dr Claire Ashton-James, one of the few pain scientists who specialise in the social aspect, has said, "We as a society are more compassionate and empathic towards people with an acute injury than we are with people with chronic pain. We would never send a bunch of flowers or a get well soon card to a person that has been suffering with chronic pain." And you know, she's right! You may well make the same choice, even though the chronic pain sufferer probably needs the flowers, love or attention more. While, for the person with the acute injury it may be painful or inconvenient, the injury will heal and, in most cases, they will get back to normal life within three months. It's the chronic pain sufferer who lives with pain for years on end.

If you're having problems at home, in work, in a toxic relationship or you are constantly stressing, worrying or overthinking about something that's going on in your life then how can you think that there will not be changes that will be happening in your body? Your social life can dictate your mood, stress levels, sleep, emotions, lifestyle and health. It could be argued that the social aspect is the most important area.

I truly believe that if you went to the best doctor, surgeon or physio in the world and they could provide you with the best treatment on the market, if the social contributing factors of your pain were not addressed as soon as you left their office, it would not be long until you were back to where you were before you went in. I see this all the time when clients come to me and say they have been to "everyone." They jump and jump between therapists, doctors, specialists and get treatments like medication, exercises, or even surgery but the social aspects are not addressed. Clients are going home after their consultations and working sixty-hour weeks, eating poorly, drinking too much alcohol, being couch potatoes or living in toxic environments. This sort of lifestyle is all too common nowadays, along with less movement, less sunlight, more stress anxiety and more depression. Chronic pain is getting worse as time goes on, not better. You'd think that, because of technology and new pharmacological interventions, chronic pain would be on the decline but the sad reality is that it's not. So, it's time to start looking at pain from a broader perspective. Treatments need to be personal, and the social aspects need to be considered.

The social side of pain is gaining momentum thankfully. Scientists and doctors who specialise in pain are starting to take notice. Social scientists agree that the social side of pain has a huge role in the pain experience. So much so that some social pain scientists are recommending a change in the official definition of pain to include a social aspect. There is always a social element to your pain, no question. Your social life may have influenced your pain from the beginning or it may have become more of a factor since your pain experience started. The longer that you are suffering the more your social life is affected.

There are many overlaps between each of the biological, psychological and social domains. These three areas do not work independently of each other. They are mixed up and deeply intertwined with each other. The biopsychosocial model is more like a bowl of spaghetti than three separate entities.

We could talk about how living or working in a stressful environment can influence pain but we have spoken about this in previous chapters. We know that too much stress sensitises your system. We know that living in constant stress due to your social surroundings can suppress your immune system, and make you be more susceptible to getting injured, having flare-ups and having more episodes of pain. Yes, stress at work, long hours, deadlines, negative people, and problems at home are all technically social aspects that influence pain. But they have been covered already in different chapters.

So, in this chapter we are going to focus on the deeper social aspects of pain: how you are perceived in the world and how you perceive yourself in the world. I'm talking about your response to pain in society and society's response to you.

We will touch on how pain affects your relationships, not just at home but also with work, friends, and healthcare practitioners: support networks around you and those who are not around you anymore. You may or may not have thought about this. What I see in my clinic is roughly 50% of my clients are unaware of the deeper effects. I think they all know on some level and they may have thought about it superficially from time to time but never really dived deep into the effects of pain and how their social life has changed.

All of these are unspoken aspects of chronic pain. Not unspoken because it's an unwritten rule: "The first rule of social pain is don't talk about social pain." No, I mean it just isn't spoken about because frankly very few people know about social pain and its effects. Take it from me, there are not too many psychologists or psychotherapists that specialise in pain.

There are no medications or physio exercises that will sort out your social problems. Reading this chapter will hopefully help you see this. There is no silver bullet that will wipe away the social element of your pain either. Medication may give you some short-term relief but it's not going to resolve your environment. It just kicks the can down the road and doesn't sort anything out.

Reflection is needed on this topic, but only after education. Take it in and then reflect. This will probably be the most unexplored area in your chronic pain journey so far. Just read on with an open mind.

Social role swap

We all have a social role to play, whether we like it or not. This is how society in general functions. You could be a teacher, a student, a parent, a boss, or a police officer. Whatever the role, we play parts that are expected of us in whatever situation we are in. William Shakespeare once said, "All the world's a stage, and all the men and women merely players: They have their exits, and their entrances; And one man in his time plays many parts." In each role you play, your behaviour will change to suit it. You could be a fun-loving dad at home, always messing and joking with the kids, but when you are at work you will be a lot more serious and professional.

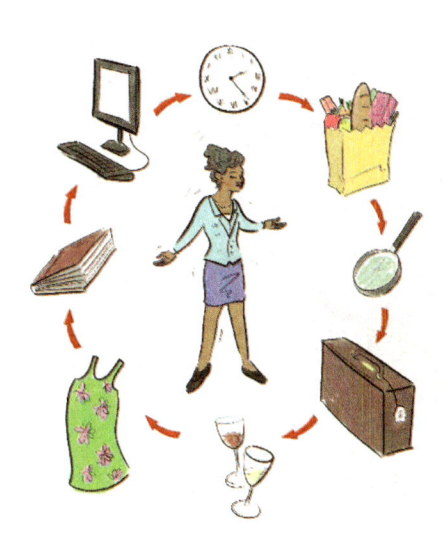

Social roles create structure in society. With each social role comes a set of expectations and behaviour. Mothers care and show love to their young. Police officers support local communities, build relationships and combat crime.

In our house my fiancé likes to find jobs for me to do. I have adopted the social role of the DIY guy. She loves to buy flat pack furniture and leave it there until I put it together. There's not even a conversation where she politely asks, "Kieran, would you mind putting together this flat pack dining table that I bought." She will just say, "I got us a new dining table." When I walk into the dining room, all I can see is a rectangular box in the corner of the room. I spend three hours getting annoyed trying to follow instructions that don't make any sense. I'm not even any good at being the DIY guy but somehow, I have adopted this role and my behaviours have changed to play this role.

The Stanford Prison Experiment is a great example of how we conform to the social role that is expected of us. This experiment was so incredible that they made a movie about it. (SPOILER ALER: If you haven't watched the movie, skip the next two paragraphs and watch it.)

Scientists at the University of Stanford wanted to find out if the brutality reported among guards in American prisons was due to the sadistic personalities of the guards or more to do with the prison environment that they were in. So they set up a fake prison on college campus. After advertising for volunteers to take part in an experiment, they split up the twenty-one participants into two groups: eleven guards and ten prisoners. The guards would work in eight-hour shifts while the prisoners would be assigned cells and a cellmate. Prisoners were given ID numbers and their names were taken away in order to make them feel anonymous. They wore a prison uniform, which was a smock, and which had their ID number on it.

Within hours of the experiment starting, the guards started to harass the prisoners. They would wake them up in the middle of the night blowing their whistles, getting the prisoners to line up for head counts. They would give the prisoners physical punishments like push-ups or give them boring tasks to do. Prisoners started to rebel on the second morning by taking their numbers off and barricading themselves into their rooms. The guards called for reinforcements and used fire extinguishers in order to get the prisoners to back down. As a punishment, they took their beds away. Many prisoners started to conform to prison rules after this and even started to snitch on other prisoners breaking the rules in order to get special treatment from the guards. The prisoners became more submissive as time went on and the guards became more aggressive. The experiment was intended to run for two weeks but it was terminated after six days due to the emotional breakdowns of prisoners, and the excessive aggression of the guards. It was a really amazing study and an example of how we play the roles expected of us in order to keep a society functioning.

Playing multiple roles

Studies have shown that having a greater number of valued social roles is related to higher levels of self-esteem and overall wellbeing, and fewer psychological symptoms such as depression and anxiety.[121]

You may cherish the role you have or may not cherish it. Some people who are suffering with pain may not be able to fulfil their role anymore because their pain is too debilitating. A mother may not be able to nurture her kids the way she would like to. She might not be able to work because sitting causes too much pain. When these roles cannot be fulfilled, a social role swap can take place. It may start off as a brief swap to help out, but when the pain doesn't get better things don't go back to the way they were. It can be a relief that someone is helping you in this situation or, depending on the role and how much you cherish it, it can be difficult to allow someone to take over this role.

The more you value the role you play, the harder it will be on you emotionally when a spouse or a colleague takes it over, for example, if a father has to a take over his wife's previous responsibilities in the household or vice versa.

Generally, parents really value their role and the thought of handing over part of that role can be a tough pill to swallow. Your self-esteem can take a huge blow, feelings of inadequacy can manifest and mood can change as a result. We know that these changes can influence pain and feed the problem. This creates another pain loop (pain – disability – mood – pain).[122] But the majority of us play multiple roles in society, such as a parent at home, a tennis coach at our local tennis club, the dispenser of advice to a friend, or a manager at work.

Social role swaps are unlikely to happen in isolation. They can, but more often than not, when a person cannot fulfil one role due to pain, it's likely that the pain is interfering with other aspects of their life as well, such as career, family, friendships or hobbies. You could be a person that everyone relied on and now you're in too much pain to help others. This is surprisingly common in my clinic. Even those who are in terrible chronic pain do not want to give up their role. They continue to put others first, even when they really aren't fit even to deal with their own issues.

Those who do give up this role tend to hide away rather than being seen to be weak. They struggle with being seen in a vulnerable position. One client, "Sarah," was suffering with severe back pain as a consequence of a car crash a number of years earlier. Her role within her circle was being the person who looked after everyone. When they had problems, they went to Sarah. Sarah always gave the best advice and came up with the right solutions. She would regularly help out with babysitting, book spa weekends away and organise nights out with the girls. But now she had a problem. She was suffering terribly with her back. Her friends still called her up and asked her to help out with babysitting so they could have nights out with their husbands. What they didn't realise was how badly Sarah was suffering. She didn't want to tell anybody. They knew that she was in pain, but she would always brush it off. She didn't want anyone to know how she was addicted to the pain medication, how little sleep she was getting or how her marriage was in turmoil because of the pain she was in. All because she didn't want to be seen as the vulnerable one. She had a role to play and she was sticking to it.

Reasoning with Sarah was difficult. It was more like a negotiation. But how could she ever truly be able to help others if she couldn't help herself? I tried to reassure her she would be able to resume this role again in the future when she got herself back in a better place but for now, she needed to take a break away from being the go-to girl in the group and put herself first for once. Eventually she reluctantly agreed. She took the time out to work on herself and now she is back playing that role again like a champion.

At this point we are just acknowledging that these roles play a factor. If your pain is getting worse due to a role that you are fulfilling, you should accept help if it is offered, to help ease the burden in the short term. That would be a start. Speak to your friends and tell them about your situation. If they are your friends they will understand and show support to you. Chronic pain is invisible. People won't know how badly you are suffering unless you tell them. In the final chapter we will find a way to help you plan for getting your social role(s) back. But if your pain is getting worse and you feel you cannot fulfil a role you need to listen to your body, stop taking on more roles for now and put yourself first.

How pain affects intimate relationships

Relationships can be tough enough, without living with persistent pain. So, when you throw pain into your everyday life it can make or break a relationship. Chronic pain will have impacts on relationships in one form or another. Your life will be disrupted. You may not be able to do the things that you did before as a couple. You may need a social role swap at home where your partner takes over some duties around the house. Date nights, holidays and even your sex life can be affected.

Many of my patients report that their sex lives have been interrupted; the pain sufferer can begin to fear sex as it may be too much of a challenge.[123] Also, the sex drive can be affected as, if you are living in fight-or-flight mode, your libido can be reduced. Certain painkillers and anti-depressants can also diminish your sex drive. All of these factors can reduce the intimacy in relationships. Your relationship can become more distant. You or your partner could see a lowering of self-esteem or self-worth.

Studies indicate that not only is chronic pain associated with problems in marital relationships but also heightened distress and physical symptoms in spouses as well.[124] "These effects are related less to the existence of a chronic pain problem per se and more to patients' and spouses' way of coping with the situation." Studies show that the involvement of your spouse in the treatment process improves marital satisfaction among chronic pain patients; their support-seeking needs are best satisfied through the involvement of their spouses in the process of treatment.[125]

So, a better plan for how to cope with the situation is needed. Who is going to take up which roles in the house? Get a plan written down so everyone is clear on who does what. But remember that, if your spouse is taking up these new roles, this is part of a short to medium term strategy. Your plan isn't for your spouse to do everything so you can relax and put your feet up. Your spouse is going to take up these roles in order to free up more time for you to make the changes that are needed for you to get back to optimal health. We will speak about this more in the final chapter.

A career with pain

In 2016 it was estimated that ill health costs the UK economy £100 billion annually, with musculoskeletal conditions being the second highest cause of sickness absence.[126] Strategies like pain meds and sick leave can be implemented in the short term but they aren't sustainable. If pain persists, these strategies are usually not enough. Many people have to leave their jobs as their pain is too much for them to be able to perform their day-to-day duties.

Among those who are able to continue with their work, many of them do not disclose their situation for fear of losing their job. I believe these are legitimate concerns. There is a perception that pain sufferers would not be able to handle as much work as a non-pain sufferer. A non-pain sufferer in general would perhaps have fewer sick days, be able to do more physical work and be less fatigued.

There is clearly a stigma when it comes to people who suffer with chronic pain in the workplace. And maybe you can understand why people think this way. The vast majority of the general population doesn't understand pain. They think that it is only due to tissue health, so when they see a colleague suffering with pain and no clear injury, they may wonder if that person is making it up to get out of work or responsibility. When you are not looking like you are in pain, they may question whether you are in pain at all. "You don't look like you're hurting."

So, what should pain sufferers do in the workplace? Speaking with management and telling them of your condition is one approach, but you may not know how they will react. Will they be empathetic to your situation or, deep down, will they think that you are looking for an easy ride and don't want to adopt any responsibility? Promotion prospects could be hindered and there is always the fear of job loss. These are all legitimate concerns to have when you are in pain. If you don't fully understand your pain, how do you expect someone else to?

There seems to be a long way to go before there is a clear consensus about what the right thing to do is. The right thing to do can mean different things to different people. If you're relying on that job to feed your family, you would argue the right thing to do is to make sure you feed your family; you don't want to jeopardise that by telling your employer about your condition. On the flip side, your employer hired you and is paying you to do a job; if that cannot be fulfilled, what is the right thing to do in this situation? Whatever the situation, it's another stress that you have to deal with on a daily basis and if you're in a job with a deadline and goals being set it makes it all the more difficult. If it's possible, the best solution is to try to build a support network around you.

As difficult as it may seem, speaking to management and advising them of your situation is the best solution in most cases. By not telling colleagues or management you run the risk of being labelled as lazy if you are having a bad flare-up, or your colleagues may become resentful because you cannot come into work. Also, negative moods can lead to negative judgement from others. If you're in pain, you may be oblivious to your mood or behaviour. Your attention span may be reduced on bad days. If your colleagues don't know about your pain, how will they understand?

If more people are told about your situation, then more people can empathise with you. You want empathy, not sympathy; you don't want people to feel sorry for you, you just want people to understand your situation better. A network of support around you can help you thrive. This cannot happen if you remain silent. But this is job-dependent. Unfortunately, given the stress and demands of jobs in the world we live in, this is not realistic in all cases. Employers can also feel deceived that you haven't disclosed this information if you were already suffering when you were hired – and maybe they have a point.

Chronic pain is correlated with unemployment and negative occupational outcomes.[127] As a result of chronic pain many people are forced into poverty due to them not being able to hold down a job. In a UK study, two thirds of chronic pain sufferers who were questioned said that they would not disclose their condition to employers due to the fear of not getting a job or losing their job.[128]

I have clients who have unfortunately stopped working altogether due to pain. Other clients have thriving careers despite their pain sometimes being debilitating. The difference is either that they're self-employed and able to work their own hours or they have a more supportive work environment where their colleagues understand their situation better. If the job itself is clearly aggravating the situation there is only so long that you will be able to tolerate the pain. So, speaking to your superiors is the only way to help come up with a solution to the situation.

If there isn't a solution to be found perhaps you might have to consider a leave of absence or finding a different job. I don't say this lightly either. I know how hard it can be to find a job and I know that bills have to be paid. But on the other hand, if your pain is too debilitating and it's not getting better, then a decision is going to have to be made at some point. You may be in a situation where you have another member of the house working full-time so the bills can be paid. You might not have the luxury of this and you could be a single parent. Really there is not one solution for all.

There isn't a solution to this in sight and educating managers more about pain would help; but that is a long shot and I can't see many companies adopting this type of education. Perhaps in big organisations they might, but certainly not in the small to medium-sized companies. It's a complex topic and not one with a clear answer. Each situation has its own issues.

Hobbies

Living in such a busy world, it's hard to find time for that escape. People tend to have many different things going on in their lives, including work, our kids, school, and relationship conflicts, plus a seemingly endless list of other minor stressors. People rarely find time for themselves.

We know that hobbies are therapeutic. They reduce stress and anxiety. They lower your blood pressure.[129] In some cases, they keep you socially involved. In other cases, they provide some form of exercise. This can help cleanse you of all of life's stresses. Almost like going to see a priest for confession and cleansing your soul, you are cleansing your mind by relaxing and escaping. It's really important that you find a way to continue your hobby. England football legend Paul Gascoigne, who is well known for his problems off the pitch, once said that while he was on the pitch all of his problems went away. "For that time on the turf, I was free."

Hobbies are a way to escape, to reduce stress and to make us happier. But they are often one of the first things that are reduced or dropped when pain develops.

If your hobby was power-lifting then obviously there's no real way that you can do that. But what can you do? Can you do a similar, less aggressive movement and start from there? This is where finding a good physiotherapist in your area can help. I wish this book could give you the answers you are looking for, but that cannot be done without a consultation. My point is though that there is always something you can do on some level so you don't just give up your hobbies.

Alternatively, maybe you didn't give up your hobby because you were in pain. Perhaps it was because you just couldn't find the time to fit it in anymore. Maintaining a good quality of life is vital to recovering from a chronic condition. I expect you already know that if your quality of life suffers, you will end up suffering.

I would argue that when suffering with pain, maintaining some level of interest in your hobby is as important or in some cases more important than doing specific exercises provided by your physio. By dropping your hobby, you are giving up on something that gives you meaning, and that gives you fulfilment and joy in your life. What's left over is resentment, lower mood, and the feeling of being excluded. This can be the start of the process of self-isolation.

It's so important to have things to look forward to. I had a client a couple of years ago called "Helen." She was heavily involved in gymnastics until she had a skiing accident which led to her being bedridden for two months. After she got back to her feet, she was suffering with back pain. She completely gave up all her interest in gymnastics. She never went to see the girls perform or tried to get on the mats. For one year she avoided the gym. Why? Because she wouldn't have been able to do the things that she was able to do before her pain. Even though she missed it terribly, she avoided it. She hadn't even considered the idea that she could get involved in a lesser capacity. Instead, she thought if she couldn't get on the mats there was no point in going at all.

Not being able to do the things that give you meaning has such a negative effect on your mood, emotions and ultimately your pain. After we spoke and came up with a plan for her to just go back inside the gym, be in that environment and help out a little, her whole face changed. The only reason she hadn't gone back was that no one had ever suggested it.

With my clients I will always focus not on what they can't do, but what they can do. It's a quick mind-set change; immediately they are thinking differently and more positively. In Helen's case, she now thought of all the things that she could help out with in the gymnastics clubs. Suddenly she had a more positive outlook on things. This induced a change in mood and a feeling there was light at the end of the tunnel.

Setting some goals is hugely important; we will talk more in depth about how to tackle this in the progressive loading section of the final chapter.

If you don't have a hobby, this should give you the encouragement to find one. It doesn't have to start with a sociable hobby. Just picking up a book and reading for six minutes a day can reduce stress.[130] A study from the *Journal of Health Psychology* found that gardening can improve your mood and reduce the stress hormone cortisol.[131] The same goes for yoga or dancing. The main thing is to find something that you are interested in, something that you would look forward to and make some time to do. The evidence is there to show you the benefits; it's just up to you to put yourself first. If you're looking to unwind what better way to do it than doing it with something you love?

Is there perceived injustice in your pain?

"Justice will not be served until those who are unaffected are as outraged as those who are" – Benjamin Franklin

I think most people like to think that the world should be fair and just, that everything in the world should be balanced out. If you do something good then you should get something good in return.

But the sad reality is that it's just not. Bad things happen to good people and good things happen to bad people all the time. The world isn't fair – far from it. If it was fair, we wouldn't have cancer, poverty, wrongful convictions or any other of the catastrophes that happen all around this planet. Life can be unfortunate and it can be tough at times. It's rarely balanced. But despite all of these potential injustices, we like to think that these bad things will never happen to people who don't deserve it. So, when a trauma like an assault or a road traffic accident ends with you being hurt, you may question why this has happened to you. You may think, "I didn't deserve this."

When we talk about perceived injustice, what do we mean? The dictionary describes it as a lack of fairness or justice. Perceived injustice (PI) is a phrase that can anger people. It can be misinterpreted as fake injustice or made-up injustices. But all perceived injustice means is that it's injustice from your perspective. I will admit that when I first heard this term, I immediately thought that this was a dodgy term that could easily be taken the wrong way. But it's just about how you see the world and the injustice based on your experiences, thoughts and emotions – nobody else's. So, it has to be called perceived injustice.

According to Dominic Harmon, professor of anaesthesiology in Limerick, the greatest predictor of chronic pain is injustice.[132] Previously it was thought that catastrophising was the greatest predictor of persistent pain. "Now we believe it to be injustice."

Injustices around the world in general can spark emotions. Personal injustices will anger and frustrate. In fact, anger and frustration are heavily linked to injustice. This anger or frustration can be hidden and not picked up on by healthcare professionals if the right questions aren't asked. The relationship between perceived injustice and pain isn't widely known but this phenomenon is more common with chronic pain sufferers than you might think. Certainly, in my training or research it's not something that has cropped up many times – because this process acts unconsciously. Psychotherapists or psychologists will be more versed on the subject than your regular doctor or local physiotherapist. But let's face it, how many people would go to speak to a psychotherapist or psychologist when it comes to pain? Not very many in my experience. So, it's unlikely that the healthcare professionals you generally deal with will ever be able to pick up on this and put two and two together.

Typically, perceived injustice will manifest from unnecessary suffering as a result of somebody else's actions.[133] It can be a result of the trauma where the perpetrator hasn't taken responsibility for the incident, or it can be a result of medical negligence whereby you feel let down by the medical professional such as your doctor, surgeon or the system in general. It doesn't usually start at the time of the incident. It usually develops when things don't get better. This makes it more difficult to resolve because by the time the connection is picked up (if it ever is) it's usually years after the initial trauma.

A lack of understanding and acknowledgment from family or friends can also leave you feeling injustice. "People don't know how badly I'm suffering"; "It's not fair." Anger, bitterness, resentfulness and frustrations can manifest because of these feelings.

In all of these cases it is important for you to get the acknowledgment that you have been wronged. From your perspective, people need to know what you have been through and what you are still going through, especially if there is no visible injury. If there's no visible injury it's harder for people to see your suffering; this can lead to an increase in pain behaviour, to demonstrate to other people how much pain you are in. If people see how badly you are suffering, then they may see how much you have been wronged. There is a degree to which you need to hold onto your symptoms until you get the justice you feel you deserve. It's important to note that this isn't a conscious thought and is more attributed to unconscious thoughts and behaviours.[134]

Dr Jonathan Douglas, a clinical psychologist from Canada, explains how this concept works: "My injury proves that what you did was horribly wrong. If I get better, it's like I'm letting you off the hook! So... how can I get better, when my injury is the proof of what's been done to me, and **my injury is proof that my anger and bitterness is justified.** " In one of his lectures, he explains how crazy it is that we would make ourselves worse off unconsciously. Nonetheless you can get stuck in this sense of "justified bitterness."

Greater perceived injustice equates to greater pain behaviour.[135] This makes sense because you need to show the world that you have been wronged. If there is no pain behaviour, how would they ever know? Perceived injustice is highly correlated to catastrophising. We spoke about catastrophising and how that is one of the greatest predictors of persistent pain in the psychological chapter.

In Dr Douglas's research, of patients who were still in pain two years after their accidents, 95% were the people not at fault from the accident. You would expect by the law of averages that it would be somewhere around the 50/50 mark. There is no way of predicting who was going to be in more or less pain after an RTA accident between the person responsible for the accident and the victim. What does that tell us? It tells us that there is definitely merit in this theory.

Some people may argue that the victim might be in "pain" because they are going though legal proceedings and perhaps because they see an easy pay-out. But thought processes like this are part of the problem. Insurance companies can be deeply cynical when it comes to paying out compensation. They can leave victims having to jump through hoops seeing multiple physicians to prove that they have been injured.

These claims and court cases don't happen overnight either, so when a victim is left injured after an accident and you have medical professionals assessing you to see if you're actually injured, what do you think the victim is going to do?

The effect of lawyers on recovery has been well documented, and it is consistently associated with worse pain outcomes, greater disability and poorer psychological functioning.[136] If you need your symptoms to prove your case, how are you ever going to get rid of them?

I'll repeat, the greater the perceived injustice, the greater the pain experience.[137] We spoke before about how the brain is a conditioning machine and that we are creatures of habit. We can get conditioned into behaving that way, and as we hold onto these injustices, our behaviour stays the same; unconscious behaviours, unconscious thought processes and unconscious actions. Injustice becomes familiar. You can become comfortable with being in pain or injustice. Over time you change until this can become part of your identity. As we think back to the identity chapter, we know that our behaviours and actions will derive from our identity.

The cost of this is huge. It needs to be identified because it seriously interferes with your recovery, social life, work, relationships, hobbies and more. You may consciously think that you want to get rid of your pain but your unconscious is following a totally different strategy. It's an internal conflict between your conscious and your unconscious mind and something that you will be totally unaware of. We operate unconsciously 90% of the time so there's only ever going to be one winner there.[138]

It can sometimes be easier to forgive the perpetrator than to forgive the insurance company who was supposed to have your back. You may have got your justice with regards to the initial incident, but there could be unresolved anger or bitterness that has grown after the incident.

People prefer to punish perpetrators rather than compensate victims.[139] If you feel have been treated unjustly by a medical professional, the likelihood of getting any retribution is low. At the end of the day, this is from your perspective; they might have a different view on it if they have been following protocol. If it really was medical negligence, you might have a case. But usually it's not medical negligence; it's just the healthcare system in general with long wait times and a lack of suitable treatment. This is certainly the way it is in Ireland anyway. Large parts of the healthcare system are so busy with huge waiting lists, and this can certainly help stall recovery and promote injustice. Up to 61% of chronic pain patients have injustice in their lives and healthcare has been shown to be the greatest source of the injustice.[140]

Even when you get the right treatment, it has been shown that people don't comply with treatments if they feel there is injustice with their pain.[141] They need to hold onto their symptoms to show how they have been wronged, and this will inhibit recovery. "It's your fault I'm not getting better. So, to prove that you have wronged me I'm not going to get better for you." It's like drinking poison and expecting someone else to suffer.

Dr Michael Sullivan, another clinical psychologist from Canada, is leading the line when it comes to perceived injustice with respect to pain and disability. He has published over 200 peer-reviewed papers. In his research, he has found that high scores on perceptions of injustice are correlated with pain catastrophising, fear of movement, and depression. Perceived injustices are also an indicator of poor rehabilitation outcomes and prolonged work absences. Perceptions of injustice not only interfere with physical recovery after injury, they also negatively impact recovery of the mental health problems that might arise after a traumatic injury.[142]

He continues to say that "Injury severity was only associated with appraisals of blame/unfairness, but not perceptions of severity and irreparability of losses sustained. Appraisals of blame and unfairness are dictating the severity of the trauma and not the injury itself. That is really something to behold."

Dr Sullivan has created a short questionnaire that has been shown to do a better job at predicting the outcome of persistent pain than the injury itself. Take a minute to fill out this questionnaire; if you score above 28 then there is some injustice that will need to be investigated.

When injuries happen, they can have profound effects on our lives. This scale was designed to assess how your injury has affected your life.

Listed below are twelve statements describing different thoughts and feelings that you may experience when you think about your injury. Using the following scale, please indicate how frequently you experience these thoughts and feelings when you think about your injury.

0 – never   **1** – rarely   **2** – sometimes   **3** – often   **4** – all the time

1. Most people don't understand how severe my condition is.

2. My life will never be the same.

3. I am suffering because of someone else's negligence.

4. No one should have to live this way.

5. I just want to have my life back.

6. I feel that this has affected me in a permanent way.

7. It all seems so unfair.

8. I worry that my condition is not being taken seriously.

9. Nothing will ever make up for all that I have gone through.

10. I feel as if I have been robbed of something very precious.

11. I am troubled by fears that I may never achieve my dreams.

12. I can't believe this has happened to me.

...*Total*

(Copyright Dr M. Sullivan 2002)

If perceived injustice is playing a role in your ongoing suffering, then it's important that it is identified. Generally, it doesn't work itself out, and the longer it goes on, the more your life is affected and the more resentful and bitter you can become. It doesn't do you or anyone around you any good, so take some time and sit with this and think whether this is something you can work on. If you're waiting for the world to be fair to you, then you're in for a long wait. As much as we think or want everything to be balanced out, it just doesn't work this way. It's time to take control of your situation and start putting yourself first. If you're living in a perpetual world of injustice, you are the abuser. You're abusing yourself by becoming angry, frustrated, bitter or resentful because the world hasn't been fair to you. By holding onto this you can and will hold onto your symptoms, which will lead to not just your recovery being affected but also your life in general.

I mean it in the nicest possible way when I say the world is not fair. You need to dust yourself down and work on yourself. You have the power to change the way you think. Letting go and forgiving is the only way you will ever be able to get justice for yourself. Attributing fault to someone, or something (e.g. an animal or environmental feature), other than oneself is frequently associated with poorer coping with illness.[143]

There may be a lot of anger, frustration, bitterness or resentment built up because of your current circumstances and you may be well entitled to feel all of those things. However, it doesn't do you or anyone around you any good. It affects your relationships with family, society and healthcare when you fail to move on with your life. Accept what has happened and look forward to a better tomorrow. As Jordan Peterson says, "be better than the person you were yesterday." By living in the past and not letting go, you stay in an endless cycle of reliving those emotions and experiences from the past. Whatever happened in the past is in the past! It has happened and it's done. There is nothing you can do about it now. You are reliving the past today by holding on to these emotions and not letting go. The brain is experiencing the past over and over as you replay it in your mind.

So, let's revisit the Benjamin Franklin quote: "Justice will not be served until those who are unaffected are as outraged as those who are." I would have to disagree with this statement, because if you're waiting for other people to be as outraged as you, you are in for a long wait. Work on yourself; you cannot control what others think or do.

On that note, if you feel you have been wronged in the past and you don't want to let go of this injustice, I would recommend speaking to a psychotherapist or a psychologist on this matter. This book isn't designed to help you with those deep-rooted feeling and emotions. But if it can bring you awareness that these emotions can influence your pain and affect your recovery then that's good enough for me.

What do you gain from being in pain?

I believe that this is the most controversial topic in the book. It's probably the hardest thing to discuss with my clients (if I have to), along with the pain medication conversation. It has created conflict in the past. This is because the mere suggestion that someone is benefitting from pain can easily offend. But in order to resolve a complex issue, difficult questions must be asked. I said at the start that I'm not trying to make friends with this book and some people might get offended reading some parts because perhaps some areas may be difficult to acknowledge. All I ask is for you to read this part with an open mind and be honest with yourself. Because, in some senses everyone benefits from being in pain.

I accept that is a controversial statement, but it's true. It all depends how much. Pain will mostly be a disadvantage but there are some benefits. The question is, are these benefits stalling your recovery? It's something that requires honesty not just with me (in my consultations) but with yourself. We call this benefit a "secondary gain." And again, this is another concept that works on an unconscious level. So don't worry; I'm not suggesting that you're sitting at home scheming about how you are benefitting from your condition; although some recent studies have shown that it can be done on a conscious level too.[144]

Secondary gain is benefiting by not reaching a goal or solving a problem. Primary gains are those that connect to the original cause of the pain such as not walking because you injured your ankle; so, you are not walking on it in case you make it worse. This is the primary gain to the injury. Secondary gains are a result of the injury. So one might be that you get the day off work because of the injured ankle. This concept is largely influenced by Sigmund Freud. He believed that secondary gains were unconscious needs and desires that we have and are unaware of. Initially this concept was scorned as another one of Freud's crazy theories.

But then his theory gained traction and eventually, in the 1980s, it was adopted in the Diagnostic and Statistical Manual of Mental Disorders (DSM). Today, we can use it to help us understand why someone isn't getting better no matter what interventions have been attempted. It can apply if a client is stuck and isn't motivated to do any of the things that will benefit them or help them on their road to recovery. I've had clients in the past where I could not understand why they wouldn't do even the simplest of tasks, like basic exercises: five-minute meditations, gentle walks or reducing their processed food intake and trying to eat more healthily, all designed to help them improve their pain. I used to feel I was banging my head on a brick wall in frustration.

I began to research this area and came across the concept that some people don't want to get better. They are in the clinic because, consciously, they *do* want to get better, but unconsciously, they have other motivations. Their unconscious mind wants to remain in pain because there are other benefits that they receive while being in pain.[145]

We have all experienced benefits from being in pain at some point in our lives. Some are big, some are small. For instance, if you sprained your ankle, you might get a day off school or get out of going to mass at 10 a.m. on a Sunday. They may seem small benefits, but they can feel big at the time. But what would motivate you to remain in pain in the long term? Surely nothing can be worth being in chronic pain and stopping you from recovering? To understand this as a therapist I really need to understand my client. I need to get to know them and build a relationship first. I would need to build a rapport, and trust would need to be established before the topic was approached. This is why, in a lot of cases, the public system fails. It's not because of the quality of the physician or therapist; it's about the amount of time they have to give to their patients. How could you ever get to know someone in ten to twenty minutes – if you're lucky enough to even get that?

The more I get to know my clients the more I can envision what they are going through. I try to find out what a typical day is like for them. I go through this from the time they get out of bed: when they have their breakfast, daily chores, work, exercise and everything in between. Sometimes I get a look of confusion when I ask such unusual questions but I'm trying to build a profile of their life. I am interested in seeing what responsibilities, obligations, and behaviours they have on a day-to-day basis.

I will admit that I am not asking these questions purely to find out if they have any secondary gains but the information they give me can be useful in determining whether there are any. The primary goal for me is to work out if the person is under a lot of stress, how physical their day is, and how well they sleep.

Secondary gains that are completely stalling recovery aren't that common but are occasionally an obstacle. As I said, this information is useful either way, and if I feel there are any blockages as we progress through our treatment plan, I will revert back to these questions. I may even ask what a typical day was like for them when they weren't in pain and compare this to identify any differences or benefits to being in pain now. This could mean going back twenty years in some cases. Pain could have served a purpose back then by protecting you from a job you hated or a life you wanted to avoid. The pain could have been serving a purpose at one point. This may give us a reason for why you may not want to recover.

"Lisa" was a client of mine who raised five children on her own while her husband went to work and left her to do all the household chores as well as school runs, football practice, dance lessons etc. When he got home from "a hard day's graft," the house was clean, dinner was cooked and the clothes were washed and put away. He put his feet up and had a beer as he had had a "hard day" and Lisa clearly hadn't. We all know that raising five kids is easy, right? When Lisa fell off her bike and injured her back, she was in so much pain from the injury that she couldn't even get out of bed.

As he felt sorry for her, her husband started to help out around the house. He got home from work and cooked the dinner and even the kids helped out with the chores.

Lisa received so much care and love from her family. Although she was in pain, she finally was able to get a full night's sleep. She even lay in while her husband got the kids ready for school. Over three months or so Lisa became less incapacitated and was able to get up and move about the house a bit more. But she was still in a lot of pain and wasn't able to do anything for any long periods without increases of pain. She went down the medical route, got MRIs and injections and so on, but her doctors were all saying that they didn't see anything major in her scans.

The help, love and attention were something that Lisa didn't want to give up because she had been under enormous pressure and stress before the injury, so this is where her recovery stalled. She spoke about how pain was getting in the way of her life but once she started to go to her physio, she had no motivation to do any of the exercises that would benefit her. To be honest, I could see why she wouldn't want to get better. Who would want to go back to that stressful life where she was taken for granted and unappreciated? So, this self-sabotaging behaviour kicked in unconsciously. The emotional part of her brain saw benefits to being in pain. If she got better, she would go back to stress, misery and being an unappreciated chauffeur, cleaner and cook who got no gratification, love or attention. She consciously wanted to get better, but perhaps her brain was subconsciously trying to protect her from her previous life.

This unconscious/conscious conflict is the most common type of secondary gain. People usually don't recognise that they are gaining from their pain.

You can become comfortable in, and familiar with your pain situation. You may not have any responsibility or any social obligations anymore. Pain is a great excuse to get out of doing things you don't enjoy that you were previously obligated to do. Especially if you're an introvert, pain can be a way to not feel pressured into going to places that make you feel uncomfortable anyway. Or maybe the disability benefit you receive would have to be given up and you would have to go and get a job again. The thought of this can create anxiety and fear, which would be another good reason to remain in pain. Becoming well and getting back to optimal health could mean that this excuse is gone and all of these obligations would have to be filled again. It may even mean that you have to come up with another excuse not to have sex with your partner.

Perhaps it would mean that you have to go back to a stressful job with long hours and a boss who gives you a hard time. These are all good reasons for you to stay sick. Because, when you are sick you ironically feel safe and secure at home with all the love and care you may be given. It's the lesser of two evils in the mind of your protective brain. You may be getting something that you never received before and something that you always longed for. Becoming well might end up meaning that you don't get this love and nurturing anymore. This could be the price you pay for becoming well again.

But this self-sabotaging behaviour is interfering with all the good things in life. The only way you will get over this is by digging deep and asking yourself some serious questions. Start off by writing down all the things that suck about being in pain. This should be easy to do. It could be not being able to work in a job you love, it could be not being able to play with your kids or grandkids or even going out to meet friends for a meal. Write down as many things as possible, from the most emotionally important to the least.

Then I want you to make a list of all the benefits of being in pain. What would you have to give up if you were to get back to optimal health? These are difficult questions to ask yourself. But you need to be honest with yourself. It may be embarrassing to you to write it down, but remember it's not for anyone else's eyes. You can always rip it up and throw it in the bin afterwards. There will definitely be some benefits, even if they don't seem that significant. Whatever benefits you get from being in pain, imagine what it would be like to lose them. What if the benefits stopped? How does that feel? How does that sit with you? Does it feel scary? Do you feel anxious or worried about not receiving love or attention anymore? Would you feel comfortable being pain-free and living a normal life with all the responsibilities and stresses that go along with that? These could all be triggers for self-sabotaging behaviours.

As I have said many times, the priority of the brain is always safety. If you feel safe feeling like this and if there is a threat from getting better, the brain can block us from moving forward as it is trying to protect us. Making a list of the things you're missing out on is pivotal. Hold on to the things that are emotionally important to you and use that as motivation. Don't just hold these things in your mind. Write them down and put a list up on your bedroom door or your fridge so you regularly see it.

Pain is familiar. Familiarity is safety, no matter how destructive it is. The unknown is scary. Pain can motivate you to stay away from the unfamiliar, unknown and keep you in a painful but familiar world.

Social isolation

Human beings are social animals, we have been from the beginning of our species. There are many upsides to this. Probably the most obvious reason is for survival purposes. There is safety in numbers. Being part of a group helps us do things that we couldn't do on our own. By cooperating with others, we can hunt, fight off predators and build civilisations. At the end of the day, a group is more powerful and intelligent than an individual. Being part of a tribe gives you protection from predators and from other tribes. Being part of a larger group has reproductive advantages as well. The bigger the group, the more chances of finding a mate. I'm sure you've heard the old African proverb "it takes a village to raise a child." This is still true, even if it is more so in developing countries than the West. Living in a group has the advantage of kids being educated by many different people who all have different skill sets. Some could be good at hunting; others make better clothing or tools. Being part of a group allows the young to be able to develop their skills under the watchful eye of elders.

So, we know the importance of social interaction but what happens if we isolate from each other? Social isolation is common in people suffering from chronic pain. You may want to shy away from the world because you feel that you are a burden on others or you may be embarrassed that you cannot do the things that you were able to do in the past. Or perhaps you had a certain role in your group or family and you cannot fulfil that role anymore as the pain is too much.

It could also be a stress response. Life at home away from the world may seem easier and the best option for yourself and everybody else. This may be a good short-term strategy but to social animals who have so much neural activity during social encounters this will have consequences. Unfortunately, social media interaction doesn't count. We don't have the same neural connections through screens that we do with face-to-face encounters.

Before Covid most research on social isolation was done on the elderly. What was found was that the more socially isolated the subjects were, the greater the cognitive decline, with loneliness increasing the risk of dementia up to 40%.[146] During lockdown in the pandemic the demand for anti-depressants went up by 21%.[147] Many of these were for people who were shut off from the world and isolated, including the young, middle aged and the elderly. Not being able to socialise with friends, play their favourite sports, or see loved ones had enormous effects on their emotional wellbeing. Many reported suffering with higher levels of depression, anxiety or lower self-esteem.

Studies have also been conducted on prisoners subject to solitary confinement. Solitary confinement constitutes spending up to 23 hours a day in a 12 x 10-foot prison cell, with no other interaction with humans. The remaining hour or so is spent in a yard, usually on their own. This is typically designed for the most dangerous types of prisoners who have committed the most heinous crimes, but not always. In some cases, prisoners can be put into solitary confinement for stepping out of line in prison or for protective reasons. In some cases, it can even happen due to understaffing.

Over the years it has become subject to controversy, as research suggests spending this much time on your own is a form of psychological torture. This form of punishment leads to increased anxiety, self-harm and suicides. Prisoners struggle to socialise with other inmates after they are moved back into the general population. In a large study of 32,000 people the people that were socially isolated showed brain loss in the temporal region (which processes sounds and helps encode memory), the frontal lobe (which is involved in attention, planning and complex cognitive tasks) and the hippocampus (involved with memory).[148] Social isolation significantly increased a person's risk of premature death from all causes, a risk that may rival those of smoking, obesity, and physical inactivity.[149]

Even for an introvert, socially isolating still has consequences. Although introverts feel more comfortable being on their own, studies conducted during the Covid-19 pandemic showed that isolation was a predictor of more severe loneliness, anxiety, and depression experienced as a result of pandemic-related changes. So regardless of whether you are an introvert or extrovert, you still need social interaction. Being social is far more taxing for an introvert and uses up more energy, with longer recovery time than for an extrovert.[150] But it is still essential. You just don't need to do it as frequently. But abstaining from socialising altogether is not a good idea for your overall health. This just feeds the pain beast and contributes to a sensitised nervous system. Being on your own also gives the brain this feeling of vulnerability. Remember, we are a lot safer in a group. Being isolated will increase your brain's natural sensitivity to threat. This could lead to anxiety, an overactive immune system and even more pain.

When we have social interactions in face-to-face encounters there is a lot of neural activity in the brain. Brain scans conducted on two people socialising showed that areas of both of their brains were simultaneously activated while they were engaged in conversation.[151] It is almost as if they were connected and synchronised with each other. Social interaction increases the release of the hormone oxytocin (the love hormone) which can decrease cortisol levels and enact a parasympathetic response. This explains why a hug or touch can make you feel better, loved and supported.

The great thing about the brain is that with neuroplasticity the brain can change in a positive way. By becoming more social these brain areas can tighten and strengthen again. In terms of pain, improvements in social isolation accounted for significant improvements in self-reported emotional and physical functioning.[152] Just surround yourself with people that you love and care about and more importantly people that care about you and your best interests. Don't surround yourself with toxic people who will only stress you out and encourage you to socially isolate more.

If social situations are challenging for you, you have the power to dictate how much socialising you do. Pick quality over quantity. It doesn't have to be going out for dinner or for a day shopping to reap the benefits. Calling over to a neighbour for a cup of tea is more than enough to get started. Then scale up from there in your own time.

Social exclusion

We have spoken about the importance of being part of a social group or tribe. We know how crucial it has been to the survival of our species over millions of years. So, what would happen if we were suddenly ostracised, rejected or excluded from our tribe (friends, family)? A feeling of being excluded or rejected is common to many of my clients.

Many of them report not being invited to social events or activities. These clients understand that there is no malice intended by their friends or family and that it's most likely due to them not being able to participate due to their pain. What's the point in inviting you if you cannot participate? But that doesn't prevent them from feeling excluded all the same.

On the flip side of that, because pain demands your attention, this can impair your judgment on other social aspects such as showing empathy or being able to interact as you would usually be able to. And this can have an effect on you. People may feel that you are not listening, paying attention or being present during the social interaction. This may motivate people to exclude you from future outings if they come to think that you don't want to be there in the first place. They may not know the true reason for your lack of attention. If you put yourself in their shoes, perhaps you have seemed rude through no fault of theirs or yours.

Hearing stories of where their friends or family went on a hike, to watch a football match or out for dinner can make pain sufferers feel inadequate, worthless or excluded. In other words, it can "hurt." When we say something hurts, what do we mean? Usually, we would say if you injured yourself, it would "hurt" or it was "painful." But coincidentally the same terms can be used for social suffering. We say a break-up was "painful" or the loss of a loved one "hurts." It's not a coincidence that these terms are shared. There is more of a relationship between social pain and physical pain than we think. There is now evidence that social and physical pain share many of the same brain regions.[153]

The physical pain model whereby tissue damage or potential tissue can result in pain as a warning sign or protective mechanism has now been applied to evolutionary models of social pain. An incredibly interesting study was conducted at University College Los Angeles (UCLA) by Professor Matthew Lieberman. They put participants into MRI machines to play a game of virtual ball tossing (cyberball) and monitored their brain activity during the game. The participants were told they would be playing against two other participants in different laboratories. What the participant didn't know was that the other "two participants" were being controlled by the scientist conducting the study in the same lab.

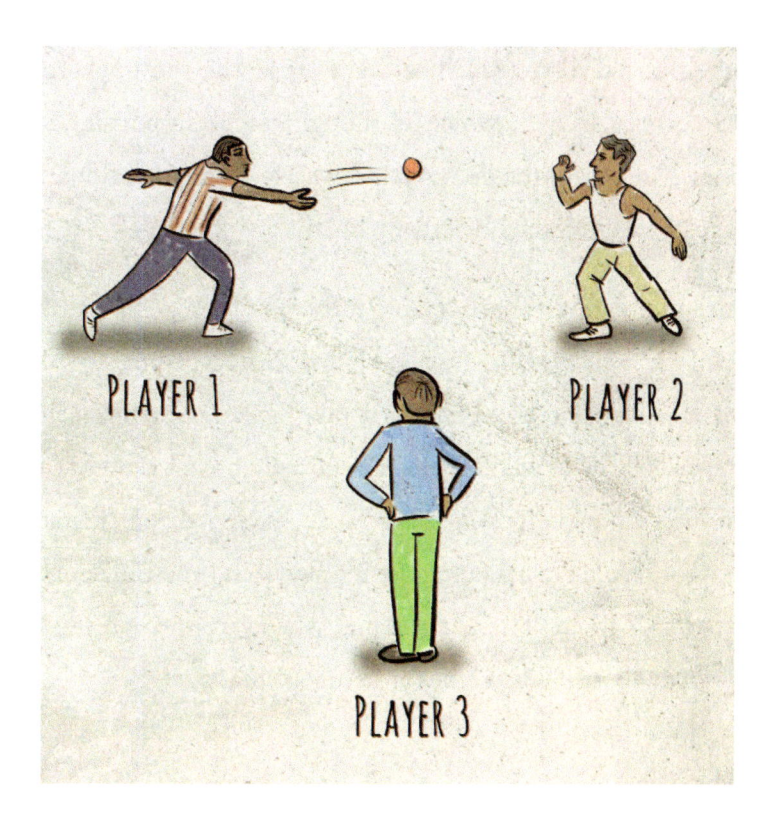

It started off with two rounds of just tossing the ball to each other. When the ball came to the participant, they had the choice of who to throw the ball to. Pretty boring game in all fairness. But in Round 3 things got interesting. The other two scientists never threw the ball to the participant. They kept throwing it back to each other and never gave it to him or her again, totally excluding him or her from the game.

At the end of the round the participants were given a painful stimulus and told to rate their pain. The results showed that the more social distress the participant felt because of being excluded from the game, the more pain they reported. The experiment also found that the activity in regions of the brain that are active during physical pain were also active during their social distress. These were areas like the dorsal anterior cingulate cortex (dACC), which is thought to be important for pain processing,[154] and the insula, which is active during noxious stimuli. This suggests that social pain actually hurts.

Even more interestingly, participants who were then given paracetamol or Tylenol reported feeling less excluded. So according to Matthew Lieberman, "The same painkiller that takes away your headache takes away your heartache as well." Even in a subsequent variation of the game where it was financially beneficial to be excluded, participants still preferred not to be. Participants lost money each time they got the ball thrown towards them. The participants who were thrown the ball the least, or not at all, still felt worse for being excluded.[155]

Have you ever not been able to go somewhere because of your pain? It may be for a walk with your friends or it could be out for dinner for a birthday party. Not being able to go and having that feeling of being excluded can create this activity in your brain, especially if you subsequently hear all the stories about the great times everybody had.

Not feeling part of this can make that difficult to hear and may result in you withdrawing more socially to avoid hearing these stories in the future. The more social exclusion or rejection you get, the more you will avoid people, and the lonelier you will become. It's like a self-fulfilling prophecy. You are protecting yourself from the emotional pain in the short term but in the medium to long term you are just fuelling the problem.

In general, as a society we are becoming less sociable. Ironically, even with technology, we are less connected than ever. There is less community than ever before. We know less about our neighbours than fifty years ago; we are having smaller families and we have fewer close friends that we can rely on. One in five men and one in ten females report having no close friends.[156] Our social circles are getting smaller as each generation passes. At the same time, chronic pain is on the rise.

So, it is not unreasonable to assume that not being involved in social activities that you have joined in the past can create pain activity in the brain. If these brain regions are more active during perceived social threat, then your brain obviously thinks that this area is important.

Only you can know whether this affected you. Social inclusion and acceptance are essential to survival. Remember that, in evolutionary terms, the more sociable and bigger your community is, the more protection we have and the safer and more secure your brain will feel.

Our brains are programmed to keep us safe. So, it makes sense that there will be overlaps in these regions in the brain where there is perceived threat involved, be it physical, social or emotional threat.

Has your pain been validated?

Validation is the acceptance of someone's thoughts, feelings and emotions. Invalidation is the opposite. It's a form of emotional or psychological abuse that happens across many sectors of society. If you're a chronic pain sufferer, the chances are that your condition hasn't been validated somewhere down the line. At some point someone will have acted as if they don't believe you, played down your condition or said that your feelings were wrong. Many of my clients report not being believed, heard or listened to. Often, they say they have been made to feel like they are exaggerating or that the pain is just in their head. Sometimes it's on purpose but most of the time the invalidator isn't aware that they are invalidating. Invalidation can come in many forms of communication; a few examples are in the box below:

Type of communication	Invalidating	Validating
Verbal	"You're overreacting, you don't look like you're in pain, it can't be that bad, man up."	"That must be awful, I'm sorry you have to go through this."
Body language	Rolling eyes, showing confusion, smirking.	Nodding, eye contact, holding hands.
Behaviours	Looking at your watch, not paying attention, doing something else while you're trying to speak to them.	Listening, showing interest in what they are saying, repeating what they say.

Validation vs invalidation

Invalidation has consequences. It often leads to emotional distancing, conflict, and disruption in relationships, as well as feelings of loneliness, worthlessness, confusion, and inferiority in the affected individual. These relationships are not just those at home but those in society and healthcare too.[157]

When it comes to pain, people who have received low levels of validation showed higher levels of pain sensitivity, and likewise people who were shown higher levels of validation reported lower levels of pain sensitivity.[158]

Validation isn't necessarily agreeing with the person. You may have different thoughts or feelings on the matter but you can still listen to and empathise with them without judgement. To validate a person is to listen and acknowledge how the person feels and let them know it's okay to feel that way.

I have split the topic of validation/invalidation into two separate areas. The first area I want to talk about is the healthcare system. When we have pain, usually the first place we go to is our local GP. The GP is the first port of call when it comes to pain or disability. So, invalidation here isn't a good start. This is where you would expect to be heard and understood the most. But clients of mine regularly tell me that they feel that their GP doesn't listen to them.

Again, I don't want it to sound like I'm bashing doctors. I'm aware I only ever hear the bad stories about doctors and healthcare in general. I'm not getting the stories about situations where they have been great and how they have really helped. My clients are in pain and have usually had bad experiences with the healthcare system. In my experience the story I hear from my clients is that, "My GP is not listening to me. He/she just provides painkillers and I'm out the door, until it's time for a refill of my meds."

I have an anecdotal story of my own experience with a doctor when I was in the military. I walked into the surgery where the doctor greeted me and asked me to sit down. He asked me what was wrong. As soon as I started to tell him what happened, he swivelled himself to the right to type into his desktop computer. If he could see me at all it would be out of the corner of his eye. When I started explaining to him what had happened and why I was in his office, he began slowly typing what I was telling him with his two index fingers into a keypad. It was actually painful to watch how slow he was at typing as he circled around each letter before he pressed the letter on the keypad. It was actually laughable how bad he was at typing but he still wasn't even facing in my direction. At one point he asked me to slow down so he could catch up with his typing. Thank God it was nothing more serious than an ankle sprain, but if this was how he was operating I wouldn't have wanted to take anything more serious to him. Who knows? I certainly wouldn't have felt validated, heard or listened to if I had.

I am not taking anybody's side on this. I'm just playing devil's advocate and trying to look at everything objectively. But I would expect this to be the case in some situations within healthcare.

Not everyone is trying to invalidate you. But that isn't to say that you haven't felt invalidated. Feelings aren't right or wrong. They are a reflection of your thoughts, experiences, and perceptions. Just because the invalidator isn't intentionally trying to invalidate you, it doesn't mean they aren't invalidating either.

Playing devil's advocate

In primary care there is very little time for patients and doctors to build a relationship and have meaningful rapport. Healthcare staff can have up to five patients per hour.

By contrast, like most other private sector therapists I have one client per hour for a consultation. I am able to give the client my full attention to get to know them and hear their story. The public system staff don't have this luxury. You're in and out before you even get comfortable on the chair. A study conducted on GPs in Ireland between 2010 and 2018 showed that the average consultation between a GP and their patient was 14.1 minutes. The average amount of issues was two and a half. Is that enough time for you to tell your GP what's going on in your life, get an assessment and a treatment plan for each problem? I would say no, as it could sometimes take the whole first appointment to go through a thorough assessment, especially with something as complex as persistent pain.

We might count ourselves lucky in Ireland. This report suggests the 14.1-minute average time frame is substantially longer than the UK's average of a mere 11.7 minutes.[159] The same study suggests that there is an increased workload on GPs due to a lack of manpower which in turn is due to many older doctors retiring and young graduates emigrating. This isn't just a problem in Ireland and the UK as shortages in medical staff continue to be reported worldwide.[160] Some countries have it worse than others. The UK and Ireland are somewhere around the middle. Sweden for instance has the longest average consultation time at 22 minutes whereas Bangladesh bottoms the list at an outrageous 48 seconds per consult.[161] Imagine how invalidated you would feel then.

Regardless of where you are I believe it's not enough time to really get the full picture. It's no wonder sometimes you feel you're not being heard. I would feel like that too. The point I'm trying to make is that, if this is your experience, then it might not be that the doctor, physio or specialist wasn't listening to you. It may have been that they only have x amount of time to briefly hear your story and prescribe some medication and/or a referral before they have to see the next person.

And I am not saying this is okay. Far from it, but it is likely not the practitioner at fault; it's the system. Obviously, you're going to have some poor-quality healthcare staff somewhere within the system but you will find that in any industry or organisation. However, in general, the system is overstretched and understaffed.

Sometimes I don't agree with what my clients are saying. It's not about being right or wrong, it's about listening, accepting what they are saying as real and trying to see it from their point of view. If there are things that I don't agree with I will address it in due course: maybe in a few sessions down the road. Do your healthcare staff get that luxury? Of course they don't! They will need to disagree if they feel you are wrong within that 14.1-minute time frame as they may not see you again for months on end. That process will obviously come across as invalidating.

There is a lot to be said for having the time to properly hear your patient's full history. Pretty much everyone in long-term pain has a complicated history.

We don't just bend over and throw our backs out. If a client tells me such a story I immediately think, "Okay, what are you not telling me?" I will go in detail through everything such as stress, poor sleep, family history, toxic work/living environment, overwork, stifled recoveries, poor mental health, and too much or not enough exercise. In my opinion, all of this should be discussed within a consultation when you are dealing with pain or disability. It has to be because these are the most common influencers of pain.

My consultations are almost like an interview. I want to know everything about my clients. To me the answer to their pain is in their story. I want to know everything. From their activities, routines, lifestyle, stressors to movement quality. Almost as far as what they had for breakfast. But in the current Western model there is too much emphasis on imaging and not enough time spent on patient history.

In one study,[162] scientists decided to see what the best method of diagnosis was. There were three diagnostic tools. The first group could only diagnose through a detailed patient history, the second through physical assessment and the third through investigators (MRIs, X-rays, bloods). The first group with a high emphasis on patient history resulted in a correct diagnosis 78% of the time. The physical assessment group were only correct 8% of the time and investigations group were correct 13% of the time.

When patient history was combined with a physical examination and investigation, that correct diagnosis rate increased to 98%. This study suggests that a multifaceted approach is needed in making a medical diagnosis. With all of that in mind, 14.1 minutes clearly isn't enough, even if we excluded imaging as an MRI or X-ray would usually not be done in a GP consultation. A "full" history and physical examination could never be done in that time frame. We can only get a proper history with time and time is not what the health system has.

In a large global study by the *British Medical Journal*,[163] it was suggested that "doctors feel less productive and competent at managing complex multimorbid (living with two or more chronic illnesses) patients in those settings with short consultation lengths." This review also found that "a short consultation length was responsible for driving polypharmacy (patient taking two or more medications), overuse of antibiotics and poor communication with patients."

It's clear as day that a big contributing factor to poor patient/doctor communication is a lack of time and this can also lead to a patient not feeling heard or validated.

Until the system can get enough staff to be able to manage the right amount of people and give the right amount of time required to see each patient properly, I don't see this changing. You might blame doctors or healthcare staff for invalidating you but perhaps they are doing the best they can and just playing the hand they were dealt.

Trusting your healthcare provider

Another factor for pain-invalidation within healthcare is poor patient-physician communication. Of course, some of this poor communication will come down to time but there are certainly skills that could be acquired to improve patient-physician relationships.

This comes down to a lack of education in empathy or validation training. Evidence indicates that pain patients are often dissatisfied with the communication and feel misunderstood or patronised.[164] Validation training, a form of empathetic response that communicates that what a patient experiences is accepted as true, has been suggested as an appropriate method for improving communication with patients suffering pain. More empathy and validation training can increase patient-physician communication and allow patients to feel more accepted, and thus more satisfied with their care.[165] The problem with providing adequate training is that it remains a challenge, as no given technique is currently regarded as the method-of-choice, some require considerable time to master, and many deal only indirectly with emotional aspects of communication.[166]

There is usually some level of trust in healthcare to begin with. You don't automatically distrust a medical professional, especially when their job is to help you in the first place. It's not as if you're meeting a doctor in a dark alleyway for advice on how to deal with your back pain. You're meeting your healthcare practitioner in a room within a vicinity where there are many other healthcare staff who are all working together for one objective: to help people. So, there is a natural level of trust to begin with and rightly so. There is so much natural trust in healthcare that, in marketing, green is perceived as a trusting colour. Green evokes a feeling of abundance and is associated with refreshment and peace, rest and security.[167] Many doctors even use green in their offices to put patients at ease.[168]

It's when trust is lost that outcomes are affected. This goes across all healthcare from medical to psychology to fitness. "Patients reported more beneficial health behaviours, less symptoms and higher quality of life and to be more satisfied with treatment when they had higher trust in their health care professional."[169]

For many of my clients, their level of trust in healthcare has been diminished over time. This can be from misdiagnosis, poor communication, invalidation, or a procedure or operation that hasn't turned out as planned.

A lack of trust in your healthcare provider can also have consequences for patients' treatment satisfaction, health behaviours, symptom severity and quality of life. It can also result in patients not being compliant with treatment. Why would you do something if you have lost trust in the person treating you? The intention of the provider is to help but if the trust is lost, negative outcomes are increased. There can also be a nocebo effect, from the anticipation of negative effects due to the lack of trust in the provider or system.

This can also be a barrier for patients to seek therapy for pain management and rehabilitation.[170] We don't want people who are suffering to avoid looking for help because they are afraid of being invalidated again.[171]

"Trust in the healer is essential to healing itself" – Brody, H., 1992

There is plenty of evidence that communication skills would help resolve these problems. So, who's at fault here? Is it the education curriculum that hasn't put enough emphasis on communication skills in universities? Is it the healthcare system that hasn't provided the adequate training to their staff? Or is it the individual who hasn't upskilled themselves in order to be able to communicate better with their patients? Whatever the reason for the invalidation, we need to improve this where we can, whether it be with better education for staff or more time for patient consultations or at the very least raising awareness on this topic.

If you are having trust issues with your medical provider, something needs to be done. If it's a physiotherapist, you can always find a new one. There are plenty of them around and, from my experience not every therapist is suited to every patient anyway. I think every physio will admit that. If it's your doctor, it may be a little bit more difficult to do this. The way things are in Ireland you cannot easily change physician. So, speaking to him/her about your concerns and how you are feeling is certainly better than not saying anything and continuing to distrust them. As I said, good communication between patient and physician is the bedrock of trust. Don't forget your doctor is there to help you and you will need their help.

Trust in this relationship is essential to recovery.

The second part of this is validation in your social circle. Are you suffering with chronic pain, but feeling invalidated at home, work, with friends or society?

One main reason for invalidation within society ironically is reassurance. Reassurance minimises a person's feelings or experiences. This is mostly true with loved ones. They feel they are helping the situation by downplaying your condition to make you feel better. This is often done by people who are genuinely trying to make things better. Certainly, Irish culture involves trying to make light of everything. We like to make the situation better in an instant. So, when a loved one, friend or family member tells us what they are going through, instead of listening and showing empathy to them we try to make them feel better in that moment.

This reassurance doesn't make the situation any better – all it does is invalidate the recipient. People may be uncomfortable with your vulnerability, and it makes sense to them to try to cheer you up. But we now know that this type of reassurance does not decrease negative affect and may be perceived as not taking the symptoms seriously.[172] Dr Brené Brown is a research professor at the University of Houston Graduate

College of Social Work who has written several books in this area. In her research, she talks about how we as a society try to make things better in an instant. But we rarely succeed. Instead, she says we should learn to listen and empathise with the person who is talking with us.

Validation from a partner or family member can be strengthened by education. This can help your significant other, family member or close friends to understand what you are going though. Having a knowledge in the subject can lead to more understanding of your condition, which in turn may bring down the level of any tension, frustration or resentment that may be going on in the relationship. We spoke earlier about how powerful words can be. Having a loved one change their language to a more validating choice of words can increase the strength of the relationship, and reduce pain catastrophising.[173]

The whole point of this book is to help educate not just you, but the people around you. Get them to read the book too. (But make sure they buy their own copy, ha ha! Only kidding, but do pass this book around to as many people as you think will read it.) The more people in your circle who understand pain, the more validation you will get, and the more understanding and empathy you will receive.

If we can learn how to validate the pain sufferer there are many positive outcomes. In couples where the partner provided higher levels of validation, patients were much more likely to engage in disclosure and much less likely to report a sense of support entitlement. Also, higher levels of validation were not related to patient reports of pain or symptoms of anxiety or depression.[174]

Interventions designed to teach family members or partners how to validate pain-related thoughts and feelings may improve family relationships and patient outcomes.[175]

In my opinion, if a partner or family member understands pain in a little bit more detail, it is easier to show this validation. Having a linear view of pain can have a negative effect and your partner may show some signs of not really recognising your pain, which can lead the pain sufferer becoming resentful in the relationship.

Coping with invalidation

Others may dismiss your story more intentionally; they may believe you have other intentions like malingering or exaggerating for financial gain. Or perhaps they just don't care about you being in pain. The harsh truth is that some people just don't really care about others. These people are out there unfortunately. We just have to accept that people have their own problems and some people don't care about yours.

Coping with invalidation can be tough. As I said, a chronic pain sufferer will have been subject to invalidation in several areas of their life. That is a certainty. When this happens, the typical response will be the desire to defend yourself. This can lead to anger, frustration, bitterness and/or resentment. And, there's an argument that you would be justified – but it doesn't do you any good. Sure, it's important to stick up for yourself when the time is right but you shouldn't be relying on what others think in determining your own self-worth. Becoming bitter or resentful towards a system or a person only hurts you more.

There may be areas where you need to grow, and become strong or more resilient yourself. We can run into emotional problems and become victims when we rely too heavily on external validation. Your internal validation is what matters. A victim mentality will not allow you to progress. Don't be a victim and don't blame others for making you feel this way. You are responsible for how you feel. Feeling invalidated is not nice but you have the power to change how you feel. You can decide to address the invalidation with your loved one or health professional.

If someone is invalidating you, this can trigger a fight-or-flight response which in turn can lead to emotional distress and increased pain. The brain detects a threat so it will act accordingly in the only way it knows how when it perceives danger. When you are in fight-or-flight mode, you will either act aggressively or defensively. This can start conflict or lead to you becoming fearful about bringing up the topic again. Neither are beneficial to you for your recovery.

So, a sense of invalidation can be caused by either your social circle or the healthcare system. If you want to improve you need both of these groups on your side. You can't do it alone. If you could, you wouldn't be reading this book. If there is any resentment or blame towards either group, it will inhibit your recovery. Building a good support network around you and perhaps building a thicker skin yourself will only serve you well for when the time arises.

Not addressing the invalidation will bring up resentment and bitterness towards the person or the system. So, address it. Don't leave it bottled up. You don't need to create conflict or do it aggressively. You can address the person assertively. Remember that your feelings aren't right or wrong; they are real.

So, identify if you have been invalidated and address it. But firstly, ask yourself, who is this person? Does this person's opinion even matter? This is a choice you have to make, because sometimes it's not even worth sharing your feelings with somebody who is not that important. And, if they're not important enough to speak to them, why even bother allowing that person to dictate how you feel? Generally, the closer you are to the person, the more important they will be in this process.

If the person isn't that close to you in your social circle, then perhaps it's not worth the time or energy of having this conversation. If on consideration you do feel that this is worth your time and effort, bring it up calmly and explain how you feel your feelings were invalidated.

Most of the time people will be receptive and emotionally willing to change. They will usually try not to invalidate you again. Emotionally intelligent and stable people do not repeatedly invalidate you. If they do, then they most likely have their own issues. Just move on with your life.

At the end of the day, you know what's important. You don't need someone else to validate you or dictate your own self-worth. The only person who can validate you is yourself.

If a doctor or a healthcare provider has invalidated you in the past, you may bring it to their attention if you want to, but if you don't, don't hold onto it and become resentful or bitter. This resentment or bitterness only hurts you. It doesn't hurt them. You are only shooting yourself in the foot by allowing somebody else's actions to dictate how you feel. You know what's true and know your feelings are real. It's easy to become resentful and bitter towards the whole healthcare system because of a few individuals – but remember you need the healthcare system to help you recover. You may have had some bad experiences in the past but there are a lot of great doctors and healthcare staff out there who truly care about you and how you feel.

I'm saying all of this to help you understand that people in healthcare or in your social circle don't usually have an agenda or the intention of invalidating you.

Remember that your feelings are valid. Your feelings are reflections of your thoughts and experiences. You are not crazy and this is not "all in your head."

NOTES

_____

_____

_____

_____

_____

_____

_____

_____

_____

_____

_____

_____

_____

_____

_____

_____

_____

_____

_____

_____

Chapter 7

Sleep

Pain sufferers almost all suffer with sleep issues. In fact, a 2015 National Sleep Foundation poll found that two in three chronic pain patients suffer from recurring sleep disruptions.[176] When the light is turned off, and the curtains are drawn, everything in your room is silent except for your body. Pain is the only thing that will have your attention. This uncomfortable feeling makes it difficult to get to sleep, and even when you finally do, just rolling over in the bed, pain wakes you up again. This often happens multiple times a night, disrupting the quality of our sleep and making it truly difficult to get back to sleep again. When the morning finally comes around you don't feel rested or recuperated.

One of the greatest mysteries in the scientific world over centuries was the purpose of spending so much time doing nothing. Every night every person on this planet goes into a state of unconsciousness and paralysis. There have been many theories as to why this happens but even now today it's not fully understood. Some suggest that, by relaxing, lowering our heart rate, we are conserving energy for when we need it most during the day. Other theories suggest that we sleep as a way to stop us exploring at night and getting attacked by predators. Probably the most well supported theory suggests that we heal, recover and recuperate while we are in the land of nod. The latter is probably the most accurate but the other two theories could be part of the process too.

Before we lived in a world polluted with artificial light, we had a relatively simple life. This mainly consisted of farming your own crops, catching and killing your dinner, reproducing, and avoiding catching the plague, if you could call that a simple life. Maybe not. But it was a simple life in the sense that it wasn't as superficial or complex as it is now. It wasn't as busy. Everybody wasn't in a rush to go somewhere. We didn't live in a world where you "needed" the latest and greatest gadgets, and where family and community were still the important thing. We didn't focus on career and status as a way to establish if we were worthy persons. Life was slower and "simpler." We worked during the day and rested at night.

However, from the turn of the industrial revolution, people started to get increasingly time sensitive. Time was money, and when the sun went down, it meant that little work could be conducted due to the lack of visibility. Many forms of artificial light were introduced to help fight the darkness, such as open fires, candles and gas lanterns, but they all had limitations. After Thomas Edison invented the lightbulb, life would never be the same again, especially when it came to sleep. Culturally things started to change. Now we could work through the night, have sports venues open after dark, and bars and restaurants could stay open until they wanted to. "Thanks to Edison, sunset no longer meant the end of your social life; instead, it marked the beginning of it."[177]

Edison had a "sleep less, work more" mentality. He said that no one needed more than three or four hours of sleep per night. He regarded sleep as a "waste of time." In today's modern world, many people would have a similar thought process. Time is money and time in between the sheets could be better used to get some work done. But if Thomas Edison was right and sleep was just a waste of time, how did Mother Nature get it so wrong? Consider the fact that most animals on the planet sleep – surely it must be important? We have evolved over hundreds of millions of years from being reptiles to monkeys to humans. Throughout that whole evolutionary period spanning hundreds of millions of years, natural selection never found a better or more efficient alternative to sleep. Even though we are at our most vulnerable from predators when we are in la-la land, we still sleep for approximately seven to nine hours each night. Surely, it's more important than Thomas Edison thought it was?

I think Allan Rechtschaffen summed it up when he wrote "If sleep does not serve an absolutely vital function, then it is the biggest mistake the evolutionary process has ever made." It turns out that that Allan Rechtschaffen was right and Thomas Edison was very wrong.

Previously, we always thought of sleep as just our brain's way of recharging or pressing the reset button for a while. Thanks to the neuroscience revolution in recent decades and the birth of a new sleep science, scientists now understand that sleep affects everything in our body: tissue health, cell growth, cognitive performance, sport performance, cardiovascular health, stress levels, digestion, fertility, immune function, emotional wellbeing, mood, metabolism and, most importantly for this book, "pain." Literally everything in the body is affected by a good or bad night's sleep.[178]

Sleep science

Although there still isn't a proper consensus on why we sleep, it looks like sleep is the single most important thing we can do for our health. We will keep this all in the context of pain; although the wider subject of sleep health is incredibly interesting, I don't want to veer too far from the topic here.

To understand why it's important to sleep and what the relationship is with pain, I believe it's important to understand how these mechanisms work, even just on a basic level. As you know by now, I believe knowledge on a subject removes the excuse of ignorance. Now, you cannot say to yourself that you didn't realise sleep was so important.

Knowing how sleep or a lack of it can have a dramatic influence on your overall health can change your thought process and behaviour when it comes to good sleep hygiene. When I speak about sleep hygiene, I don't mean having a shower before you go to bed. Sleep hygiene is just good sleep habits. But we will speak about this a little later.

The sleep cycle

Sleep science has evolved slowly over time: so slowly in fact, that it's considered a new science even today. Up until the 1960s, sleep was just considered a way for your brain to reset. But then a discovery was made through the use of an electroencephalography (EEG) machine. What was found was that not all sleep was the same. Sleep wasn't as passive as previously thought. In different times during the night there was a significant difference in electrical activity going on in the human brain. In 1968, two researchers, Allan Rechtschaffen and Anthony Kales, published the first guideline for determining sleep stages; it is still used today. The discovery that not all sleep was the same gave scientists some evidence that there was more to sleep than just recharging your batteries. Today scientists can use a number of tools to evaluate sleep. The four main ones are EEG, to evaluate electrical activity in the brain, electromyography (EMG), to measure muscle tone, as muscle tone is different in sleeping and waking states, electro-oculography (EOG) to measure eye movement, and of course the MRI scanner to take detailed images inside the body.

A sleep cycle is broken up into five phases. There are four Non-Rapid Eye Movement (NREM) phases and one rapid eye movement (REM) phase. NREM sleep is subdivided into four categories, NREM 1–4. The names of these phases come from observing the flickering in the eyes of the test subjects during rapid eye movement sleep.

Each sleep stage has a different role. N1 is transitioning from wakefulness to sleep; if you were woken at this stage, you would often think you hadn't been asleep at all. In N2, your heart rate drops and your body temperature cools. (Your core body temperature needs to cool down in order for you to fall asleep. That's why it's easier to fall asleep in a cool room than a hot room.)

N3 and N4 are considered the deepest parts of your sleep. This stage is your body's restorative stage as it repairs and regrows its tissues, builds bone and muscle, and strengthens the immune system.[179] If you are feeling ill, you will spend more time in this phase for obvious reasons.[180]

Then we have arguably the most famous stage, your REM sleep. This sleep stage is associated with dreaming. When we pass into this stage, we go into a state of paralysis. Muscles will lose their tone everywhere except the eyes and diaphragm. It appears this is a preventive measure the brain takes in order to prevent you from acting out your dreams – the last thing I want to do is to kick my fiancé as I score the winner for Ireland in the World Cup final. REM sleep is very different physiologically to NREM sleep. EEG machines show that the electrical activity during REM is similar to that in a waking state. There are also some studies that show that, after learning new skills throughout the previous day, the brainwaves in REM show similar activity when you are sleeping as when you were learning that new skill. It is almost as if you are replaying what you have learned over and over while you are asleep.[181] This phase is also thought to be important for brain development. Most adults spend approximately 20–25% of a full night's sleep in REM sleep but an infant spends up to 50%. This is presumably because of all the new learning and growth that is happening as a child.

Additionally, REM sleep is critical for regulating your emotions, consolidation of memories, problem solving and overall heightening general creativity.[182]

As you can see, all sleep stages are important in their own right, REM and deep NREM sleep in particular. They are also the most fragile part of your sleep as they are the easiest to disrupt.

Stimulants like caffeine can affect how deeply you can sleep. Any caffeine taken up to six hours before bedtime can lead to a significant increase of sleep disruptions through the night.[183] You may be one of those people who can fall asleep even after an espresso late in the evening but that doesn't mean you'll be able to move into your deep N3 stage as well as you should.

While alcohol can shorten the time it takes to fall asleep, it actually affects the quality of your sleep. It blocks access to your REM sleep and, without you knowing it, you wake more times during the night. You may sleep deeper in the earlier part of the night but the second half of the night is filled with lighter stage N2 sleep.[184] This is contrary to what we want, which is more REM sleep in the second half of the night.

Opioid medications significantly reduce your deep NREM and REM sleep.[185] Although you may feel drowsy, ironically, opioids can block deep NREM and REM sleep and you spend more time in NREM 2 sleep. Sleep can be much lighter and more broken. And it can be a vicious cycle because, if you don't get full restorative sleep this can amplify pain as a result the next day. This means that a night of poor sleep can lead to increased opioid consumption the next day.[186]

Anti-depressants are also known for disrupting sleep. Most anti-depressants work by helping the serotonin system. Serotonin, a.k.a. "the happy hormone," is also an arousal neurotransmitter, one of many that is produced to wake you up in the morning. Serotonin functions to promote wakefulness and to inhibit REM sleep.[187]

So, although having more serotonin in the brain may help you feel better, it can also disrupt your sleep[188] by keeping you more alert.[189]

This leads us onto sleeping tablets. You may be shocked to know that taking sleeping tablets does not encourage natural restorative sleep.[190] Sleeping tablets are classed as sedatives/hypnotics; they work by turning off your cortex (the outer wrinkly part of your brain), which helps you go into a state of unconsciousness. But there is one key problem here. Sedation is not real sleep. Many things are happening when you are asleep; it's not just a case of switching off when you close your eyes. Many parts of the brain are highly active throughout the night and just sedating yourself doesn't allow your brain to do the restorative work at the level it usually can. One key reason to this is that pretty much all sleeping tablets cause either decreased REM or suppressed REM. There is also an increase in the lighter NREM 2.[191] Matthew Walker, professor of neuroscience and psychology at the University of California, says that "from the science I have seen there are no upsides to taking sleeping pills and many downsides including increased risk of cancer and death." Walker goes on to say that "many GPs don't even know this information because they are on average only provided with two hours of sleep education during GP training school." A third of our life sleeping compared with two hours of training. That seems reasonable!

The brain's internal timepiece

What!? Our brain has its own clock? Yes, we have an internal clock called the circadian rhythm (CR) which is situated in a place called the suprachiasmatic nucleus located in the hypothalamus. This internal timepiece is set up to synchronise with the day/night cycle and follows a 24–25-hour clock pattern. When the sun comes up, this clock initiates arousal hormones and neurotransmitters such as serotonin, dopamine, cortisol and noradrenaline to wake us up and make us alert. When darkness falls, the hormone melatonin is released to make us feel drowsy and initiate sleep. (There are many neurotransmitters that are released to wake you up but only one (melatonin) to put us to sleep.)

This system is triggered by sensory information such as light and heat from the sun, which is picked up through our eyes and skin and communicated to our internal timepiece. What's cool is that this internal timepiece continuously recalibrates with seasonal changes to make sure it stays on track. This recalibration happens when we travel across time zones and get jetlag. The light and heat is absorbed through your eyes and skin in the new time zone, and the recalibration begins. Jetlag is extreme recalibration though, and not something that is recommended on a regular basis. This recalibration happens on a smaller daily cycle too. In the past we would need this system to follow the day/night cycle, as summertime is longer than wintertime. But nowadays that system is easily manipulated by artificial light and blackout blinds. Life has changed over the last few hundred years. Our daily schedules do not correlate with sunrise and sunset anymore. This is why our circadian rhythms can get confused or manipulated to some degree.[192]

As there is so much artificial light all around us now, it can be more difficult for the initiation of melatonin to happen as the brain thinks it's always daytime. Prior to the invention of the lightbulb, when the sun went down, we would naturally get this release of melatonin and sleep was initiated. I think it's important to note that we did use artificial light for hundreds of thousands of years in the form of campfires – but that was nothing compared to the light pollution we deal with in modern society. Red light at eye level has been show to help with initiating sleep, which is speculated to be because of the role of campfires throughout human history.[193]

Nowadays, we can stay up and watch TV, we can go to the gym or even eat at a restaurant after dark. All of these luxuries are a testament to how much modern technology has advanced and how lucky we are to be born in this era. There was a time when we didn't have the luxury of being able to walk into a room, flip on a switch and have instant light. This amazing advance in technology changes our physiology though. Because now we have the power to have light whenever we want, it affects the time when our natural release of melatonin will happen. If the sun goes down at 8 p.m. the secretion of melatonin will be suppressed if you are in a lit-up area.

What's really interesting though is that, if we get away from all the artificial light, our body naturally synchronises to the natural day/night time again; in some studies when people have been taken away from all this artificial light altogether, they felt tired two hours before their usual bedtime due to their natural release of melatonin.[194]

Sleep cycle

As I said, a sleep episode begins with a short period of N1 progressing through to light N2 (most of your sleep is spent here), followed by your deepest N3 and N4 phases and finally we cycle back down through the stages until you're almost awake until we enter REM sleep. However, we don't remain in REM sleep the remainder of the night, we cycle between stages of NREM and REM throughout the night.

A full night's sleep consists of 4–6 cycles of these five phases. Each cycle on average lasts approximately 90 minutes. Each of these phases has a different role to play within the sleep cycle as we saw above.

You might be wondering why I'm bothering explaining the cycles of sleep to you. Why is all of this important? Well, when you don't get enough sleep at night, you're not just reducing the amount of sleep you're getting. It's the type of sleep you're missing out on.

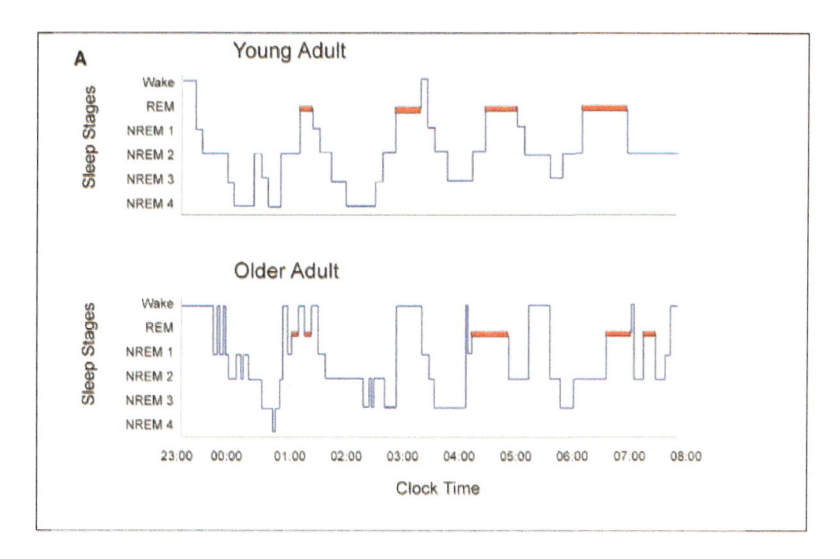

If you're usually asleep for six hours or less, I'd like to ask you right now to use your fingers and cover up the far-right quarter of the diagram above. Do that before you read on.

Here you can see that, if you are only getting six hours of sleep every night, you're not just missing out on a quarter of your total sleep, but up to 75% of your REM sleep. Let that sink in. We've already spoken about the importance of REM sleep in your brain and body's restoration – not just physically, but, psychologically, cognitively and emotionally.

Under normal circumstances, giving yourself at least a seven-hour sleep opportunity (time asleep) is critical to optimal health. Otherwise, you will just build up sleep debt that cannot be paid off. You cannot under-sleep and then hope to be able to catch up on it at the weekends.[195] It doesn't work like that. Once your sleep is lost, it's lost forever, regardless of whether you sleep twenty hours at the weekend. A consistent seven to nine hours' sleep every night is important to avoid any sleep deprivation.

Sleep deprivation

In the dictionary, "deprivation" is defined as a lack of something that is considered to be a necessity. A full night's sleep is a necessity. We know that a full night's sleep consists of 4–6 cycles of five phases of sleep and somewhere between seven and nine hours. This includes adequate deep NREM and REM sleep. A lack of any of the 4–6 cycles of the five phases will be considered deprivation. So, it's not just time slept. You can give yourself the correct sleep opportunity but how high is the quality of your sleep?

There is also some debate around whether we need less sleep as we get older. Many older people report being able to sleep less and the quality of their sleep not being what it used to be. Although there doesn't appear to be a consensus on this, the evidence points not towards older adults having a reduced sleep need, "but rather, an impaired ability to register and/or generate that unmet sleep need."[196]

Sleep is an important factor in your body's constant attempt to maintain homeostasis. Being sleep-deprived can put things out of balance. A common example of this and one that we will all have definitely experienced at some point is being in a bit of a mood following a poor night's sleep. You can be cranky, ratty, sharp or aggressive all because you didn't have a good night's sleep. This is largely due to an overactive amygdala (an area of the brain that is responsible for negative emotion) after a night where you are deprived of REM sleep. As little as one night of sleep deprivation triggers a 60% amplification in the amygdala, relative to a normal night of sleep.[197] Unsurprisingly, morning mood improves when REM-sleep is intact.[198]

Another example of sleep deprivation effecting homeostasis is how sleep affects your energy levels the next day. Energy systems can be lowered, you get tired more easily during the day and you may not be as productive. One reason for this is glycogen levels. Glycogen is involved in storing energy in the brain and muscles and liver, and glycogen levels have been shown to decrease during wakefulness. The longer you're awake the more glycogen you will use. Then, when you don't have deep restful sleep those glycogen levels are depleted and so the cycle continues.[199]

But these are just two obvious examples. You know when you're moody and you know when you have low energy, and you can probably easily put two and two together. But what's going on under the hood that you may not be as consciously aware of when homeostasis is out of whack?

You are also almost twice as likely to get injured if you have less than eight hours sleep before an activity.[200] This continues to get worse the less sleep you get. The lower the sleep length, the higher the injury risk.

One system that is dramatically affected by sleep deprivation is your immune system.[201] Poor sleep quality increases your body's production of proinflammatory cells. Inflammation is our friend, but we don't want inflammation there when we don't need it. Having high inflammation in our brain and body can develop into chronic conditions or development of disease as discussed earlier.

Incidentally, strangely enough, too much sleep can also induce high levels of proinflammatory cells. For people who sleep ten hours or more this can actually aggravate chronic inflammation more than people who sleep less than seven hours. So there should also be a balance when it comes to sleep.

I won't say more about high inflammation markers here, as we have already spoken about the effects of having high proinflammatory markers back in Chapter 4. If you want, go back and have another read of that to refresh your memory.

Pain processing

Another area you probably won't be aware of is our brain's pain processing and natural painkiller system. Not every noxious stimulus needs to be turned into pain. If you can remember back to Chapter Two, we spoke about nociceptors, which are our body's danger detectors. If there is potential danger these nociceptors will fire off and tell the brain there is danger. But you don't want the firing of these nociceptors turning into pain if they don't have to.[202]

When our brain receives information from the nociceptors, it has the ability to process, evaluate and make sense of what's going on. If the brain decides that this stimulus isn't a threat it can release some of its own natural opioid pain killers to dampen down the sensitive information. Pain scientist David Butler describes this process as "the drug cabinet in the brain." But again, sleep deprivation affects this system. Regions of the brain that are responsible for evaluating and making sense of these stimuli shift in effective evaluation and poor decision making, resulting in amplification of pain.

You can think about it like this. A man walks into a shop with a gun on his belt. The shopkeeper who didn't have a good night's sleep takes one look at the gun, screams and runs out of the shop. The other shopkeeper who did have a good night's sleep serves the policeman and the policeman calmly leaves. The difference between the two shopkeepers is how the information was processed. Both shopkeepers saw the same gun but processed that information differently. The first shopkeeper perceived danger and the second didn't. Sleep deprivation does this to the brain's evaluation of stimuli. The tired brain may not evaluate the information as well as a well-rested brain and, as a result, pain can be amplified.

The endocrine system

Furthermore, sleep deprivation affects the control centre for the endocrine system. The endocrine system is the system that controls your glands and hormones. This system has a direct relationship with the nervous system. I'll spare you the name of the control centre. Anyway, this control centre controls the release of many hormones in the body.

One particularly important hormone in the context of pain is cortisol. When cortisol is released from the control centre, it moves your body into a fight-or-flight response. This is a good system when we need it to happen.

The growth hormone that is responsible for the growth of muscles, bones and immune function is mostly released during your deep N3 phase of sleep[203] so, if you're not accessing this phase of your sleep, it won't be released as efficiently.

Cortisol suppresses the growth hormone. If you have high levels of cortisol, then accessing N3 sleep will be more difficult and the secretion of the growth hormone will be inhibited. This makes it harder to recover and repair tissue. Cortisol also suppresses the immune system, and, again, immune function is optimised during N3 and N4 deep sleep.

Cortisol is an important and vital survival hormone, and it probably gets a bad reputation (as discussed in Chapter 2).

However, to briefly summarise, too much cortisol being released has physiological and psychological repercussions. For starters you are more likely to be in fight-or-flight mode, which is physiologically demanding on the body. If your immune function is suppressed, it is going to make it harder to recover, repair and fight off infection. You will find it difficult to sleep and access your deeper NREM and REM stages of sleep. And we know at this point the many other issues that can arise with sleep deprivation.

There is a lot more to it than we have time for here. But for me, the areas we've discussed have the strongest impact on pain influencing systems.

These systems don't work independently of each other, by the way. I am just trying to split it up and break it down as best I can to show you what can happen when you are sleep-deprived. All of these changes are happening whether you are feeling symptoms in those areas or not. If you are sleep-deprived the only symptom you may have is pain. You may not even feel sleep-deprived. But not getting adequate fully restful sleep is affecting many systems that have an influence on pain.

Sleep broadly serves to maintain homeostasis and good quality sleep is the single greatest thing we can do to restore homeostasis in our brain and body. You need to make sleep a priority, if it's not already one.

The chicken or the egg?

Pain and poor-quality sleep are often bidirectional, meaning they are often present together, with one setting off the other. In fact, sleep complaints are present in 67–88% of chronic pain disorders and at least 50% of individuals with insomnia suffer with chronic pain.[204]

Logic might lead you to assume that poor sleep quality starts with the onset of pain, but surprisingly, sleep impairments are a stronger, more reliable predictor of pain than pain is of sleep impairments.[205] It's difficult to measure sleep before pain onset because it's already happened, so you'll just have to rely on your memory. But when you think back, make sure you factor in your level of sleep opportunity, meaning how long you are actually asleep. Don't include time in bed as time slept. Factor in sleep quality too. Did you feel refreshed in the morning? How often did you take sedatives such as alcohol, medications or marijuana? Did it take you long to fall asleep? Was your mind racing in bed? Perhaps your sleep routine wasn't as good as you thought. This could be a factor in the original development of your pain. It doesn't have to be the sole factor, but if you haven't been getting quality sleep over time, it's fair to say that it has contributed on some level. This will usually not be factored in when you are being diagnosed. It will usually be diagnosed according to the thing you were doing when the pain started or the results on a scan. It's difficult to factor in sleep because there is no way to measure it as a contributory factor. We can only use scientific evidence to consider whether it has played a role.

Sleep changes after pain onset are much easier to measure, because pain is very good at making us aware of what's going on in our body. To be fair, that's its job. When the room is dark and silent the only thing that you can feel is the pain you are experiencing. It's difficult to think of something else. When you roll over in the middle of the night you know you rolled over. When you get up to go to the toilet, you feel and remember every step. It's much easier to measure than how you slept, because pain demands your attention. You know how many times you have been awake and how long it took to get back to sleep. It's easier to compare nights when you slept well and nights when you slept badly. You may have noticed that when you don't sleep very well your pain tends to be worse the next day.

Long-term studies consistently suggest that chronic pain is a significant predictor of development of sleep problems in the future.[206] So, which is it? Is it the chicken or the egg? Has your sleep been disrupted because of your pain? Or, are you in pain because of your poor-quality sleep?

Conclusion

I hope this section has been a bit of an eye opener, excuse the pun. The relationship between chronic pain and sleep is self-reinforcing, as sleep can be affected by chronic pain, but it can also modulate the pain experience.

An important part of our recovery plan in the final chapter will be to help you get adequate sleep because sleep is a painkiller in itself. Getting consistent natural sleep increases your pain threshold, which puts it on a par with analgesics such as aspirin, acetaminophen and ibuprofen; and REM sleep is an antinociceptive (a reduction in sensitivity to pain).[207] Additionally, several large prospective studies suggest that good sleep increases the chance that chronic pain will reduce over time.[208] You just need to engage in behaviours that promote sleep. We will discuss that more later. For optimal health, good quality sleep is a necessity and this is non-negotiable. There's no way around it.

NOTES

Chapter 8

Your Pain Map

Up until now I have been talking about what influences pain and I have encouraged you to take notes at the end of each chapter. Now it's time to put all your note-taking to good use.

In this chapter we will discuss how you can put these influences together to show you how these influencers have affected your pain. I will use some illustrations and analogies to give you a better understanding of how this model works. What's good about looking at pain from this perspective is that it is scientific but also very logical. But what I love the most about it is that it's very personal to you and your life – nobody else's. It doesn't matter if you have a twin brother or sister with the same type of pain symptoms. The influences and stressors will be different. Unless of course you have had the exact same life, thoughts, physical activities, beliefs, diet or sleep, which is impossible.

When a client's eyes are opened up to what pain really is, it usually gives them a bit of hope that there is light at the end of the tunnel and also that enthusiasm to make the kinds of changes that are necessary to finally become pain-free. If you haven't done this by now don't worry. This chapter will aim to bring clarity to how all of this works. My hope is that I will inspire that enthusiasm to make changes in your life.

There will definitely be areas of your life that influence your pain more than others. This is true whether it started with a physical trauma, a stressful part of your life or poor lifestyle. Not all influencers are created equal. At this point we just want to lay them all out, and put them into context so we can logically see how and why they are influencing your pain.

Mapping out your pain

So now we are moving on to the part where we start to map your pain. This simple but excellent illustration brings your influencers to life. Using the notes that you have been taking, this is your chance to map your own pain, taking into account everything you have learned in this book that is relevant to your pain.

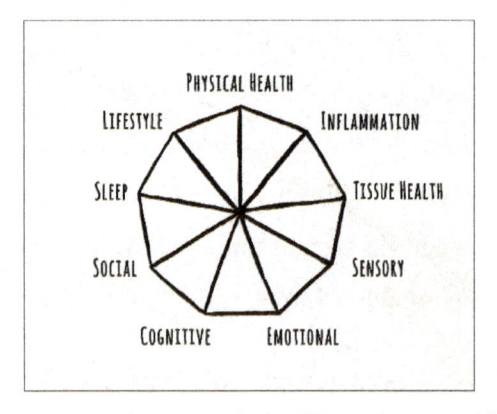

Images care of P.A. Morand, a.k.a. "The Back Pain Coach"

The image above shows an nonagon with nine different areas around it, all of which have been discussed in the book. Using a scale ranging from 0 to 10, I want you to put a score in each area, with 0 meaning it's not influencing your pain at all and 10 meaning it is influencing it hugely. For example, if I was highly stressed, I would hypothetically put an 8/10 on the stress area, and draw a dot 8/10 of the way from the centre to the edge. Then continue to do this on all remaining areas and finally join the dots until you have an image like the examples below.

Then mark out your respective pain map and this will give you a visual of the areas that we need to work on.

Physical health – Are there any comorbidities that are affecting your health, like obesity, diabetes, respiratory issues, heart conditions?

Tissue health – This includes injuries, deformities, nerve impingement, disc prolapse, arthritis, illnesses, and diseases (such as cancer, MS, and Parkinson's). How is your overall physical fitness and conditioning?

Social – Are there any social aspects that could be influencing your pain? How has your social life changed? Consider work, family, hobbies, friends, social exclusion, social isolation, validation and relationships (especially in relation to your spouse and healthcare providers).

Lifestyle – This relates to diet, water intake, medication, narcotics, smoking, alcohol intake, exercise or just your all-round quality of life.

Sleep – Sleep could and probably should be under the lifestyle category but it needs its own category just so you are clear about how vital it is.

Are you getting the recommended seven to nine hours of sleep consistently? What is the quality of that sleep like? Is it being affected by medications (including sleeping pills)?

Cognitive – What were your thoughts and beliefs around your understanding of your pain before you read this book? I hope I'm at least giving you some new things to think about and ways to question your beliefs. Make sure you mark what your limiting beliefs were before reading this book.

Emotional – This is about anxiety, depression, general day to day stresses, mood, fear and worry (about, for instance, movement, exercise, and potential surgery).

Sensory – How sensitised do you think your nervous system is? Does gentle movement cause pain? Are you in constant pain or are you only in pain after physical activity or exercise? Does it take much activity to experience pain?

Inflammation – How much of a role do you think inflammation is playing in your pain? Is there untreated acute inflammation? Are there any chronic inflammatory issues, or auto immune conditions? All of these are most likely going to be high on the scale, especially if they are a regular occurrence. How often you do feel things are inflamed? Sometimes it can be difficult to know if there is inflammation because it doesn't always swell up. One way you can check for increased inflammation is to see if there is temperature in the area, increased puffiness, redness or pain. But chronic inflammation doesn't always show these signs. Also, if you are taking anti-inflammatories, do they work? If you're not getting any relief from them, perhaps inflammation isn't too high on the scale.

Ankle sprain

Let's look at some hypothetical cases. It's important to note that, with any condition the influencers could be higher or lower on the scale or there could be some other contributing factors in your case that I have not included. As I already said, pain is a personal experience and no two people have the same pain experience, nor are they influenced the same way.

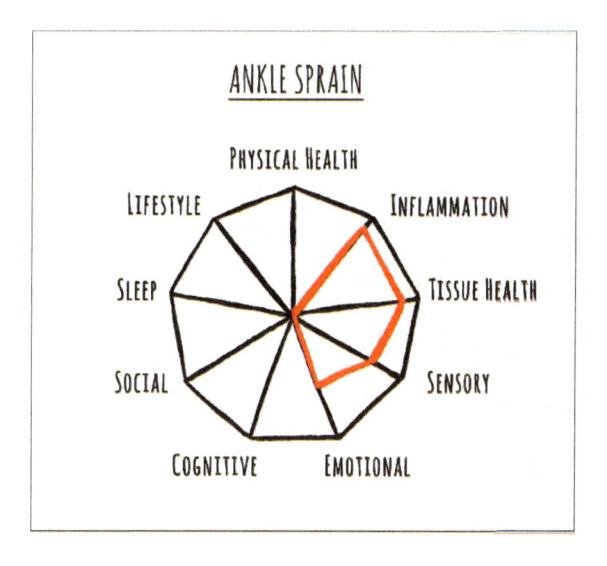

In the first image here, we have a common ankle sprain. This is unlikely to be you if you are reading this book but I'm sure you've had a soft tissue injury at some point in your life that you can relate to. Generally, your experience of an acute injury is influenced by the tissue damage itself, the sensory nerves that become sensitised due to the injury, and the inflammation that occurs to protect the area. Also there is always some sort of an emotion related to the injury. For example, this person may be worried or fearful that something sinister is the cause of their pain; or they may be afraid to bear weight in case of making the injury worse. The timeframe with this should be up to three months. If it's any longer, it's less likely to be related to the tissue damage as all tissue should heal within this period. You could also logged in a bit of sleep and lifestyle just to illustrate that will play a role in acute injuries too. The overall health of the tissue will be affected by how well you recover and how healthily you live your life, as discussed in previous chapters.

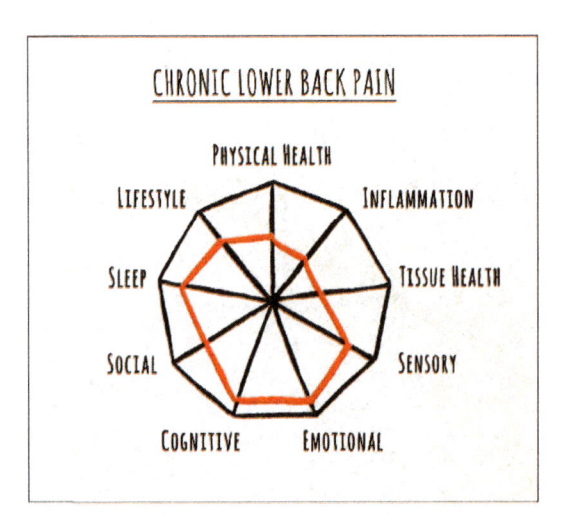

Chronic lower back pain

Probably the most common complaint I get in my clinic is lower back pain. In all honesty, it's usually not that difficult to resolve. Yes, there are some cases for which it can be really difficult to resolve, but for most people who suffer with lower back pain it can be easily resolved if treated correctly. About 90% of people will suffer with lower back pain at some point in their life and the vast majority go on to live happy normal lives free from pain. In my experience it's mainly due to doing too much too soon, daily habits, poor movement, muscle guarding, fear of movement, negative limiting beliefs or poor lifestyle. It could involve all or some of these influencers.

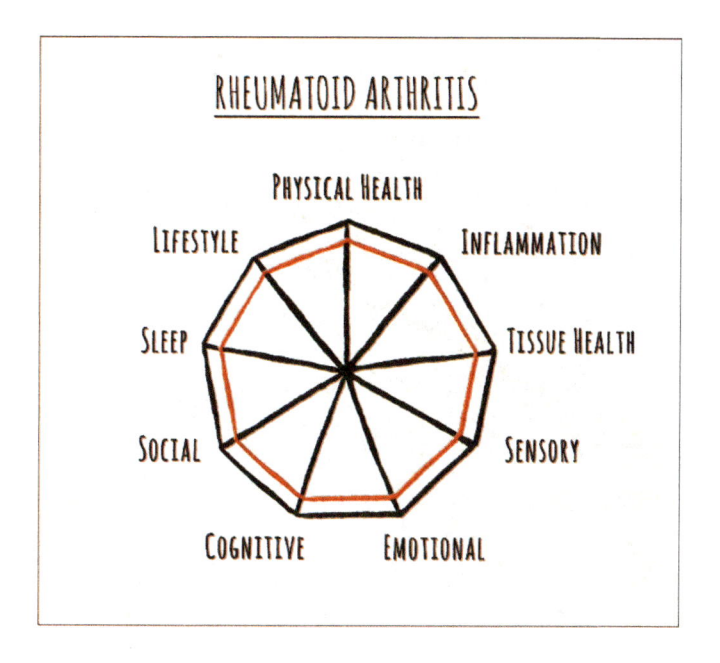

Rheumatoid arthritis

In this image, we have a representation of someone suffering from an inflammatory condition such as rheumatoid arthritis. In these conditions, as you can see, many people score high in many aspects of the chart. Flare-ups come in waves and often across multiple joints in the body. When the flare-ups come, they can be debilitating, which in turn affects all stressors on the chart. This is primarily an immune condition but so many different influencers are at play here, even though they may be secondary to the immune condition. Using a biopsychosocial approach is crucial as it helps strengthen the immune system through such things as improving sleep, reducing stress, exercising at comfortable levels and just improving overall health, which has been shown to improve conditions like these. So, even in severe debilitating conditions there are still many avenues to go down and improve.

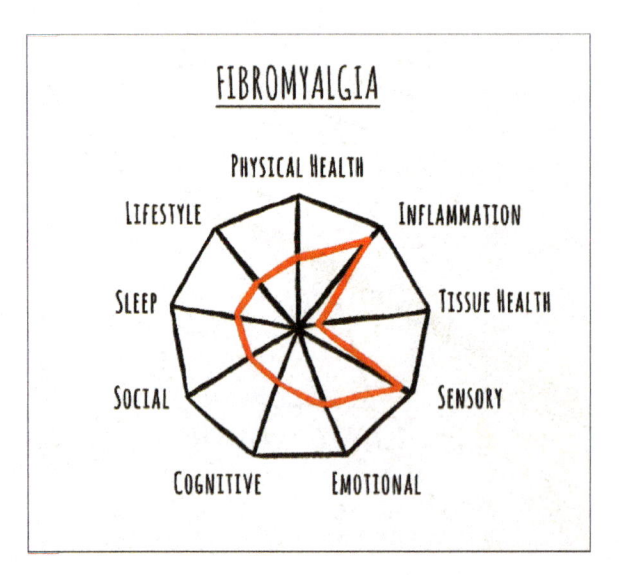

Fibromyalgia

Fibromyalgia is often seen as a made-up condition. I don't know where or why this started, as it's very real. Perhaps because it's an invisible condition, it gets this false reputation. At least if you have rheumatoid arthritis (I say this with tongue in cheek), you may see physical symptoms such as joint deformity. But often with fibromyalgia there are no visible symptoms – just widespread pain, fatigue, gastrointestinal issues and often emotional components. Pain scientists believe it may be caused by a malfunctioning nervous system and can often start off when you have a trauma (emotional or physical) and your system is compromised around that time.[209] There is also a new concept regarding fibromyalgia pioneered by Dr Asaf Klaff Weissman who is citing fibromyalgia as a neuroimmune condition. He explains it to be like "a dysfunctional interaction between the immune system and nervous system whereby aberrations in the immune system cause a release of chemicals that sensitise nociceptors." This results in developments of conditions like fibromyalgia and some autoimmune diseases.

Emotional, physical, and sexual abuse during childhood are considered high risk factors for fibromyalgia, as well as genetics, obesity, and chronic stress. Fibromyalgia is also more prevalent in females than males,[210] with the ratio being approximately 9:1.[211]

To my knowledge there isn't one ideal treatment for this as yet – what is recommended is to find ways to calm the nervous system down. Again, using a personalised biopsychosocial approach covers many ways to calm down the nervous system rather than just focusing on one treatment. One person I would recommend listening to is Bronnie Thompson, who is a pain scientist who also suffers with the condition. I think she's a great source of information because I feel she has an invested interest in it combined with a biopsychosocial approach.

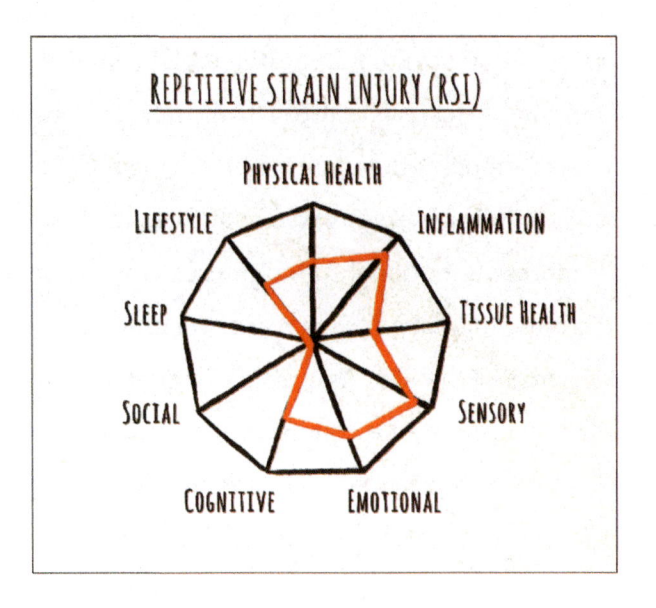

Repetitive strain injury (RSI)

Our last example is an RSI. These are mainly influenced by physical components. Unsurprisingly they arise from doing repetitive movements. The best-known versions are tennis or golfer's elbow. But it can happen in many areas of the body. Some include plantar fasciitis, Achilles' tendonitis, recurring hamstring injuries or even general back pain. When we're looking at RSIs we have to take into account what's causing the pain. As you can see in the image, inflammation and sensory issues are big influencers. So how do we change that? First, work on desensitising the area and reducing inflammation. Then work on physical conditioning to be able to manage the amount of activity you can do with that part of the body. This will all be explained in more detail in the next chapter.

This was just a visual to show you how all pain is different and the approach needs to be personalised to the individual. I hope you are beginning to see the importance of understanding your pain and treating it using a full lifestyle approach.

Chapter 9

Putting It All Together

I want you to go back to the time leading up to when you were first in pain and write down any pre-pain stressors that were going on in your life. We have discussed all the potential stressors in the book so far and you have hopefully taken notes. It doesn't matter how big or how small the stressors were – just compile them in a list for now and we will sort them out later in this chapter.

It doesn't matter how long it has been since you first were in pain. If they haven't been addressed, perhaps they could be one of the main reasons why you are still in pain. Maybe they have been resolved, but I want you to identify them and write them down anyway, and we will decide if they are worth addressing as a priority in a bit.

If your pain started from a trauma such as a car crash or a bad fall the pre-pain stressors won't be as important but there's still no harm in going back to them. Maybe they are not at the forefront of your mind. Again, that doesn't mean they don't exist anymore. This is why you need to go back to the time when you were first in pain, to make a list of all stressors from a physical, psychological, emotional and social point of view.

Next, it's time to write down the post-pain stressors.

These are newer stressors that have come after the pain or injury came along. They include anything that manifested after the injury happened but is now contributing to the problem. These might include medication, deconditioning/fitness level, scars, sensitisation, fear, worry, poor sleep, negative expectations, negative beliefs, stress, financial problems, or disability.

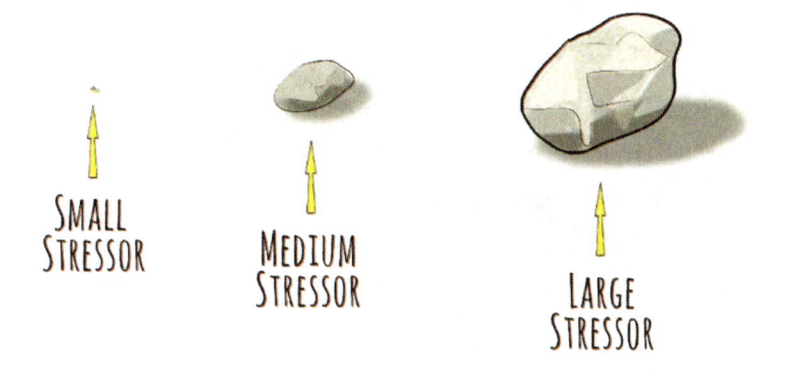

SMALL STRESSOR

MEDIUM STRESSOR

LARGE STRESSOR

Now that you have all your pre- and post-pain influencers written down, we are going to split your stressors up into three separate categories.

1. Small stressors – these are small influencers that make a minor demand on the body: something that is physically, psychologically, or

emotionally demanding that you are dealing with occasionally. This can be represented by a grain of sand.

2. Medium stressors – these are medium demands on your body: something that is physically, psychologically, or emotionally demanding that you are dealing with multiple times per week. This can be represented by a pebble.

3. Large stressors – these place a high demand on your body, physically, psychologically or emotionally: things you are dealing with on a daily basis without much emotional or physical recovery. This can be represented by a stone.

In this analogy the glass represents your body. The sand, pebbles and stones represent your influencers/stressors and the water level signifies how well you're coping with the influencers/stressors.

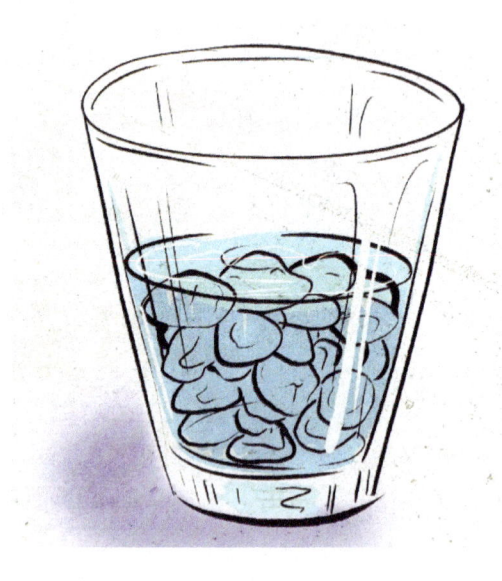

Your glass will have some water in it to begin with. Even the most basic survival functions such as breathing, walking and eating place a demand or stress on the body. So, there will always be water. The day you have no water in your glass, trust me – you won't need to worry about trying to resolve your pain. As the famous endocrinologist Hans Selye once said, "The absence of stress is death."

A stone obviously holds more weight and size; it's obvious if you have a stone in your glass the water levels will rise significantly. These are the stressors we want to focus on first to see if we can change them because they hold more weight.

Then we have the pebbles. The pebbles aren't as bad as the stone but still have substance to them which will push up the water level, especially if there are multiple pebbles. After we focus on the stones, or if we cannot change the stones, then we will focus on the pebbles.

Finally, we have the grains of sand. These are smaller stressors and less important, but even so, if there are many grains of sand, they can be important, especially if the water level is just on the rim of the glass. It may only take a few grains of sand to make the glass overflow.

We are capable of managing stones and pebbles; we don't need to take them out altogether. The problem is that, if the stones and pebbles are in your glass long-term, it doesn't leave much room for any other sand, stones or pebbles. Life will always throw new stones and pebbles in your glass, so you don't want unresolved stones to stay in your glass.

Sometimes a pebble can turn into a stone, for instance if you start doing more physical work for a period or perhaps taking on more responsibility at work. Any increase of a stressor will change the size of the object in the glass, thus raising the water level in the glass.

If you have too many stones or pebbles in your glass, eventually your glass of water is going to overflow. When the glass cannot tolerate any more stressors, it will overflow and that's when pain is experienced. Pain is communication and it's designed to tell you your glass is overflowing so you should do something about it. But here's the problem; if the right number of stones or pebbles aren't taken out of the glass, the water will continue to overflow.

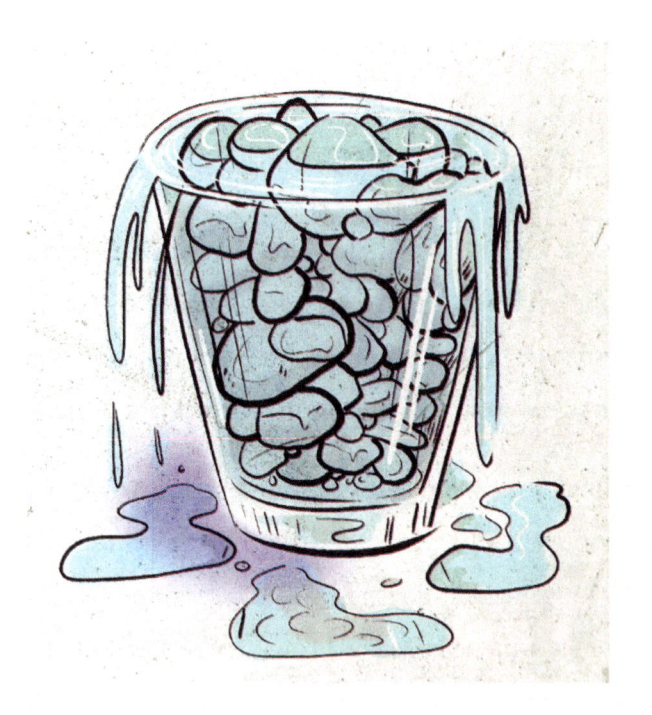

When we don't fully understand why the glass is overflowing this can lead to poor movement, fear, worry or anxiety, which will increase the number of stones or pebbles being thrown in the glass. Then, even if you take out the original pebbles or stones from the glass, you're left with lots of new pebbles and stones and the water keeps overflowing. This can be even more confusing. For example, imagine you injured yourself and a stone was put into your glass representing the physical injury. Then, as a result of that, you have maladaptive behaviours such as poor movement, fear, anxiety about movement, deconditioning, poor mood and poor sleep quality. All of these are a result of the initial injury and carry their own stones and pebbles. When the tissue injury heals, as it will do within three months, the new pebbles and stones remain.

This is why I want you to make a list of your pre-pain stressors and your post-pain stressors – so we can ensure we address the stones and pebbles that are keeping the glass overflowing.

The idea is that you want to keep the water levels relatively balanced. Sometimes you'll have more stones and pebbles in your glass as you go through life, but that's normal and we are built to cope with that. But what we're not built to cope with is constant stressors and demands, without taking any of the stressors out of the glass.

Every person is different and some people are more resilient than others. Some people have bigger glasses and are able to handle more influencers without any problems. You should never compare your glass to others. Just be grateful that you have water in your glass.

When we take personality into the equation, people who score higher in neuroticism will generally have less room to work with in the glass.[212] So what may be perceived as a grain of sand for someone who scores low in neuroticism will end up being a pebble or a stone for someone who scores high in neuroticism. These people tend to catastrophise, which can bring the level of water up higher for something that another person may see as less sinister.

Once we have done this we will start to work on two things.

Looking at the whole glass (the biopsychosocial model)

I have given you a wide variety of conditions for a reason. I wanted to demonstrate to you first of all that all pain is different and influenced by many different types of stressors. No two people's pain are the same and hopefully I have been able to get this across to you. So, with that in mind, it makes sense that not all treatments will be the same. It wouldn't be logical to approach all pain the same way even if the symptoms were similar.

This is why I believe that every treatment should be personal, specific and tailored towards each individual from the beginning. It doesn't always need to be to the level of detail of which I'm speaking now but it should at least be observed through the same biopsychosocial lens. Of course, if it's an ankle sprain, it is less likely there will be major psychosocial issues contributing to the pain, but if we're dealing with something that is persisting for an extended period of time, then it's important to observe it from a broader perspective.

To observe through the biopsychosocial lens, the practitioner needs to have a deeper grasp of the complex phenomenon that is pain. And I'm not so sure the average practitioner does.

Every practitioner has their viewpoint and their methodology, be it massage, manipulations, acupuncture, medication, exercise or one of the many other forms of manual therapy. All of these approaches used individually have a therapeutic effect, but using them on their own has limitations, especially when it comes to persistent pain.

Let's put that into context with regards to the chronic lower back pain individual mentioned above. If a physio used massage and exercise as a way of treating the chronic lower back pain without addressing the other stressors, the treatment is less likely to have long-term benefits because there are other aspects that are contributing to the pain.

There is nothing wrong with the treatment per se, it's just limited to the physical aspects. An integrated approach involving all three areas of the biopsychosocial model will have more of a chance of leading to sustained long-term results.

The biopsychosocial model isn't a treatment. It's an observation point. A therapist can use whatever methodology they want to achieve their patients' goals, once all areas of the person's life are considered.

Take me for instance. Good quality movement, strength and conditioning is my main methodology and is how I like to treat clients. And yes, you could say I am biased towards this; but I use this approach within a biopsychosocial framework. My end goal is to get my clients conditioned for whatever it is they do in their life and for them to have better quality movement more often during the day. But this may not be achieved through conditioning and movement exercises alone. There may be other psychosocial factors that limit my end goal for them. If these other non-physical influencers aren't addressed, then my end goal may not be possible. I can't force someone to move better if their body is telling them not to move.

You don't need a psychologist or a psychotherapist to be able to identify psychosocial factors in pain. You just need to find a practitioner who looks at pain from a less biomedical model and more of a biopsychosocial model. Moreover, if better questions are asked by the practitioner, then psychosocial aspects can be identified and treated as long as it's within the scope of practice.

I personally have trained in Cognitive Behavioural Therapy and many other practitioners have trained in other psychological treatments. But I also have no problem referring patients to psychologists, psychotherapists, or counsellors if I have identified something that is outside the area of my expertise. This is how the system should work for chronic pain: a crossover approach where practitioners from psychological and physical backgrounds can work together. Instead, most pain is treated with a biomedical model.

As the famous quote by Abraham Maslow goes, "If the only tool you have is a hammer, you tend to see every problem as a nail." I firmly believe that, when treating a client from a biopsychosocial point of view, you have much more than a hammer at your disposal. It's like the Swiss army knife of approaches as there are many different ways to treat a condition.

The whole point of this book is to empower you to help yourself by figuring out what is contributing to your pain. At least now you can make a more informed decision on where to go from here. This may be to apply the changes suggested in the next chapter, find a new therapist with a biopsychosocial point of view or maybe addressing deeper emotional issues you might need to work through with some form of counselling.

Becoming more informed and educated leads to you making better decisions for yourself. You don't have to rely on others to tell you what to do for you. We're at a stage now where your biological, psychological and social aspects have been identified.

Now, who's ready for a plan to move forward?

Chapter 10

Optimise Yourself for Recovery

Many pain sufferers want to move ahead with the rehab exercises without putting themselves in a state to recover. It's tempting to push ahead with exercises or activity because this gives the illusion that you are moving towards something.

But what if your body doesn't want exercise? What if your body isn't in a receptive state? In this case, exercises are just going to aggravate it further, which can in turn discourage you from exercise in the future.

The first part of this chapter is all about how you can optimise yourself and put your body in the best position to recover. The foundation needs to be set to build a solid recovery plan. Without a good foundation, no building will survive any adverse conditions.

Pain acceptance

Before you move forward, you have to accept where you are now. This is not a negotiation, it's a prerequisite. It's impossible to ever move forward if you're stuck in the past. Accepting your pain, regardless of its magnitude, as well as the impact on your life, or the changes it has brought upon you, is an essential step towards improvement.

Pain acceptance isn't a nice term. Many people, myself included, don't like the word "acceptance." It's almost like you're accepting defeat. But I assure you that's not true. Pain acceptance is the process of stopping the struggle and accepting that this is the way it is, at least for now.

Chronic pain can sometimes be like being in quicksand. The more you struggle, the worse it gets. It's best to accept that whatever has happened in your life has led you to here and now you're in quicksand. So, are you going to keep fighting and sinking deeper, or are you going to accept that you're here now and stop the struggle to find a better way out?

This is not defeat. It's more like you're calling it a draw. Shake hands, get on better terms with your pain, and work together to overcome it. For some this might mean that you learn better ways to live with your pain. For others it means accepting what has happened in the past has happened, forgiving and getting on with your life.

You may even need to *redefine what you consider normal for yourself.*[213] Perhaps stop holding onto the old you. You might argue that it's easy for me to say that. I understand that it's easier said than done. I recognise that accepting your circumstances can be challenging, particularly if you're facing impending court proceedings, experiencing invalidation in your environment, or have lost your sense of identity;

but you need to do it, whether that means coming to terms with it on your own or with the help of a professional.

Acceptance and commitment therapy (ACT) is a type of psychotherapy that emphasises acceptance as a way to deal with negative thoughts, feelings, symptoms or circumstances. But pain acceptance isn't about your own mindset. Educating yourself and others around you can also facilitate acceptance.[214]

"Greater acceptance of pain is associated with reports of lower pain intensity, less pain-related anxiety and avoidance, less depression, less physical and psychosocial disability, more daily uptime, and better work status."[215]

Accepting your situation may be a bitter pill to swallow, but it's a much better pill to swallow than a lifetime on pain medication.

Changing your daily habits

A habit, as defined by the Oxford Dictionary, is something you do frequently and almost unconsciously. But how do we alter actions we perform without even being aware of them? The first step is identifying your current habits.

Remember, a habit is essentially a network of brain connections that have become so familiar that they function seamlessly without conscious thought. Through repeated practice, these habits have been ingrained in your brain, transforming into efficient pathways. Your brain has become an expert at executing these habits. Habits encompass a wide range of behaviours, from how you rise out of bed in the morning to how you lift an object from the ground, and even how you perceive certain thoughts.

By now, you should have a list of "stones, pebbles" or actions that contribute to filling your glass. Our goal is to pinpoint habits that no longer serve your wellbeing and work on changing them. Instead of relying on those deeply entrenched habit "superhighways" that are no longer helpful, we aim to create new, healthier pathways or "forest trails" of behaviours that do serve your needs. Eventually, through intention and repetition, we want to turn these beneficial behaviours into habit "superhighways."

In the sections that follow, you'll find a list of ways to alter the contents of your "glass of water." Some strategies will focus on expanding the glass's capacity, while others will involve removing some of the metaphorical stones and pebbles from the glass. One remarkable aspect of this approach is its versatility. There are numerous areas that can be enhanced. If you encounter difficulty in changing one aspect, you can shift your focus to another, knowing that progress in one area can positively influence others over time. Remember, the brain has changed over time to get you to this point. So, in order to get to where you want to go, change is imperative. As Einstein famously remarked, "The definition of insanity is doing the same thing over and over again and expecting different results." Change is essential to recovery.

This transformation involves modifying your behaviours, thoughts, emotions, movements, education, and, crucially, the way your brain generates pain. It all begins with a resolute decision and unwavering commitment to initiate change. Education serves as a catalyst, reshaping your thought processes and even altering the interpretation and perception of experiences. By embracing change, you pave the way for a renewed perspective and improved wellbeing.

Improving your breathing

When we try to improve our health, most try to change the things that we can survive the longest without – mainly exercising, food quality or water intake. Few people ever consider trying to improve the very thing that, if we stopped doing it for three minutes, would lead to death. If you have been suffering with pain for a long period and nobody has ever mentioned breathing until now, you have missed a big opportunity for change.

First of all, it's so easy to implement, as it can be done right away. You don't need any equipment or to get yourself into gym gear. You can do it in bed, in the car, while watching television or even exercising, and best of all, it's free. All it takes is just a little self-awareness and some discipline. Just a few minutes a day is enough to seriously improve your health.

There are two main reasons why good quality breathing is important for health. The first will be to optimise your breath. This focuses on reducing the number of breaths you take per minute. If you counted more than twelve breaths per minute in the test you took in Chapter 3, here is a breathing exercise you can implement that will help reduce the number of breaths you take throughout your day.

There are many breathing techniques from a wide range of breathing coaches. I am just going to keep things simple for you. Some breathing coaches overcomplicate things with breathing drills, but for a novice, what's really important is to be able to access deep diaphragmatic breathing.

For best results you should do this exercise twice a day. If you are not breathing diaphragmatically comfortably, with twelve breaths or fewer per minute, then your breathing exercises should be in the goals/plan we will create later.

Lie down on a bed or sit upright with your back on a chair. Put one hand on your chest and one hand on your belly. Set a timer for one minute to begin with. As time goes on and you start to become better at this, you can increase it to two to three minutes twice a day. There is absolutely no harm in doing this for longer if you want to. In fact, it will only benefit you more, but I'm realistic and I understand that people will generally only allocate a few minutes a day to breathing exercises. Start your timer on your first inhale. Inhale for six seconds and exhale for six seconds. Ensure that your belly hand is rising first and not your chest hand. If you are a very dominant chest breather, this may be difficult to begin with, but don't get frustrated. You can gently tap your belly with your hand to increase your body's awareness of where you are trying to breathe into. Some people will be able to belly breathe straight away, but for others it can take a few attempts, so don't get frustrated. Just be patient.

Once you can access your belly breathing and you have mastered the inhale and exhale, we can progress this exercise by putting both hands across your lower ribs with your fingers pointing towards each other across your belly. Put a bit of pressure on your bottom ribs as if you're slightly pushing them in.

Now you're going to do the same breathing technique, inhaling for six seconds and exhaling for six seconds. You're still watching your belly rising first, the only difference this time is that you are encouraging your ribs to subtly flare outwards during the inhale. When we breathe and our lungs fill up with air, it is just like blowing up a balloon, whereby the air is filling up in a 360-degree direction. Sometimes, when people belly breathe, the only focus is on their belly rising first. To know that you are properly doing diaphragmatic breathing, there needs to be a rise in (intra-abdominal) pressure the whole way around. Just like when you're blowing up a balloon. This is why you have your hands on your ribs: to make sure of this. If you feel you aren't flaring your ribcage outwards then I suggest putting pressure on one side at a time and focusing on trying to breathe into that area. Then do the same on the other side. When you feel both sides rising comfortably, revisit the breathing exercise. In time you won't need to place one hand on your belly and the other on your chest. You will be able to do this automatically and comfortably.

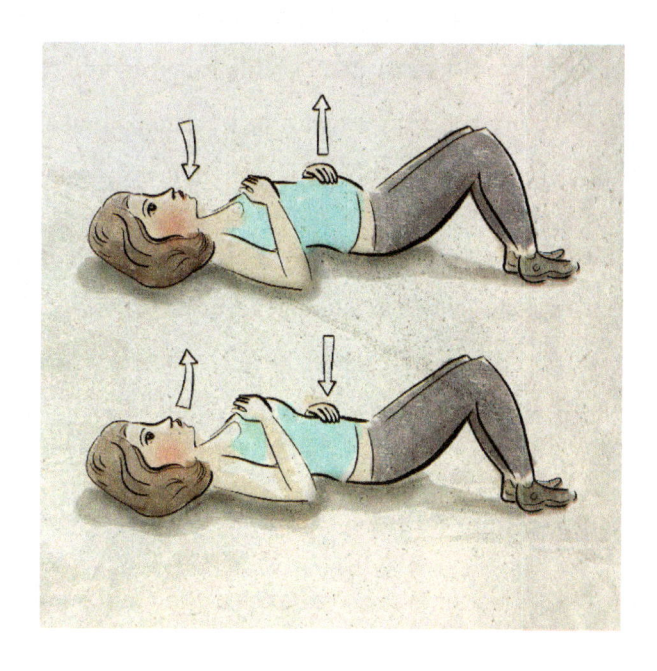

Learning this diaphragmatic breathing means we can stimulate the vagus nerve. When you stimulate the vagus nerve, this lowers the heart rate and calms down your nervous system. This not only helps with the efficiency of your breathing but also puts you in a state of rest and digestion or safety which will be an important capability to possess later in this chapter.

Improving your sleep

What if I was to tell you that I had a pill that reduced pain, reduced the risk of injury, helped fight off cancer, heart disease and Alzheimer's, improved your mood, improved your athletic performance and improved your cognitive function? Also, this magic pill has absolutely no side effects and it's free without a prescription. Would you take it? You're damn right you would. In fact, if this magic pill was advertised on the television there would be a queue a mile long outside the pharmacy to get it. This amazing pill isn't a result of pharmacological innovation though. It's something that everybody has at their disposal: sleep.

Since the 1960s, as a society we sleep 1–2 hours less per night.[216] Some people wear their sleep loss as a badge of honour,[217] as if it's something to be proud of. I wonder why that is? Perhaps there's a perception that people who sleep are lazy and people who sleep less are better workers. This kind of thought process is not only wrong, but it almost certainly also sets you up for an unhealthy life.

We now know that patients who improved their quality of sleep saw significant improvement in their pain score and quality of life.[218] This is something that you can start to work on straight away. Bear in mind this isn't a quick fix – but when you start to make these changes, they can have lasting effects. Furthermore, sleep deprivation studies have shown that in healthy volunteers, poor sleep lowers the pain threshold, whereas recovery sleep after sleep deprivation increases the pain threshold. [219]

Remember that sleep and pain have a bidirectional relationship. Improving your sleep hygiene starts at home; here are some steps that you can take to help with a better night's sleep.

Better sleep hygiene[220]

• First, try going to bed at the same time and waking up at the same time. Regularity is key. Even if you have a bad night's sleep, get up at the same time every day. I know it will be tough to do, especially if you're very tired after a poor night's sleep, but you need to expose yourself to natural light early in the morning in order to get that release of the sleep-inducing hormone melatonin at the right time at night.

• No caffeine after 3 p.m. This is a tough one and one I struggled with myself at the beginning, but try to not to have caffeine after lunchtime. This can be a challenge, especially if you are a coffee lover like myself or if you have had a poor night's sleep the previous night and you need to function for work. Up to 50% of the caffeine is still in your system six hours after ingestion and it can take up to ten hours to completely get caffeine out of the bloodstream. If you are a fragile sleeper, the closer you have it to your bedtime the more it will affect your ability to fall asleep and it will also affect the quality of the sleep, and how well you access that deep phase 3 restorative sleep. If you think that it doesn't affect your sleep, it will still have an effect on your sleep quality without you knowing it.

• **Alcohol**. As I said, alcohol is a sedative. It can help you fall asleep faster but it greatly affects the quality of your sleep, blocking your REM phases and leaving your night littered with more awake time. As much as you feel you deserve your glass of wine or bottle of beer after a long day, know that it's affecting your sleep. I don't want to come across as a buzzkill and take all the fun out of the world. These are just the facts. Try to limit your alcohol intake and don't have it too close to bedtime.[221]

• **Exercise**. We already spoke about how important exercise is for getting a good night's sleep. Trying to get regular exercise helps with how fast you go to sleep and also how deeply you sleep. For people with sleep problems, long-term exercise improves sleep onset and sleep quality. This is something that changes over time. However, don't expect to get a great night's sleep after your first day of exercise.[222] We also need to know how much to exercise because there is also the fear that over-exercising can increase pain levels. That is a fair concern and probably something that has affected you in the past. I will talk about this during the progressive loading section later on.

• **Make your room colder.** Your body needs to drop its core temperature by up to one degree Celsius or two to three degrees Fahrenheit in order to fall asleep; sleeping in a hot room can make this harder to do. Open a window if it's not too noisy or use a lighter blanket if you can. I don't want you to be shivering in bed though. According to sleep scientist Matthew Walker, having a hot bath late at night helps with sleep onset because when you get out of the bath there is a "massive dump of heat" which helps with sleep onset.

• **Don't eat two to three hours before bedtime.** Your blood sugar levels are naturally higher at night-time. One of the reasons for this is that the release of melatonin slows down the secretion of insulin in the pancreas.[223] As evening time sets in, if your circadian rhythm is optimised, melatonin will start to be released two to three hours before bedtime. This binds to receptors in the pancreas and this reduces the secretion of insulin by the pancreas. Insulin helps control your blood sugar level. When your blood sugar levels are too high, insulin is released by the pancreas which brings them back down to a safer level.[224] Eating too close to your bedtime spikes your blood sugar levels and there isn't the same release of insulin to bring them back down. This can increase sleep disturbance levels and will affect how well you access your deeper restorative sleep phases. Very few people eat a salad when late night snacking. Usually, it's something quick and tasty after a long day and the chances are it will have a higher sugar content. Just make sure it's not too close to your bedtime as timing is a modifiable risk factor for nocturnal awakenings and disrupted sleep.[225]

• **Dim the lights in the house one hour prior to your bedtime.** If the lights are shining, your brain still thinks it's daytime, so it will make it more difficult to release that all-important melatonin. For most of human history it was easy for us to get that natural release of melatonin. For the most part we lived outside and when the sun went down our brain would release the sleep hormone. Now we mostly live inside surrounded by artificial light, which sends a signal to the brain that it's daytime, which confuses the brain and affects it release of melatonin. To help combat this and promote the release of melatonin, try to limit your exposure to artificial light. There are several things you can do like dimming lights, turning on blue light filters on laptops and phones, and not watching TV or using your phone in bed.

• **Get your bedroom associated with sleep time.** If you're used to being awake in your bedroom, then you have created a habitual way of keeping your brain awake. If you've ever heard the story of how Pavlov conditioned his dog to salivate to the sound of a bell, in a similar way your brain can create associations between your bed and awake time.

The more you're in bed awake, the more your brain associates bed with wakefulness. It could get to a stage where you go into your room and your brain says, "Oh, this is where I think, this is where I worry, or this is where I plan." As a result of this association, the brain releases the hormones and neurotransmitters that assist with this.

To combat this and change the association between your bed and wakefulness, you need to disassociate bed and wakefulness. If you're not asleep within twenty minutes, get up and do something different. Don't go back downstairs and start watching television again or start needlessly scrolling on your phone. All you're doing is confusing your brain with artificial light again which will affect your melatonin secretion. Go into a different room with a dim light and read a book, do a crossword or do some journaling. Then when you start to feel sleepy again, go back to bed and try to fall asleep. Keep repeating this process until you fall asleep, and keep repeating this process every night until you change the association between your bedroom and sleep.[226]

• **The anxious brain.** We have all been there, when you're trying to go to sleep but can't because you have a lot on your mind. Your mind is racing when thinking about what needs to be done tomorrow, deadlines at work, bills that need to be paid or something that somebody said to you. Being in a state of worry pushes you into a fight-or-flight response, releasing cortisol or adrenaline which is not helpful when trying to fall asleep. These hormones are released for situations when things need to be done, not when you're doing the opposite.

Your brain is always trying to come up with solutions to problems. Worry is like a cue from the brain to figure out a solution to an unresolved problem. During the day, life is filled with other noise like family life, work or hobbies and if the cue (worry) from the brain to find a resolution to an unresolved problem is brought up it can easily be pushed to the back of your mind because there are other things that need to be done at that moment.

Bedtime might be the only time to actually process or actively think or resolve problems. However, it isn't helpful to do this at 2 a.m.

So, you have essentially taught your brain that the time to worry is in bed.

Good sleep hygiene is important but if you have multiple unresolved problems in your life that are keeping you awake at night, it can still make it very difficult to fall asleep because the brain wants to find solutions to the problems. Your brain is a processing machine. Its job is to take in sensory information, process it and come up with solutions. But having loads of unresolved problems in your head it's like you have a computer with ten different tabs all trying to open up at the same time. Your brain is trying to process everything at once but the process is lagging.

An extremely effective way to combat this is to set some time aside during the day to worry.[227] This is called "deliberate worry." Deliberate worry isn't just a way to needlessly worry about things. It's a way to find solutions to problems so this doesn't have to be done at night. Write down all the problems that are unresolved and what is keeping you up at night. Then follow the same reverse engineering process that we are using to resolve your pain, breaking down your problem and setting mini goals for how you can resolve that problem. At least then there is a plan. Some problems just can't be solved in the short term, but if there are multiple things worrying you, resolving some of them will at least reduce your stress levels. From here you add in your sleep hygiene tools.

Sleeping medications don't resolve your problems. Your fears and worries will still be there when you wake up.

• **Meditation.** Another great tool to help calm the nervous system down is meditation. Meditation has been used for centuries (particularly in the East) in the context of spirituality and religion. But there have been many studies recently that have shown its effects on reducing stress, anxiety, improving sleep, giving mental clarity and promoting relaxation within the body. Just as little as three to five minutes per day has been shown to help with sleep and reduce pain. Meditation is also a great way of helping the brain catch up and load some of those lagging tabs that it's been trying to open.[228]

This leads us perfectly into our final tip.

• **Cognitive Behavioural Therapy – Insomnia** (CBT-I) is a new way to combat sleep issues. It has been shown to be as effective at treating insomnia as sleeping tablets and the results may be more durable.[229] The difference is that sleep without medication is real natural sleep, for which there is no substitute. We have already spoken about the negative effects of sleeping tablets. CBT-I treatment isn't widely available, at least it isn't in Ireland. But if you can get it then it's advisable. Today we have the luxury of being able to do video consultations online. This may be a solution if you can't find a practitioner in your area.

Getting your sleep back on track is as important as it gets when you are trying to overcome pain. This may not happen overnight (excuse the pun) and it may take you working on other pebbles or stones first before you get on top of the sleep issue. But there are some things that you will definitely be able to try straight away.

Giving yourself a better night's sleep will have a domino effect in your life like you wouldn't believe. Think about what it would do to your mood if you started to have a better night's sleep. Straight away, when you're not tired during the day, your emotions will be regulated better. You will have more energy, better cognition, improved memory, reduced risk of injury, less pain, less craving for sugar, and less likelihood of putting on weight. If you're not sleeping, your recovery is being affected.

Sun exposure

In our modern world, we are a sunlight-deprived generation in comparison to previous generations. Nowadays people are generally stuck in the office from nine to five, and even if they aren't at work, a lot of their time is spent indoors. Most public health messages of the past century have focused on the negatives of too much sun exposure. Reduction of time outdoors has been amplified by skin cancer prevention campaigns to minimise sun exposure and rightly so – but this has also brought the perception that sun exposure is bad for you. The necessity and benefits of getting natural sunlight on your skin daily are not very well publicised.

Sunlight is absolutely essential for a healthy life. Again, it's worth comparing our ancestors' life to our modern life. The reason I do this is because our body has evolved to our environment. So, it has come to rely upon things that it was exposed to through our evolution for various reasons. This includes exposure to cold water, fasting and sunlight. Nowadays, in first world countries we aren't exposed to these things the way people would have been in the past.

Regular exposure to sunlight does more than give you a lovely tan. The best-known benefit is its ability to boost the body's vitamin D production which helps strengthen our immune system and maintain healthy bones. But there are many more benefits. Sunlight has a huge effect on regulating your circadian rhythm (the body's internal clock). Our internal clock relies on sunlight to continuously recalibrate our sleep/wake cycle through the release of hormones and neurotransmitters like melatonin, serotonin and dopamine.[230] Cortisol levels that are not aligned with the sun can disrupt melatonin secretion at night and affect sleep, anxiety, mood and stress. Avoidance of sun exposure is also a risk factor for all causes of mortality and actually increases the likelihood of certain cancers. This seems totally counterintuitive to the common belief.[231]

In Scandinavian countries it's well-publicised that they get less natural sunlight than southern European countries. It's also well known that there is a higher demand for antidepressants during the winter months up there.

In fact, 8% of Swedish people suffer what is called seasonal affective disorder (SAD) or having the winter blues. This is attributed to a lack of sunlight. In Stockholm, the sun rises at 9 a.m. and sets at 3 p.m. in winter. The further north the more it decreases, to as little as four hours of sunlight. If your job is indoors, it makes it very difficult to get natural sunlight during these hours. Modern life and work styles have led to much more time spent indoors, often with lower daytime and higher evening/night-time light intensity from electrical lighting than outdoors. 90% of our time is spent indoors[232] and if you compare that to how our ancestors lived there are huge differences. The human body needs sunlight exposure to produce Vitamin D and no tablet will supplement that.

If we suddenly reduce or remove that essential natural resource for large portions of our day, there have to be consequences. And the consequences are clear: lower mood, weaker immune function, badly regulated sleep/wake cycles and increased mortality.[233]

It doesn't take much to change this. Get outside and get some sunlight on your skin. Make a conscious effort to be outside more. Just fifteen minutes a day has been shown to improve mood, boost immune function and increase energy levels.[234]

Direct sunlight on the skin stimulates mitochondria to produce melatonin on site, which works as an antioxidant. You only want melatonin in your bloodstream when you are ready to go to sleep. But you do want to have melatonin in your mitochondria to absorb the oxidative stress. To get that melatonin release in the tissue you need exposure to sunlight, specifically infra-red rays of sunlight. Infra-red rays can penetrate through clothing or windows. If you've ever felt heat from the sun through clothing or a window then you have been exposed to infra-red rays. These infra-red rays are invisible and different from UV rays are just as important.

On the flip side, there is no advantage to having more than thirty minutes of sun exposure per day so don't use this as an excuse to spend three hours at the beach. Remember there are also disadvantages that come from too much sun exposure. As with everything in life, there is a happy medium.

Have your morning coffee in the garden if it's possible, walk to work, sit outside at lunch time. From an infra-red point of view, going outside at any time is beneficial to you but for your circadian rhythm it's beneficial to get that sun exposure close to waking up in the morning. Looking in the direction of the sun is the most efficient way of absorbing the most in the shortest amount of time. This isn't to say look directly at the sun, of course! Ideally getting your exposure to sunlight before 9 a.m. is best as it helps with your circadian rhythm recalibration.

One thing that's clear is that we need sunlight to thrive. There is simply no excuse for not getting sunlight. It's free, it's readily available every day and its benefits are there for all to see. From a pain point of view, I want you to make sure you're getting adequate sun exposure because you get a boost of energy and improved mood that way. All of this will increase your motivation. Sustaining motivation is necessary when you are having a bad day, which you will have as we all do. But having a bad day when suffering with pain is a lot harder than having a bad day when not suffering with pain.

Your new identity

"Changing your identity reshapes your reality" – Dr Joe Dispenza

We have already said that our ego, self-image and identity (internal thermostat) will always keep us consistent with who we see ourselves as. "Human behaviour is based on the perception of your reality and not reality in itself."[235] How we act and behave is an outer expression of our inner self-image. If your self-image is of someone who is in pain and you cannot see yourself not being in pain, these unconscious thoughts have to be addressed internally before you can ever try to change anything externally. If we can change how you see yourself then you can change how you act and behave.

I had an interesting conversation with a friend and client of mine who happens to be a psychotherapist. I will call her Rachel for the purpose of this story. I was explaining to her about how changing your identity was important for overcoming pain and getting your life back. Rachel has had a hard life filled with abuse, bullying, addiction, failed back surgeries, and debilitating chronic pain. Rachel explained to me how for years she saw herself as Rachel, the person in pain. That was top of her list. Her chronic pain was her identity. It took over who she was until in reality it wasn't the pain that was debilitating her anymore, it was her self-image.

As a result of this self-image, her actions and behaviours aligned with who she saw herself as. Every movement, every thought and every action were those of someone who was in debilitating pain. Each movement was coupled with a groan or an expression of how bad she was feeling. Every time she was asked to do something or go somewhere, her response was to say no because she "wasn't able." She saw herself as a victim at the time, and who could blame her with all she had been through? But it wasn't helping her. When pain gets deeply rooted in your identity, pain becomes you and you become pain. It's part of who you are and no physio exercises, manipulations or surgeries are going to change that. Thinking of herself as a victim, not being able to do things because she was so disabled through pain and going through the same routine every day strengthened these disabling neural pathways in her brain. Rehearsing this same debilitating process day after day only made her better at being one thing: a person in pain.

In order to get past this, she needed to change the way she saw herself, or at least reframe how she saw herself, because it was impeding any chance she had at a happy life. At the end of the day, she was more than just Rachel the chronic pain patient. She was Rachel the psychotherapist, the teacher, the walker, the swimmer, the friend, the sister, the daughter and more recently the yoga instructor.

She realised this and worked on her inner self; she was able to start to change her outer expression. This opened up more doors for her, allowing her to take control of her life and start to overcome her pain. Today, Rachel "the chronic pain patient" was way down the list. Her actions and behaviours corresponded to who she saw herself as now and not who she had seen herself as when she was a patient. Yes, she still had pain. But pain wasn't consuming her life anymore. Her life had meaning again. She was counselling others, teaching, swimming, walking and taking yoga classes. She wasn't able to go back to the person she had been pre-pain. She knew she had limitations and she accepted that. But it didn't mean she couldn't live a fulfilling life. None of this would have been possible if she had still seen herself as Rachel the chronic pain patient.

Changing identity exercise

Let's do a little exercise now. Sit down and imagine you're looking into the future and that you are truly happy. What would your life look like? Who would you be and what would you be doing? For many people it's just the little things like playing with their kids or grandkids, getting back to work or being able to be sociable with friends. Pain may have taken some or all of that away and you just want it back.

For those who have been in pain for a long time or have had many unsuccessful treatments, it's hard to believe that you can ever get your life back, so your identity has just shifted to your new reality, with corresponding actions and behaviours. Pain makes this happen. At the end of the day, its job is to change your behaviour. But as your behaviour changes, your identity shifts to your new reality.

So, in order to get the reality back we need to change your identity to the person you want to be and align your behaviours with this person. So, if you were that person, what would you be doing? What would your day look like? How does that person act and how would they behave?

Visualisation exercise

We have spoken about how the brain doesn't know the difference between reality and illusion.[236] By vividly imagining the person you want to be, your brain is making new connections. It's creating new positive forest trails. This is your first exercise and needs to be completed every day for a month. You can start with fifteen minutes a day. If you find fifteen minutes too difficult, you can split your fifteen minutes up into two or three shorter segments. As time goes on and you get better at this you should work up to fifteen minutes in one sitting.

Imagine, visualise and put in the steps to get there!

When you visualise something, it's like the brain has experienced it. When you go to try to fulfil your goals it feels easier as you have experienced it already. Sit or lie down in a quiet room simply visualising your daily goals to begin with. Whatever your daily goals are, make the visualisation as vivid as possible. Imagine yourself doing your gentle movements, and feeling happy, safe and comfortable doing them.

Make it as realistic as possible. Visualise the places you would go and how you would act and behave. Visualise what the environment would look like. If there are any sounds, smells or other related sensations, try to conjure those up too. Make it as real as possible. Visualise what you want as if you already have it. The brain loves familiarity. When the brain doesn't feel familiar with something, its defence mechanisms may spike, leading to feelings like fear, anxiety and pain. When you have positive experiences of something, even imaginary ones, the brain is less likely to perceive it as a threat when you attempt it in reality. Repetition and rehearsing this exercise, and strengthening these forest trails, creates familiarity. And don't worry if you cannot do this straight away. With practice it will become easier. Some may see changes within the first few days and some may have to wait for over a month to see meaningful changes. Just put this into your daily goals and persist with it.

To test this theory, a scientist got three groups of basketball players together. Group A, B and C were all told to take twenty free throws and their scores were recorded. Group A were told to practice free throwing for thirty minutes per day. Group B were to do nothing at all, and group C were told to visualise taking free throws and getting them into the hoop every day for thirty minutes. Thirty days later, they were retested. Group A had improved their score by 24%, group B didn't improve at all as you would expect, but group C had improved their score by 23%.[237]

I just want to be clear; this isn't the process of imagining your way out of pain. It's just another tool that can be used to change your brain.

Not everyone has this identity issue. But if you feel this sounds like you, then I recommend starting here first. Make this a priority.

Okay, now you know the steps to put your body in a position to recover. It's time to start desensitising the system and start to build some resilience.

Movement is the key to recovery

The pain barrier line

The pain barrier line is a visual representation of how pain and the brain work. This idea is loosely based on the "Explain Pain" twin peak model, but I've added my own ideas to expand it.

In fig10a, you can see three lines: the physical activity line, the pain threshold line, and the tissue strength line. Let's break down each line:

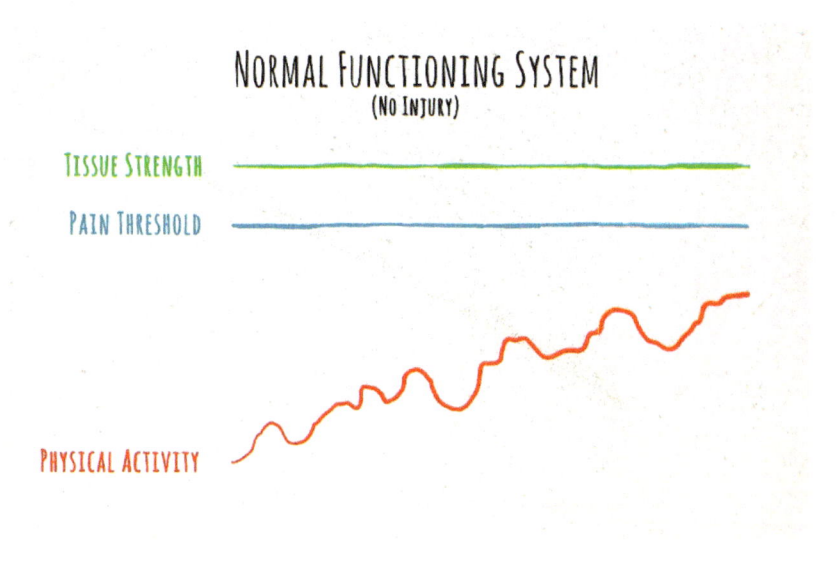

NORMAL FUNCTIONING SYSTEM
(NO INJURY)

TISSUE STRENGTH

PAIN THRESHOLD

PHYSICAL ACTIVITY

Fig 10a

The physical activity line

This line shows how much physical activity you're engaged in at a given time. When the line is higher, it means more physical demand on the body. A stable line represents a regular day without intense activity. Spikes in the line indicate aggressive movements. When the line moves up, it signifies an increased load on that day.

The pain threshold line

This line is not the same as the pain tolerance line. Pain tolerance is how much pain you can endure, while the pain threshold is the point at which your body starts feeling pain. This threshold changes constantly. Pain occurs when the physical activity line crosses the pain threshold line. For example, after a long walk, your joints might ache, even though you're not injured. This explains feeling pain without actual injury.

The tissue strength line

This line reflects your body's tissue resilience. It also fluctuates and is influenced by factors such as stress, sleep quality, and overall health. If physical activity breaches this line, injury happens. *"Injury is the inability to adapt to stress"* – Greg Lehman.

In fig 10a you can see there are no lines crossing paths, representing a normal day for a non-pain sufferer.

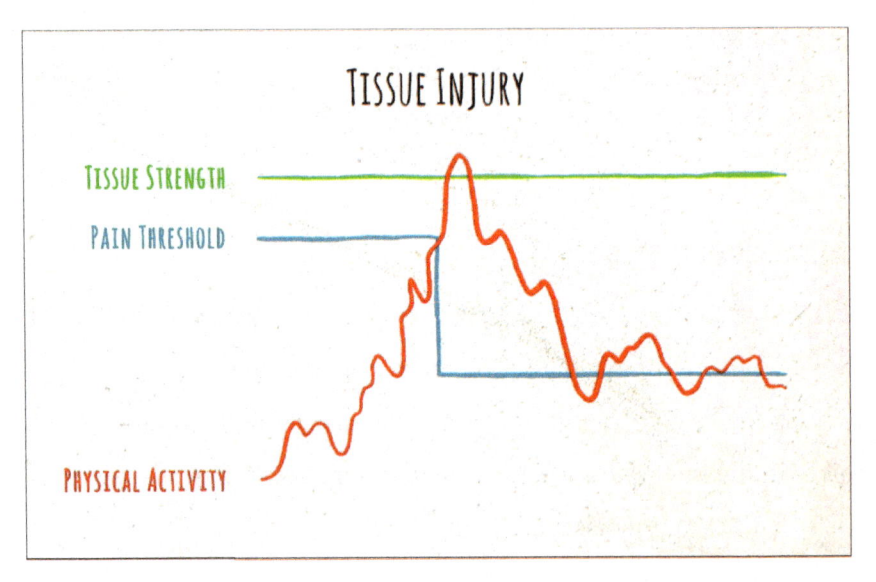

Fig 10b

In fig 10b injury is illustrated. When the physical activity line crosses both the pain threshold and tissue strength lines, injury occurs. This can lower the pain threshold line temporarily, making you aware of the injury in an attempt to prevent further damage and allow the healing process to commence. With a lowered pain threshold line, previously non-painful movements now can cause pain.

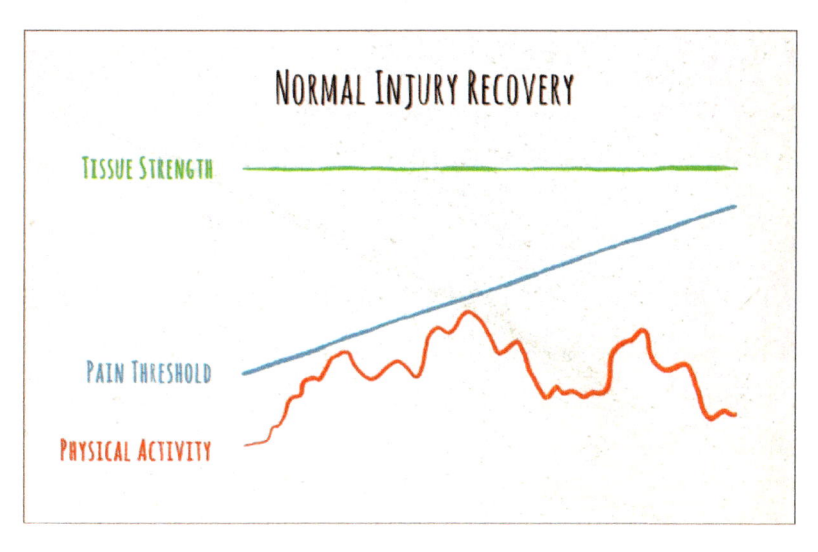

Fig 10c

Fig 10c shows that, as injured tissue heals, the pain threshold line gradually rises again. This allows more physical activity, as the body becomes less sensitised.

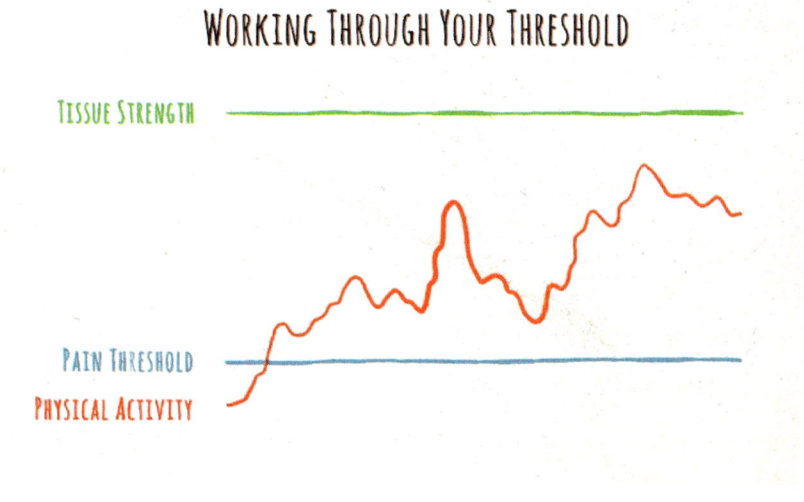

Fig 10d

However, in cases of persistent pain, the pain threshold line might not return to its original position after healing. Chronic pain means the nervous system remains sensitised, even without ongoing tissue damage (fig 10d).

Your brain prioritises safety, so anything perceived as a threat affects the pain threshold line. Negative beliefs about movement can lower this line, even if there's no actual harm. This explains how fear and stress influence a pain experience.

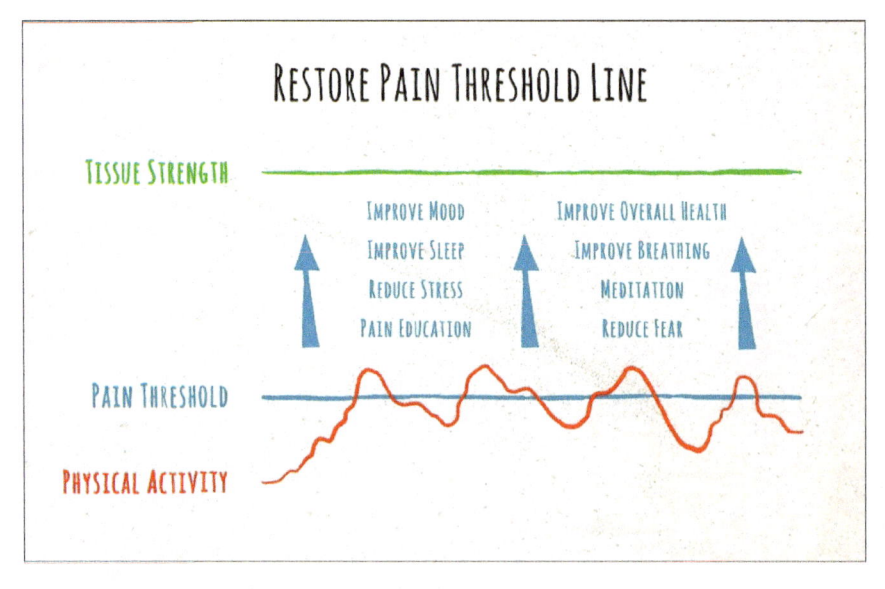

Fig 10e

To address persistent pain, a graded exposure approach is useful. Identify movements causing pain and desensitise by gradually increasing their intensity. First, work to remove some stones out of your glass like sleep issues, reducing prolonged stress levels, improved breathwork and so on to help desensitise your system and raise the pain threshold line (fig 10e). Then, slowly reintroduce movements while keeping the pain threshold line above the activity line.

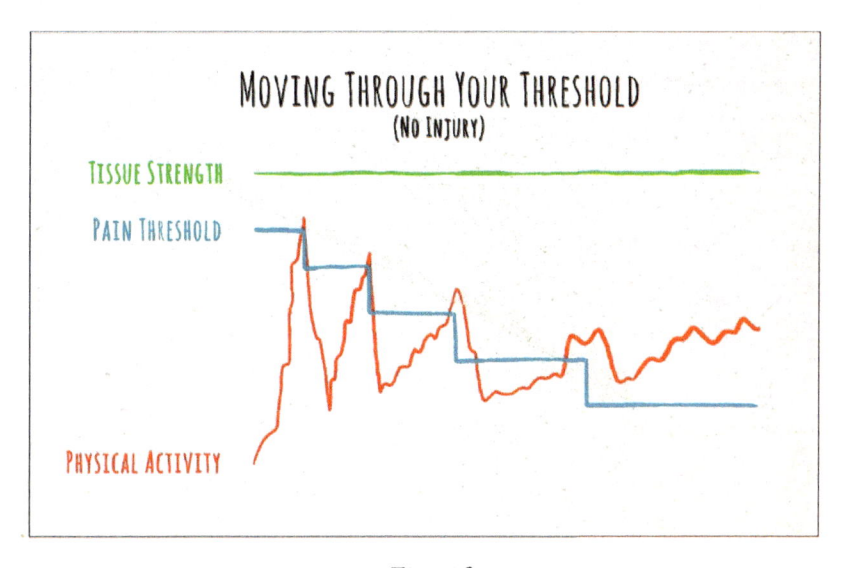

MOVING THROUGH YOUR THRESHOLD
(NO INJURY)

TISSUE STRENGTH

PAIN THRESHOLD

PHYSICAL ACTIVITY

Fig 10f

If the discomfort remains manageable, you're within the pain threshold line. If pain worsens, you might cross the line and cause sensitisation (Fig 10f).

Gentle exercises help raise the threshold line, allowing more movement. Gradually reintroduce movement and focus on controlled breathing. Avoid aggressive exercises when the threshold line is low to prevent flare-ups.

Ultimately, understanding and addressing these lines can help manage and reduce pain. They help take away insecurity, fear and worry. The lines give context and meaning to your pain in a logical sense.

A little bit of discomfort is alright. If the discomfort remains manageable, it's safe to work through it, providing they are slow and controlled movements. This means you're just testing the waters of the pain threshold line. However, if the pain worsens and continues to grow as you repeat a movement, it's a sign you might be venturing too far above the pain barrier line – essentially, you're "poking the bear." In this case, it's best to either modify the movement, scale it down, or try a different variation. "Poking the bear" could lead to more irritation and even cause your pain threshold line to drop (fig 10f).

As your pain threshold line gradually rises, you can introduce more challenging exercises (fig 10c). Movement is a cornerstone of recovery. However, movement can work against you if you don't feel safe doing it or if you believe it could be harmful. This is where the charts come into play. They help clarify that feeling pain doesn't necessarily mean you're causing physical damage. You might be sore, but you're actually safe to move. When movement causes pain, it's probably due to the pain threshold line being quite low. Now it's time to work on raising your pain threshold line back up to the tissue strength line, akin to what's illustrated in fig 10a.

Avoiding aggressive exercises or heavy lifting when your pain threshold line is low is crucial. Rapidly escalating your activity can cause the physical activity line to surge and cross over the threshold line. This triggers your nervous system to sense threat, leading to potential inflammation flare-ups and a lowered pain threshold line (fig 10g).

These flare-ups aren't ideal, as they can last from **one to seven days,** impacting your exercise routine, affecting your sleep **and mood.**

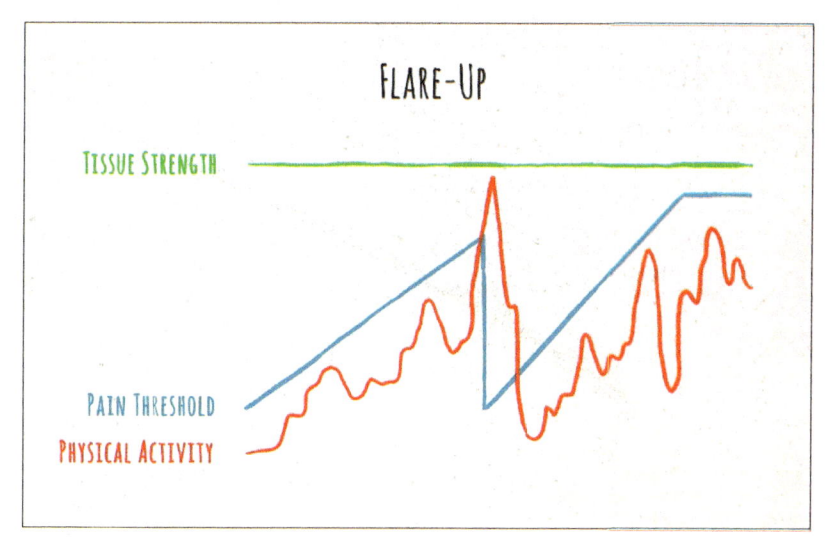

Fig 10g

Flare-ups are a common occurrence during the **recovery process. We** can't completely rule them out. Flare-ups are **particularly prevalent** among individuals dealing with persistent pain. If you **experience a flare-** up, the key is to remain calm and not lose faith. **A flare-up simply** indicates that you've crossed over your threshold line **on that specific day** (fig 10g). Your body perceives a threat and responds **with inflammation** as a protective mechanism. While flare-ups are less **than ideal, they are** not catastrophic. It might feel like you're back at **square one, but that's** not the case.

When a flare-up happens, revert to the gentle **movements you were** initially performing. Once the flare-up subsides, you **can resume your** previous progress. Utilise flare-ups as valuable information about your current status. Reflect on what activities you engaged in on that particular day that could have triggered the flare-up. Think about the analogy of the glass of water – what caused it to overflow? Consider other potential contributors to the flare-up and take precautions to prevent them from happening again. This could encompass various factors, including excessive activity on that day, stress, poor sleep, attempting something new, or performing an activity you haven't done in a while.

As you can see, when flare-ups occur, they usually don't involve damage to tissue; they happen when your physical activity line crosses over your pain threshold line. Although there are exceptions to this with conditions like rheumatoid arthritis, whereby the immune system attacks its own tissue resulting in the tissue strength line being affected, so take your condition into account.

Once the flare-up diminishes, you'll generally return to the level of progress you were at before it occurred. Remember, flare-ups are a part of the journey, and by learning from them, you'll become better equipped to manage and navigate your recovery process effectively.

By initially focusing on slow, controlled, and non-aggressive exercises, you can work below your threshold line. This gradual approach helps your threshold line rise over time, reducing the chance of flare-ups. The more flare-ups you experience, the less confident you become and the more you fear another one. And remember, the fear of movement can bring the pain threshold down again. Which is why it's best to avoid them if possible. In my experience they are more common at the beginning of the recovery as this is when your system will be at its most sensitive. As time goes on, they happen less frequently because your threshold line is higher.

Graded exposure/progressive loading

When dealing with pain, it can be challenging to determine the best exercises to start with. Giving specific recommendations for your particular issue is difficult.

To make progress, begin by identifying movements that consistently cause you pain – those that consistently worsen your discomfort. Let's take bending over as an example. When bending over triggers pain, your brain has essentially temporarily adapted itself to associate this action with threat, based on past experiences, expectations, fears, and conditioning. These experiences have created new pathways in your brain that generate pain during bending. The more you experience this pain, the stronger these pathways become, lowering your pain threshold until your body becomes conditioned to feeling pain when bending over, essentially forming superhighway connections.

While erasing these connections or memories is impossible, facing and working through negative experiences is more effective than avoiding them. Break down these experiences into smaller, more manageable versions, and create positive new experiences that your brain can use to overwrite the old negative ones. This process is similar to building new roads alongside the old ones, thus gradually replacing them. Crucially, your brain retains these negative experiences for survival reasons. Rather than erasing them, the aim is to overwrite them with new positive experiences that nonetheless somewhat resemble the old negative ones. Think of these new experiences as planting seeds of positivity in your brain's pathways. By consistently introducing positive experiences, you can eventually outweigh the older, negative ones. This process can reshape your pain experience and enhance your overall wellbeing.

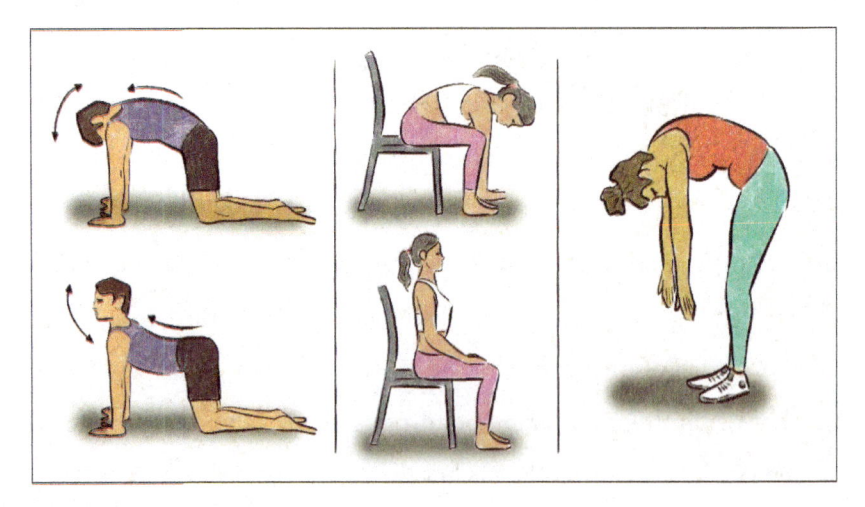

Fig 10h

Before overwriting these negative experiences, set the stage for new positive ones. Consider whether the exercise can be broken down into smaller, more manageable movements. Focus on slow nasal breathing to signal safety and relaxation, ensuring that the movement stays below your pain barrier line. Your breathwork is crucial in this process, so incorporate relaxed breathing with these movements.

So, let's break down the movements that make you uneasy. These could include actions like bending to pick something up, walking up or down stairs, lifting objects, driving, or running.

Whether you're dealing with shoulder, back, knee, or hip pain, maintaining a calm nervous system is essential for comfortable movement. Anxiety and fear can push you closer to your pain threshold line. Pairing relaxed diaphragmatic breathing with movement is a powerful way to reduce pain and elevate your pain threshold line. With a higher pain threshold line, you can engage in more activities before experiencing pain.

Feeling nervous or apprehensive about a movement indicates that negative memories are stored in your brain regarding that activity. I've listed a few examples, but remember that a physiotherapist or movement coach can provide more personalised guidance.

The best approach is to initiate movements that don't strain your joints too much – avoid starting with loaded exercises, as they might cross your pain barrier line and increase your sensitivity. Movements you're uncomfortable with are like large stones in your glass. To address this, we need to either break them down into smaller pebbles or eliminate them altogether. The process involves dissecting the challenging movement into bite-sized, more manageable versions.

Then, incorporate relaxed, slow nasal belly breathing. This type of breathing activates your parasympathetic nervous system (the "rest-and-digest" response), signalling to your nervous system that the movement is safe. By contrast, holding your breath or rapid breathing indicates potential danger. This initial step is pivotal in changing the connections in your brain and replacing those negative experiences with positive ones. Visualise the fact that you're not causing damage; you're just approaching the pain threshold line. For now, this is enough – we're in the process of altering associations, not aiming to increase strength or range of motion.

Now, how can we approach bending without straining your back too much? You could try doing it while sitting down or on all fours – such as in fig 10h. The goal is to gradually desensitise your body to the movement by executing it slowly and in a controlled manner. As your body becomes accustomed to these non-threatening movements and your pain threshold line rises with this movement, you can progress to more functional actions. Remember, repetition is key here. Neural connections don't shift immediately; you're essentially creating new forest trails of movement and safety. Be patient during this process and avoid overexertion. When pain persists for extended periods, it's better to do these movements in frequent, smaller sessions throughout the day. Thus, you are moving better more often throughout the day.

As you start moving in a safe, controlled manner, you're introducing your brain to new experiences related to those movements. Move towards discomfort, but never push through pain. As mentioned earlier, a little discomfort is okay, and is to be expected – it means you're around your pain threshold line. What we don't want is for the pain to worsen as you repeat the movement. When you perform a movement that previously caused pain, your body's familiarity with that position, and new non-threatening memories, will reduce the associated threat, decreasing the likelihood of experiencing pain.

Repetition is key to this process. A change in your pain response won't happen overnight, especially if you've been in pain for a long time. Be patient and avoid rushing. Consistency is vital; aim for three to four sessions per day at comfortable levels, with approximately ten reps at a time. Over time, your neural pathways will reshape, and your brain will create new roads and superhighways that are less likely to influence pain. As you keep practicing, these new pathways will replace the old ones. These repeated positive experiences will gradually overwrite the negative ones stored in your brain. With a desensitised brain and a raised pain threshold line, you'll have more room for activity. Remember, creating these new forest trails takes time, but your persistence will pay off. Be consistent with your movement and breathing, and you'll pave the way to a pain-free life.

You have your list of the top three pain-triggering movements. Pick one to start with, ensuring that the movement remains below your pain barrier line. If you're dealing with constant chronic pain, find a movement that doesn't worsen your condition. Incorporating a graded exposure approach to movement with relaxed diaphragmatic breathing is the next step. Begin by inhaling for six seconds and exhaling for six seconds to calm your nervous system. Once you feel composed, initiate your movement.

Goal setting

Now we have come to the application process of the book. It's been a long road and we have covered many different areas. Some will definitely be influencing your pain and others not. You should by now have identified what stones you want to take out of your glass.

So, it's time to create some goals. Goals give you direction. They orientate you in the direction you want to go. **Moving towards a goal increases your brain's natural release of dopamine, which gives motivation and helps keep you on track.**[238]

In order to move forward, you have to be very clear about where you want to go. Otherwise, you have nothing to aim for and you won't know when you have got there. It also makes it impossible to track progress if there is no goal in sight. This is where goal setting is necessary. Starting a recovery plan without a goal is like hiking with a map and compass but without knowing where the destination is. Before any journey starts, a destination needs to be ascertained. The destination is your ultimate goal. Your ultimate goal is how you would like your life to be if you didn't have pain. By now you know who or what that looks like.

So, what is your ultimate goal?

You might say that you want to be pain-free but that's not enough. You need to be very specific. The more specific the better. Just saying "my purpose is to be pain-free" is too vague. It's like saying, "I want lots of money." Why do you want lots of money?

Until you have a clear and compelling story for why you want to be pain-free you won't have your purpose. For many, the purpose isn't being pain free itself. The purpose is to be able to work, exercise or just hang out with friends. It's not the actual pain that's the problem. It's what the pain is getting in the way of. Many people say that they can live with their pain until it gets in the way of the things that gives them meaning. So, your ultimate goal should be something that gives you meaning – something that is valuable for you.

Having a valued goal builds the foundation for motivation. Advancing towards a goal releases dopamine and this can have an analgesic affect.[239] It reduces pain but also makes you feel good which is why you will seek more of it. This in turn will create a positive loop.

Specify your goals but also specify where you don't want to go, so you're terrified as well as excited to succeed. Again, this will help drive you to achieving your goal. Fear is a greater motivator than reward. So, it can also be useful to think of what you don't want your future to look like.

This could involve the idea that, if you don't make changes, you may have to get surgery or perhaps give up a job you love. Whatever it is, it's a useful thing to think about, although it's best not to dwell on it. Once you've thought about these, write them down. Any time you feel demotivated, come back to what you want to achieve or avoid. Remember, all of this is an investment into your future. No investment pays off right away. In business, it takes time for a financial investment to pay off; likewise in education it takes time and effort to acquire your university degree.

Writing your goals down and having a systemic action plan for how you are going to accomplish them will give you a much higher chance of success. A recent report released in the context of pain management revealed that setting goals led to better and more positive outcomes than treatment modalities operating without a goal.[240]

One of the more famous studies on goal setting was a 1979 Harvard study,[241] where the group of researchers found that prior to graduation:

- 84% of the entire class had set no goals at all;

- 13% of the class had set written goals but had no concrete plans;

- 3% of the class had both written goals and concrete plans.

Twenty years later, the researchers found that the 3% who had written their goals down and had concrete plans on how to achieve them were earning ten times more money than the 97% who hadn't written them down or had no concrete plans for achieving them.

It can sometimes be daunting to see a mountainous challenge ahead.

In order for your ultimate goal to not feel like an impossible task, we should break down your ultimate goal into smaller, more manageable goals.

Keep it realistic when you think about what you would like to be able to do if you weren't suffering with pain. It's difficult to give examples of ultimate goals because everyone's will be vastly different. But the regular things I hear from clients is that they would like to be able to get back to work, exercise, to go on an aeroplane or to play with their kids/grandkids. When pain gets that debilitating, it's the little things that matter to people. However, if you're quite capable of doing all of those things and more, your goal could be to do a 5k, an exercise class or even a hike.

Have a good hard think about what you would like to do. Start small, and when you achieve that you can always start the process again with a bigger long-term goal.

Once your ultimate goal is set, we have to set a timeframe, as stated above. In my example we're going to say it's six months. But it can be more or less depending on how big or small your goal is. Don't be impatient. Give yourself time. Making these changes can be challenging, because humans are habitual creatures. We don't like change. We love familiarity. Making changes isn't familiar. Moving outside our comfort zone can be uncomfortable but outside your comfort zone is where the most growth can be achieved.

Now that we have our ultimate goal and a timeframe set, let's reverse engineer it. Reverse engineering something means setting your goals and working backwards. This can help you break down the ultimate goal into smaller, more manageable steps.

The size of the goal and the timeframe will depend on how many steps or milestones have to be reached in your plan. Months and weeks are usually a simple metric to set milestones by, but you can use a more specific timeline if you would like to customise your plan.

Smaller goals make it easier to measure success. If we just focus on the ultimate goal, it may seem unattainable. Reverse engineering and creating smaller goals and milestones allow you to experience success, see progress, and maintain focus and motivation.

Because I'm working toward a six-month long-term goal, I am making six smaller shorter goals or milestones to hit.

Once your monthly goals are set, your mini goals can be further broken down to weekly goals. Again, your weekly goals are smaller and much more achievable goals. You can focus on achieving these and not your monthly or ultimate goal.

GOAL PLANNER EXAMPLE

	MONDAY	TUESDAY	WEDNESDAY	THURSDAY	FRIDAY	SATURDAY	SUNDAY
WEEK 1	Exercises (3 x 10 Reps) Sunlight (20 Mins) 2 Min Walk Sleep Hygiene	Meditation Sunlight 2 Min Walk x 2 Sleep Hygiene	Breathwork + Exercises Sunlight Sleep Hygiene	Meditation Sunlight 2 3 Min Walk Sleep Hygiene	Breathwork + Exercises Meditation Sunlight 3 Min Walk x 3 Sleep Hygiene	Breathwork + Exercises Sunlight 4 Min Walk Sleep Hygiene	Micro Goal 1 5 Min Walk Small Reward
WEEK 2	Breathwork + Exercises Meditation Sunlight Sleep Hygiene	Meditation Sunlight 7 Min Walk Sleep Hygiene	Breathwork + Exercises Meditation 7 Min Walk Sleep Hygiene	Meditation Sunlight 8 Min Walk Sleep Hygiene	Breathwork + Exercises 8 Min Walk Sleep Hygiene	Meditation	Micro Goal 2 10 Min Walk Small Reward
WEEK 3	Meditation Sunlight 11 Min Walk Sleep Hygiene	Breathwork + Exercises Sunlight 11 Min Walk Sleep Hygiene	Meditation Sunlight 12 Min Walk Sleep Hygiene	Breathwork + Exercises Sunlight 13 Min Walk Sleep Hygiene	Meditation Sunlight Sleep Hygiene	Breathwork + Exercises Sunlight 15 Min Walk Sleep Hygiene	Micro Goal 3 15 Min Walk Small Reward
WEEK 4	Breathwork + Exercises Sunlight Sleep Hygiene	Breathwork + Exercises Sunlight Sleep Hygiene	Meditation Sunlight 17 Min Walk Sleep Hygiene	Breathwork + Exercises Meditation Sunlight Sleep Hygiene	Sunlight 18 Min Walk Sleep Hygiene	Breathwork + Exercises Sunlight 19 Min Walk Sleep Hygiene	Mini Goal 1 20 Min Walk Bigger Reward

These daily goals will detail what actions you need to take in order to make the changes to your influencers. For example, if one of the main influencers of your pain is that you are highly stressed, you can add in meditation or mindfulness on three different days, and figure out ways of getting out of that stressful environment for periods during the day.

If one of the stones in your glass was poor-quality movement, add daily movements multiple times per day into your plan.

Do you need to exercise? Are you getting sufficient sunlight or improved sleep hygiene? Any of these stones can be added to your plan.

I recommend picking three different influencers that you want to work on and adding them to your action plan. Any more than three changes to your routine or habits can be very hard to keep up. Look at your pain influencer chart and pick the three areas that you feel are contributing most to your pain experience. These three areas will be a good starting point and you can slot them into your goal setting plan. If you feel you have made adequate changes and you're happy that you are keeping them up, you can always add in some other changes later on in your goal setting plan.

The beauty of having your goal plan written down is that, if you are not following your action plan you don't need to wait six months to see if you are going to achieve your goal. If you are not achieving your daily goals or weekly goals, you won't be achieving your monthly or ultimate goals and vice versa. If you are achieving your micro goals and your monthly goals you will be more likely to achieve your long-term goals.

Some people don't write down goals because of the fear of failure. This is not the time for this type of mentality. Yes, this requires work and dedication but *nothing worth having comes easy*; remember this is your life and you only get one of them. Fear of failure shouldn't be allowed to prevent you from having the best life possible.

With every rewarding goal comes failure. When someone is successful in business or sport, they often have dozens if not hundreds of failures along the way. You don't always hear about their failure; you only hear about the success, as if it was all plain sailing. Failure is a part of success. There is no success without failure. It's how you frame the failure. Thomas Edison described trying to invent the lightbulb by saying, "I have not failed. I've just found ten thousand ways that won't work."

There is room to revise and readjust your goal setting plan. It's okay to be behind, likewise it's okay to work ahead if you feel good enough to do so. The goal setting plan is modifiable. There will be days where you don't want to do your daily goals but this is when you need to think about your ultimate goal. Don't think about the sacrifice; just think about the achievement. Hold that emotion in your heart, and this will drive you forward.

Now this is extremely important. Your goal setting plan needs to be somewhere that is in your eyeline on a daily basis. You cannot leave it somewhere in a drawer for safe keeping, gathering dust. You need to be able to see your goals and plan in front of you, to hold yourself accountable. I would also tell friends or a family member about your upcoming weekly and monthly goals. This will make you more likely to not give up, as you will be accountable to them too. When writing this book, I have told many people I was doing so. So, every time I felt like giving up, which was often by the way, friends, family and even clients asked me how it was coming along. I even had a podcaster message me every now and again wondering when it would be finished so I could come on his podcast. This all gave me the kick I needed to get the laptop out and start writing again.

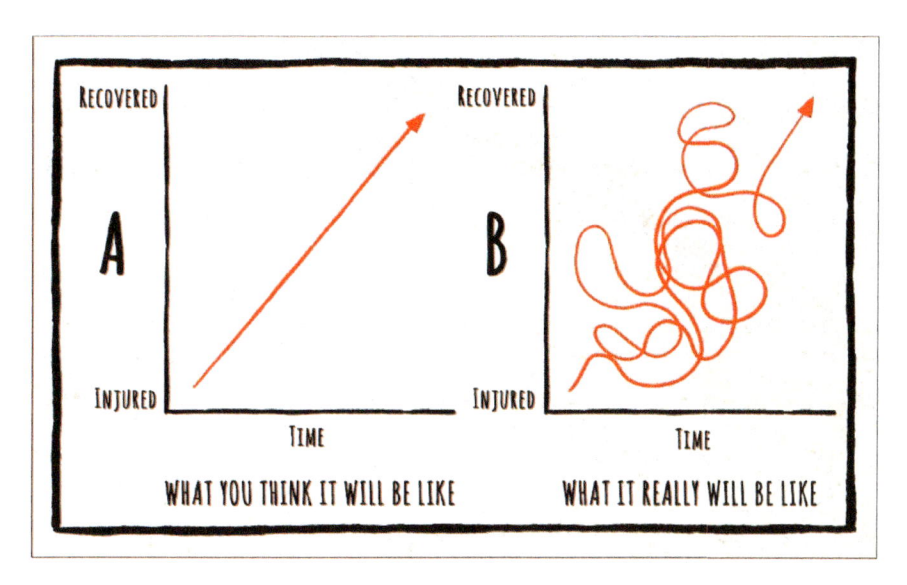

Similarly, your journey isn't going to be plain sailing. Recovery will have many ups and downs. Accept that this is the way it is and try not to analyse yourself on a daily basis, because when you have a bad day, this can cause you to lose faith.

Every goal and milestone needs a reward. I like to give myself a monthly reward when I achieve my goal and a special reward if I complete my ultimate goal in the timeframe I set out. For instance, as a reward for achieving a weekly goal, write down that you will treat yourself to a bottle of wine and a takeaway. For achieving your ultimate goal, perhaps write "I will spend 50–100 euro on something that I would never usually buy for myself."

Conclusion

Hopefully now you have a new perspective and a whole set of new tools to make the changes yourself.

You're now equipped with these tools to transform your life and break free from the grip of pain. Throughout this journey, you've learned that you're the one who can make the biggest difference in your own life. Waiting for a ready-made solution or relying solely on others should be a thing of the past.

Using the biopsychosocial approach and glass of water analogy should give you many avenues to explore.

But the key point is to make changes and stick by them. Sometimes making changes can be difficult, even when you know they can help. Making changes moves you into the unfamiliar, and the unfamiliar can be scary. *"Sometimes people would rather suffer in the familiar than make changes and move into the unknown"* – Dr Joe Dispenza.

If this is the case, my advice is to not make too many changes at once. Making changes to three stones is enough to begin with. Then, when you make changes to one or two stones and turn them into pebbles and then you can move onto other areas.

You may notice things improve quickly or it make take some time to see significant results. Don't be disheartened if it doesn't happen straight away. It takes time to change the plasticity of your nervous system. It takes time to form new habits, adopt healthy behaviours, and to reduce fear and build strength.

Tony Robbins once said that if you have two boats travelling side by side in the same direction and you adjust one of their courses by five degrees, by the end of their trip they will be in totally different places. Those small shifts in the beginning might not result in any noticeable changes straight away, but in the long term they'll make a huge difference.

I won't claim I'm giving you a panacea, a "one fix cures all" approach. Maybe there are areas of your life that need further investigation and further help. These might include unresolved traumas, sleep issues, nutrition, anxiety, depression or just general issues for which you need counselling. If so, make sure you get the help you need and remove those stones from your glass.

If you're not motivated to make changes, hold onto a goal that is emotionally important to you. Think about the outcome that you're looking for. Don't think about the sacrifice or the changes that need to be made.

Maybe you want to play with your grandkids, to be able to be sociable again or just to be able to get back into the workforce. Whatever the goal is, hold onto this and remind yourself of the future you want for yourself and the future you want to avoid.

In closing, I hope you have enjoyed reading this book as much as I have enjoyed writing it.

And remember: what has got you here, won't get you there.

Review

If you enjoyed the book, please consider leaving me a review on amazon. Leaving a review really helps more people discover this book. Thank you.

About the author

Kieran, a distinguished physical therapist and expert in human movement, passionately addresses complex chronic pain and recurring injuries. He enjoys helping people overcome challenging issues with his unique treatment style. Kieran seamlessly blends scientific expertise with practical insights, empowering individuals through engaging public speaking, writing, and clinical interventions. With a focus on holistic well-being, Kieran advocates for a healthier, more resilient individual.

In his spare time, Kieran enjoys spending time with his family and is a football enthusiast.

Notes

1 https://doi.org/10.1215/00703370-8977691

2 https://www.ncbi.nlm.nih.gov/books/NBK553030/#

3 https://uspainfoundation.org/news/research-pain-to-manage-pain/

4 Tang N.K., & Crane C., Suicidality in chronic pain: a review of the prevalence, risk factors and psychological links. Psychol Med. 2006 May;36(5):575-86. doi: 10.1017/S0033291705006859. Epub 2006 Jan 18. PMID: 16420727.

5 Whitten CE, Donovan M, Cristobal K. Treating chronic pain: new knowledge, more choices. Perm J. 2005;9(4):9-18. doi:10.7812/TPP/05-067

6 https://www.ncbi.nlm.nih.gov/pmc/articles/PMC5295184

7 Tauben DJ, Loeser JD. Pain education at the University of Washington School of Medicine. J Pain. 2013;14(5):431-437. doi:10.1016/j.jpain.2013.01.005

8 Morasco BJ, Yarborough BJ, Smith NX, et al. Higher Prescription Opioid Dose is Associated With Worse Patient-Reported Pain Outcomes and More Health Care Utilization. J Pain. 2017;18(4):437-445

9 Finnerup NB, Kuner R, Jensen TS. Neuropathic Pain: From Mechanisms to Treatment. Physiol Rev. 2021 Jan 1;101(1):259-301. doi: 10.1152/physrev.00045.2019. Epub 2020 Jun 25. PMID: 32584191

10 neurons Gulati A. Understanding neurogenesis in the adult human brain. Indian J Pharmacol. 2015;47(6):583-584. doi:10.4103/0253-7613.169598

11 https://scopeblog.stanford.edu/2022/07/15/the-science-behind-muscle-memory/

12 https://www.scientificamerican.com/article/can-visualizing-your-body-doing-something-help-you-learn-to-do-it-better/

13 https://www.ncbi.nlm.nih.gov/pmc/articles/PMC2964977/

14 Alyas F, Turner M, Connell D. MRI findings in the lumbar spines of asymptomatic, adolescent, elite tennis players. Br J Sports Med. 2007;41(11):836-841. doi:10.1136/bjsm.2007.037747

15 David Butler & Lorimer Moseley, *Explain Pain* (Noigroup Publications, 2013)

16 Dubin AE, Patapoutian A. Nociceptors: the sensors of the pain pathway. J Clin Invest. 2010;120(11):3760-3772. doi:10.1172/JCI42843.

17 https://www.ncbi.nlm.nih.gov/pmc/articles/PMC5579396/. Be it from a physical, chemical or psychological perspective.

18 https://elifesciences.org/articles/00362

19 https://pubmed.ncbi.nlm.nih.gov/34136979/
https://pubmed.ncbi.nlm.nih.gov/22659077/

20 https://www.youtube.com/watch?v=xNgQOHwsIbg

21 https://pubmed.ncbi.nlm.nih.gov/20939649/

22 Alshak, Mark N. and Joe M Das. Neuroanatomy, Sympathetic Nervous System. StatPearls, StatPearls Publishing, 8 May 2023.

23
https://www.ncbi.nlm.nih.gov/pmc/articles/PMC5137920/#:~:text=Diseases %20whose%20development%20has%20been,as%20depression%20and%20anxi ety%20disorders; increases the likelihood of injury and development of chronic pain. https://www.ncbi.nlm.nih.gov/pmc/articles/PMC5546756/

24 Sitoh, Y Y, and R D Tien. The limbic system. An overview of the anatomy and its development. Neuroimaging clinics of North America vol. 7,1 (1997): 1-10.

25 https://www.ncbi.nlm.nih.gov/pmc/articles/PMC2649674/

26 https://www.nature.com/articles/nrn2335

27 https://www.news-medical.net/news/20221025/During-sleep-the-hippocampus-and-neocortex-interact-in-ways-that-are-key-to-memory-formation.aspx#:~:text=In%20research%20published%20in%20the,novel%2C %20fleeting%20information%20into%20enduring

28 Sigurdsson, Doyère, Cain & LeDoux, 2007

29 https://www.ncbi.nlm.nih.gov/pmc/articles/PMC4495877/

30 Šimić G, Tkalčić M, Vukić V, et al. Understanding Emotions: Origins and Roles of the Amygdala. Biomolecules. 2021;11(6):823. Published 2021 May 31. doi:10.3390/biom11060823

31 https://pubmed.ncbi.nlm.nih.gov/24732922/

32
https://www.ncbi.nlm.nih.gov/pmc/articles/PMC5632999/#:~:text=The%20 amygdala%20plays%20a%20central,%2Dadrenal%20(HPA)%20axis

348

33 Jankord R, Herman JP. Limbic regulation of hypothalamo-pituitary-adrenocortical function during acute and chronic stress. Ann N Y Acad Sci. 2008;1148:64-73. doi:10.1196/annals.1410.012

34 https://pubmed.ncbi.nlm.nih.gov/2070776/

35 https://pubmed.ncbi.nlm.nih.gov/16524238/

36 mouth https://pubmed.ncbi.nlm.nih.gov/18830512/

37 https://thorax.bmj.com/content/54/10/947

38 Badawy J, Nguyen OK, Clark C, Halm EA, Makam AN. Is everyone really breathing 20 times a minute? Assessing epidemiology and variation in recorded respiratory rate in hospitalised adults. BMJ Qual Saf. 2017;26(10):832-836. doi:10.1136/bmjqs-2017-006671f

39 https://pubmed.ncbi.nlm.nih.gov/18830512/

40 https://news.stanford.edu/2020/07/21/toll-shrinking-jaws-human-health/

41 Dubin AE, Patapoutian A. Nociceptors: the sensors of the pain pathway. J Clin Invest. 2010;120(11):3760-3772

42 Dubin AE, Patapoutian A. Nociceptors: the sensors of the pain pathway. J Clin Invest. 2010;120(11):3760-3772. doi:10.1172/JCI42843

43 Mense, S. Pathophysiologie des Rückenschmerzes und seine Chronifizierung – Tierexperimentelle Daten und neue Konzepte. Pathophysiology of low back pain and the transition to the chronic state – experimental data and new concepts. Schmerz (Berlin, Germany) vol. 15,6 (2001): 413-7. doi:10.1007/s004820100002

44 https://orthoinfo.aaos.org/en/diseases--conditions/sprains-strains-and-other-soft-tissue-injuries/

45 Fleck, S J, and J E Falkel. Value of resistance training for the reduction of sports injuries. Sports medicine (Auckland, N.Z.) vol. 3,1 (1986): 61-8. doi:10.2165/00007256-198603010-00006

46 Latremoliere A, Woolf CJ. Central sensitization: a generator of pain hypersensitivity by central neural plasticity. J Pain. 2009;10(9):895-926. doi:10.1016/j.jpain.2009.06.012

47
https://www.ncbi.nlm.nih.gov/books/NBK279298/#i2137.signsofaninflamm atio

48 Verma, Vivek et al. Nociception and role of immune system in pain. *Acta neurologica Belgica* vol. 115,3 (2015): 213-20. doi:10.1007/s13760-014-0411-y

49 https://www.ncbi.nlm.nih.gov/pmc/articles/PMC3114424/

50 https://pubmed.ncbi.nlm.nih.gov/15136704/

51 https://www.ncbi.nlm.nih.gov/books/NBK493173/

52 https://www.ncbi.nlm.nih.gov/books/NBK493173/

53
https://www.betterhealth.vic.gov.au/health/conditionsandtreatments/autoimmune-disorders

54 https://www.elcaminohealth.org/stay-healthy/blog/causes-effects-of-inflammation#:~:text=Over%20time%2C%20chronic%20inflammation%20can,disease%2C%20cancer%20and%20rheumatoid%20arthritis.

55 Braund and Abbott, 2011; Stovitz and Johnston, 2003

56 https://www.ncbi.nlm.nih.gov/pmc/articles/PMC6768701/#R32

57 https://www.ncbi.nlm.nih.gov/pmc/articles/PMC6768701/#R18

58 https://www.ncbi.nlm.nih.gov/pmc/articles/PMC6768701/#R7

59 https://pubmed.ncbi.nlm.nih.gov/18721171

60 https://www.ncbi.nlm.nih.gov/books/NBK493173/

61 https://www.biotechniques.com/cell-and-tissue-biology/human-fat-storage-how-we-became-the-fat-primate/

62 Romieu I, Dossus L, Barquera S, et al. Energy balance and obesity: what are the main drivers? Cancer Causes Control. 2017;28(3):247-258. doi:10.1007/s10552-017-0869-z

63 Hall KD. Did the Food Environment Cause the Obesity Epidemic? Obesity (Silver Spring). 2018;26(1):11-13. doi:10.1002/oby.22073

64 https://www.who.int/news-room/fact-sheets/detail/obesity-and-overweight

65 https://wisevoter.com/country-rankings/most-obese-countries/

66 https://pubmed.ncbi.nlm.nih.gov/26516520/

67 https://www.nature.com/articles/s41366-020-00735-9

68
https://pubmed.ncbi.nlm.nih.gov/35386146/#:~:text=Obesity%20is%20a%20complex%20disease,association%20between%20obesity%20and%20inflammation.

69
https://pubmed.ncbi.nlm.nih.gov/35386146/#:~:text=Obesity%20is%20a%20 complex%20disease,association%20between%20obesity%20and%20inflammati on.

70 https://pubmed.ncbi.nlm.nih.gov/25185757/

71 https://pubmed.ncbi.nlm.nih.gov/25988939/

72 https://pubmed.ncbi.nlm.nih.gov/30209036

73 Riddle DL, Stratford PW

74 Body weight changes and corresponding changes in pain and function in persons with symptomatic knee osteoarthritis: a cohort study. Arthritis Care Res (Hoboken). 2013;65(1):15-22. doi:10.1002/acr.21692

75 https://pubmed.ncbi.nlm.nih.gov/27919773/

76 https://www.niaaa.nih.gov/publications/brochures-and-fact-sheets/using-alcohol-to-relieve-your-pain

77 https://www.medicalnewstoday.com/articles/sitting-down-all-day#how-long-is-too-long

78
https://www.intechopen.com/chapters/57703#:~:text=Over%20200%20years %20ago%2C%20more,is%20merely%202%E2%80%933%25.

79 https://pubmed.ncbi.nlm.nih.gov/19734238/.

80 Gatchel, Robert J et al. Fear-Avoidance Beliefs and Chronic Pain. The Journal of orthopaedic and sports physical therapy vol. 46,2 (2016): 38-43. doi:10.2519/jospt.2016.0601

81
https://www.researchgate.net/publication/262440369_Comparative_analysis _between_visual_and_computerized_photogrammetry_postural_assessment

82 Slater D, Korakakis V, O'Sullivan P, Nolan D, O'Sullivan K. Sit Up Straight: Time to Re-evaluate. J Orthop Sports Phys Ther. 2019 Aug;49(8):562-564. doi: 10.2519/jospt.2019.0610. PMID: 31366294.

83
https://www.pfizer.com/news/articles/how_genetically_related_are_we_to_ bananas

351

84 https://learn.genetics.utah.edu/content/epigenetics/rats#:~:text=It%20turns%20out%20that%20the,after%20the%20pups%20become%20adults.

85 Collier R. A short history of pain management. CMAJ. 2018;190(1):E26-E27. doi:10.1503/cmaj.109-5523

86 https://nida.nih.gov/publications/drugs-brains-behavior-science-addiction/drugs-brain

87 Wilson SH, Hellman KM, James D, Adler AC, Chandrakantan A. Mechanisms, diagnosis, prevention and management of perioperative opioid-induced hyperalgesia. Pain Manag. 2021;11(4):405-417. doi:10.2217/pmt-2020-0105

88 Mao, Jianren. Clinical Diagnosis of Opioid-Induced Hyperalgesia. Regional anesthesia and pain medicine vol. 40,6 (2015): 663-4. doi:10.1097/AAP.0000000000000317

89 Costa & McCrae, 1992a; Goldberg, 1993

90 Xi C, Zhong M, Lei X, et al. Psychometric Properties of the Chinese Version of the Neuroticism Subscale of the NEO-PI. Front Psychol. 2018;9:1454. Published 2018 Aug 17. doi:10.3389/fpsyg.2018.01454

91 Witvrouw, Erik et al. Catastrophic thinking about pain as a predictor of length of hospital stay after total knee arthroplasty: a prospective study. Knee surgery, sports traumatology, arthroscopy : official journal of the ESSKA vol. 17,10 (2009): 1189-94. doi:10.1007/s00167-009-0817-x

92 https://www.medicalnewstoday.com/articles/320844#summary

93 https://pubmed.ncbi.nlm.nih.gov/12455946/

94 https://link.springer.com/referenceworkentry/10.1007/978-3-319-28099-8_717-2

95 https://www.verywellmind.com/who-discovered-depression-1066770

96 Kirsch I. Antidepressants and the Placebo Effect. Z Psychol. 2014;222(3):128-134. doi:10.1027/2151-2604/a000176

97 https://evidence.nihr.ac.uk/alert/parents-depression-impact-their-childrens-mental-health-school-performance/#:~:text=They%20are%203%20to%204,behaviours%20could%20also%20be%20important.

98 Hidaka BH. Depression as a disease of modernity: explanations for increasing prevalence. J Affect Disord. 2012;140(3):205-214. doi:10.1016/j.jad.2011.12.036.

99 Hendrie, C. A., and Pickles, A. R. Depression as an evolutionary adaptation: implications for the development of preclinical models. Medical hypotheses vol. 72,3 (2009): 342-7. doi:10.1016/j.mehy.2008.09.053

100 https://news.emory.edu/stories/2012/02/depression_evolution.

101 Miller, Andrew H, and Charles L Raison. The role of inflammation in depression: from evolutionary imperative to modern treatment target. Nature reviews. Immunology vol. 16,1 (2016): 22-34. doi:10.1038/nri.2015.5

102 Teh CF, Zaslavsky AM, Reynolds CF 3rd, Cleary PD. Effect of depression treatment on chronic pain outcomes. Psychosom Med. 2010;72(1):61-67. doi:10.1097/PSY.0b013e3181c2a7a8

103 https://pubmed.ncbi.nlm.nih.gov/22660945/

104 https://socialwork.columbia.edu/news/groundbreaking-study-confirms-that-complicated-grief-is-not-depression-thus-requires-targeted-therapy/

105 https://www.psychologytoday.com/ie/blog/laugh-cry-live/202303/as-you-grieve-your-brain-redraws-its-neural-map

106 http://www.skilledatlife.com/how-beliefs-are-formed-and-how-to-change-them/

107 Sathyanarayana Rao TS, Asha MR, Jagannatha Rao KS, Vasudevaraju P. The biochemistry of belief. Indian J Psychiatry. 2009;51(4):239-241. doi:10.4103/0019-5545.58285

108 Wiercioch-Kuzianik, Karolina, and Przemysław Bąbel. Color Hurts. The Effect of Color on Pain Perception. Pain medicine (Malden, Mass.) vol. 20,10 (2019): 1955-1962. doi:10.1093/pm/pny285

109 https://www.psychologytoday.com/ie/blog/the-power-prime/201908/perception-is-not-reality#:~:text=Our%20perceptions%20influence%20how%20we,But%20it's%20not.

110 https://www.ncbi.nlm.nih.gov/pmc/articles/PMC4142751/

111 http://sm.stanford.edu/archive/stanmed/2008summer/spoonful_of_sugar_pi

lls.html (https://www.youtube.com/watch?v=udJ31KKXBKk); image from MRI.

112 https://pubmed.ncbi.nlm.nih.gov/12110735/.

113 Horsfall L. The Nocebo Effect. SAAD Dig. 2016 Jan;32:55-7. PMID: 27145562.

114 https://bmjopen.bmj.com/content/3/4/e002654

115 Zale EL, Ditre JW. Pain-Related Fear, Disability, and the Fear-Avoidance Model of Chronic Pain. Curr Opin Psychol. 2015;5:24-30. doi:10.1016/j.copsyc.2015.03.014

116
https://www.ncbi.nlm.nih.gov/pmc/articles/PMC2802367/#:~:text=%5B8%2C9%5D%20Beliefs%20are,Beliefs%20help%20in%20decision%2Dmaking.

117 https://www.psychologytoday.com/ie/blog/finding-purpose/201810/what-actually-is-belief-and-why-is-it-so-hard-change

118 https://www.psychologytoday.com/us/blog/true-believers/201604/the-receptive-mind

119 https://www.ncbi.nlm.nih.gov/pmc/articles/PMC2802367/

120
https://www.ncbi.nlm.nih.gov/pmc/articles/PMC2802367/#:~:text=The%20sources%20of%20beliefs%20include,Beliefs%20are%20a%20choice

121 Menaghan, 1989; Spreitzer, Snyder, & Larson, 1980; Thoits, 1991

122 Garbi Mde O, Hortense P, Gomez RR, da Silva Tde C, Castanho AC, Sousa FA. Pain intensity, disability and depression in individuals with chronic back pain. Rev Lat Am Enfermagem. 2014;22(4):569-575. doi:10.1590/0104-1169.3492.2453

123 Payne, Kimberley A et al. When sex hurts, anxiety and fear orient attention towards pain. European journal of pain (London, England) vol. 9,4 (2005): 427-36. doi:10.1016/j.ejpain.2004.10.003

124 Flor H., Turk D.C., Scholz O.B. Impact of chronic pain on the spouse: marital, emotional and physical consequences. J Psychosom Res. 1987;31(1):63-71. doi: 10.1016/0022-3999(87)90099-7. PMID: 3820147.

125 https://www.ncbi.nlm.nih.gov/pmc/articles/PMC5563879/

354

126
https://www.ons.gov.uk/employmentandlabourmarket/peopleinwork/labou
rproductivity/articles/sicknessabsenceinthelabourmarket/2016
127 https://doi.org/10.1111/kykl.12319
128 www.ncbi.nlm.nih.gov/pmc/articles/PMC6815386/.
129 https://connecthealth.org.au/enews/pursuing-a-hobby-can-improve-your-
mental-
health/#:~:text=Research%20shows%20that%20people%20with,yourself%20af
ter%20a%20busy%20day.
130 https://www.anxietycentre.com/research/reading-reduces-stress-by-68-
percent/
131 Van Den Berg, Agnes E, and Mariëtte H G Custers. Gardening promotes
neuroendocrine and affective restoration from stress. Journal of health
psychology vol. 16,1 (2011): 3-11. doi:10.1177/1359105310365577
132 https://doi.org/10.34961/researchrepository-ul.22110530.v1
133 https://www.jpain.org/article/S1526-5900(22)00027-X/fulltext
134 Ioannou LJ, Cameron PA, Gibson SJ, et al. Traumatic injury and perceived
injustice: Fault attributions matter in a "no-fault" compensation state. PLoS
One. 2017;12(6):e0178894. Published 2017 Jun 5.
doi:10.1371/journal.pone.0178894
135 Carriere JS, Sturgeon JA, Yakobov E, Kao MC, Mackey SC, Darnall BD. The
Impact of Perceived Injustice on Pain-related Outcomes: A Combined Model
Examining the Mediating Roles of Pain Acceptance and Anger in a Chronic
Pain Sample. Clin J Pain. 2018;34(8):739-747.
doi:10.1097/AJP.0000000000000602
136 https://www.ncbi.nlm.nih.gov/pmc/articles/PMC5459431/ 38-40
137 Yakobov E., Scott W., Stanish W., Dunbar M., Richardson G., Sullivan M.
The role of perceived injustice in the prediction of pain and function after
total knee arthroplasty. Pain. 2014 Oct;155(10):2040-6. doi:
10.1016/j.pain.2014.07.007. Epub 2014 Jul 24. PMID: 25064836
138 https://uxdesign.cc/the-unconscious-emotions-and-our-decision-making-
process-183002021a29
139 https://www.jneurosci.org/content/38/12/2944

140 https://www.jpain.org/article/S1526-5900(22)00027-X/fulltext#:~:text=In%20a%20naturalistic%20pain%20clinic,clinically%20relevant%20pain%2Drelated%20injustice.

141 https://www.jpain.org/article/S1526-5900(21)00005-5/pdf

142 https://www.ncbi.nlm.nih.gov/pmc/articles/PMC5459431/

143 Roesch SC, Weiner B. A meta-analytic review of coping with illness: do causal attributions matter? J Psychosom Res. 2001 Apr;50(4):205-19. doi: 10.1016/s0022-3999(01)00188-x. PMID: 11369026

144 https://www.practicalpainmanagement.com/resources/assessing-secondary-gain-chronic-pain-patients

145 Fishbain D.A., Rosomoff H.L., Cutler R.B., Rosomoff R.S.. Secondary gain concept: a review of the scientific evidence. Clin J Pain. 1995 Mar;11(1):6-21. PMID: 7787338

146 National Academies of Sciences, Engineering, and Medicine. 2020. Social Isolation and Loneliness in Older Adults: Opportunities for the Health Care System. Washington, DC: The National Academies Press

147 https://www.fiercehealthcare.com/payer/express-scripts-covid-19-driving-up-use-behavioral-health-medications

148 https://neurosciencenews.com/social-isolation-cognition-brain-20857/

149 National Academies of Sciences, Engineering, and Medicine. 2020. Social Isolation and Loneliness in Older Adults: Opportunities for the Health Care System. Washington, DC: The National Academies Press

150 https://www.health.harvard.edu/blog/the-introverts-guide-to-social-engagement-2018111415353#:~:text=Unlike%20extroverts%2C%20who%20gain%20energy,recharge%20by%20spending%20time%20alone.

151 https://www.scientificamerican.com/article/hyperscans-show-how-brains-sync-as-people-interact/#:~:text=Norihiro%20Sadato%20of%20the%20National,which%20helps%20predict%20the%20sensory

152 Bannon, Sarah et al. The role of social isolation in physical and emotional outcomes among patients with chronic pain. General hospital psychiatry vol. 69 (2021): 50–54. doi:10.1016/j.genhosppsych.2021.01.009

153 https://pubmed.ncbi.nlm.nih.gov/22551663/

154 https://www.ncbi.nlm.nih.gov/pmc/articles/PMC4017137/

155 https://www.researchgate.net/publication/6737401_When_Inclusion_Costs_and_Ostracism_Pays_Ostracism_Still_Hurts

156 American Perspectives Survey, May 2021; Gallup, 1990

157 Chang, J., 2020. What Is Psychological Invalidation? How It Happens and Its Effects | Regain. online Regain.us. Available at: <https://www.regain.us/advice/psychology/what-is-psychological-invalidation-how-it-happens-and-its-effects/

158 https://www.ncbi.nlm.nih.gov/pubmed/28850377

159 Pierse T, Barry L, Glynn L, Quinlan D, Murphy A, O'Neill C. A pilot study of the duration of GP consultations in Ireland. Pilot and Feasibility Studies. 2019;5(1):142.

160 https://bmcmededuc.biomedcentral.com/articles/10.1186/s12909-018-1155-9

161 https://bmjopen.bmj.com/content/7/10/e017902

162 https://pubmed.ncbi.nlm.nih.gov/11273467/

163 https://bmjopen.bmj.com/content/7/10/e017902

164 Cruz, Mariana et al. Patients and healthcare professionals perspectives on creating a chronic pain support line in Portugal: A qualitative study protocol. PloS one vol. 17,8 e0273213. 17 Aug. 2022, doi:10.1371/journal.pone.0273213

165 https://www.ncbi.nlm.nih.gov/pmc/articles/PMC4477266/#R1

166 https://www.healthaffairs.org/doi/10.1377/hlthaff.2009.0450

167 https://www.impactplus.com/blog/the-psychology-of-design-the-color-green

168 https://bcmj.org/blog/green-most-suitable-color-hospital-textiles

169 https://www.ncbi.nlm.nih.gov/pmc/articles/PMC5295692/. Building trust takes time and it can be lost is an instant.

170 https://www.tandfonline.com/doi/abs/10.1080/09638288.2019.1636888?journalCode=idre20.

171 https://pubmed.ncbi.nlm.nih.gov/31290347/

172 https://pubmed.ncbi.nlm.nih.gov/22396087/

173 Edmond SN, Keefe FJ. Validating pain communication: current state of the science. Pain. 2015;156(2):215-219. doi:10.1097/01.j.pain.0000460301.18207.c2

174 https://www.ncbi.nlm.nih.gov/pmc/articles/PMC4477266/#!po=19.2308

175 https://www.ncbi.nlm.nih.gov/pmc/articles/PMC4477266/#R1

176 https://vcresearch.berkeley.edu/news/sleep-loss-heightens-pain-sensitivity-dulls-brains-painkilling-response

177 David K. Randall, *Dreamland: Adventures in the Strange Science of Sleep* (Norton, 2013)

178 Medic G, Wille M, Hemels ME. Short- and long-term health consequences of sleep disruption. Nat Sci Sleep. 2017;9:151-161. Published 2017 May 19. doi:10.2147/NSS.S134864

179 https://www.ncbi.nlm.nih.gov/books/NBK526132/

180 Imeri L, Opp MR. How (and why) the immune system makes us sleep. Nat Rev Neurosci. 2009;10(3):199-210. doi:10.1038/nrn2576

181 Wamsley EJ, Stickgold R. Memory, Sleep and Dreaming: Experiencing Consolidation. Sleep Med Clin. 2011;6(1):97-108. doi:10.1016/j.jsmc.2010.12.008

182 https://www.ncbi.nlm.nih.gov/pmc/articles/PMC7181893/ Crick and Mitchison, 1983; Smith and Lapp, 1991.

183 https://www.ncbi.nlm.nih.gov/pmc/articles/PMC3805807/

184https://pubmed.ncbi.nlm.nih.gov/23347102/#:~:text=The%20onset%20of%20the%20first,in%20total%20night%20REM%20sleep

185 https://pubmed.ncbi.nlm.nih.gov/17557450/

186 https://www.ncbi.nlm.nih.gov/pubmed/15511701; https://pubmed.ncbi.nlm.nih.gov/11376911/

187 https://pubmed.ncbi.nlm.nih.gov/21459634/

188 Hobson JA. Sleep mechanisms and pathophysiology: some clinical implications of the reciprocal interaction hypothesis of sleep cycle control

189 https://www.psychiatrictimes.com/view/effects-antidepressants-sleep

190 Roehrs T, Roth T. Drug-related Sleep Stage Changes: Functional Significance and Clinical Relevance. Sleep Med Clin. 2010;5(4):559-570. doi:10.1016/j.jsmc.2010.08.002

191 https://www.ncbi.nlm.nih.gov/pmc/articles/PMC181172/

192 https://www.ncbi.nlm.nih.gov/pmc/articles/PMC3047226/

193 Lynn, Christopher Dana. Hearth and campfire influences on arterial blood pressure: defraying the costs of the social brain through fireside relaxation. Evolutionary psychology: an international journal of evolutionary approaches to psychology and behavior vol. 12,5 983-1003. 11 Nov. 2014

194 https://www.youtube.com/watch?v=G0Z6_RjLz_4

195 https://psychology.berkeley.edu/news/sleep-scientist-warns-against-walking-through-life-underslept-state

196 https://www.ncbi.nlm.nih.gov/pmc/articles/PMC5810920/

197 Yoo et al 2007

198 www.ncbi.nlm.nih.gov/pmc/articles/PMC7181893/

199 https://www.jbc.org/article/S0021-9258(20)39197-3/fulltext

200 Ped Ann. 2017;46(3):e106-e111

201 Rico-Rosillo, María Guadalupe, and Gloria Bertha Vega-Robledo. Sueño y sistema immune : Sleep and immune system. Revista alergia Mexico (Tecamachalco, Puebla, Mexico: 1993) vol. 65,2 (2018): 160-170. doi:10.29262/ram.v65i2.359

202 https://www.ncbi.nlm.nih.gov/pmc/articles/PMC3627385/

203 Van Cauter, E, and L Plat. Physiology of growth hormone secretion during sleep. The Journal of pediatrics vol. 128,5 Pt 2 (1996): S32-7. doi:10.1016/s0022-3476(96)70008-2

204 https://www.ncbi.nlm.nih.gov/pmc/articles/PMC4046588/

205 https://www.ncbi.nlm.nih.gov/pmc/articles/PMC4046588/

206 https://www.ncbi.nlm.nih.gov/pmc/articles/PMC4590120/

207 https://www.ncbi.nlm.nih.gov/pmc/articles/PMC4590120/

208 https://www.ncbi.nlm.nih.gov/pmc/articles/PMC4046588/

209 https://www.cdc.gov/arthritis/basics/fibromyalgia.htm#:~:text=Stressful%20or%20traumatic%20events%2C%20such,Illness%20(such%20as%20viral%20infections)

210 https://www.ncbi.nlm.nih.gov/pmc/articles/PMC9369187/

211 https://pubmed.ncbi.nlm.nih.gov/19954696/

212 Haas, Brian W et al. Emotional conflict and neuroticism: personality-dependent activation in the amygdala and subgenual anterior cingulate.

Behavioral neuroscience vol. 121,2 (2007): 249-56. doi:10.1037/0735-7044.121.2.249

213 https://www.ncbi.nlm.nih.gov/pmc/articles/PMC2671308/

214 https://www.ncbi.nlm.nih.gov/pmc/articles/PMC2671308/

215 McCracken, Lance M. Learning to live with the pain: acceptance of pain predicts adjustment in persons with chronic pain. Pain vol. 74,1 (1998): 21-27. doi:10.1016/S0304-3959(97)00146-2

216 https://www.rte.ie/lifestyle/living/2019/0826/1070931-studies-say-were-sleeping-two-hours-less-than-we-did-in-the-60s/

217 https://daily49er.com/opinions/2019/09/04/stop-using-lack-of-sleep-as-a-badge-of-honor-its-tiring/

218 Zambelli Z, Halstead EJ, Fidalgo AR, Dimitriou D. Good Sleep Quality Improves the Relationship Between Pain and Depression Among Individuals With Chronic Pain. Front Psychol. 2021;12:668930. Published 2021 May 7. doi:10.3389/fpsyg.2021.668930

219 https://pubmed.ncbi.nlm.nih.gov/11285053/.

220 https://sleepeducation.org/healthy-sleep/healthy-sleep-habits/

221 Thakkar, Mahesh M et al. Alcohol disrupts sleep homeostasis. Alcohol (Fayetteville, N.Y.) vol. 49,4 (2015): 299-310. doi:10.1016/j.alcohol.2014.07.019

222 https://www.sciencedirect.com/science/article/pii/S2095254614000131

223 https://www.ncbi.nlm.nih.gov/pmc/articles/PMC3645673/#:~:text=The%20pineal%20hormone%20melatonin%20exerts,glucagon%20secretion%20from%20%CE%B1%2Dcells

224 Rahman MS, Hossain KS, Das S, et al. Role of Insulin in Health and Disease: An Update. Int J Mol Sci. 2021;22(12):6403. Published 2021 Jun 15. doi:10.3390/ijms22126403

225 https://pubmed.ncbi.nlm.nih.gov/32295235/.

226 https://time.com/4680537/sleep-insomnia-bed-arousal/

227 https://nickwignall.com/how-to-fall-asleep-fast-with-deliberate-worry/

228 https://www.healthline.com/health/meditation-for-sleep#mindfulness-meditation

<u>229</u> Mitchell MD, Gehrman P, Perlis M, Umscheid CA. Comparative effectiveness of cognitive behavioral therapy for insomnia: a systematic review. BMC Fam Pract. 2012;13:40. Published 2012 May 25. doi:10.1186/1471-2296-13-40

<u>230</u> https://www.ncbi.nlm.nih.gov/pmc/articles/PMC6751071/

<u>231</u> https://pubmed.ncbi.nlm.nih.gov/24690623/

<u>232</u>https://pubmed.ncbi.nlm.nih.gov/18625986/#:~:text=About%2090%25%20of %20our%20time,allergies%2C%20asthma%20and%20lung%20cancer

<u>233</u> https://www.ncbi.nlm.nih.gov/pmc/articles/PMC7400257/

<u>234</u> https://pubmed.ncbi.nlm.nih.gov/29904370/

<u>235</u> (Keedy et al 2014).

<u>236</u> Increased likelihood when visualisation and health message are combined; https://pubmed.ncbi.nlm.nih.gov/24124985/.

<u>237</u> https://www.philcicio.com/power-of-visualization/

<u>238</u> https://www.nature.com/articles/d41586-019-01589- 6?utm_medium=affiliate&utm_source=commission_junction&utm_campaign =CONR_PF018_ECOM_GL_PHSS_ALWYS_DEEPLINK&utm_content=tex tlink&utm_term=PID100041175&CJEVENT=c0b5b0b77af711ee830f61c10a1 8b8fc

<u>239</u> Wood, Patrick B. Role of central dopamine in pain and analgesia. Expert review of neurotherapeutics vol. 8,5 (2008): 781-97. doi:10.1586/14737175.8.5.781

<u>240</u> Gardner, Tania et al. Goal setting practice in chronic low back pain. What is current practice and is it affected by beliefs and attitudes? Physiotherapy theory and practice vol. 34,10 (2018): 795-805. doi:10.1080/09593985.2018.1425785

<u>241</u> https://rapidbi.com/harvard-yale-written-goals-study-fact-or-fiction/

Printed in Great Britain
by Amazon

39374410R00208

GW01191495

Deadly Secrets

Robert Tenison

This edition published by Chiringuito Books, 5 Langdon Road, Bromley, BR2 9JS

First published 2009 by New Generation Publishing

A CIP catalogue record for this book is available from the British Library.

Depósito Legal: SE-4159-2009

ISBN: 978-0-9563132-1-8

Cover design by Ewout Meijer of 1Bureau (www.1Bureau.nl).

Bound and printed in Spain by Publidisa, Seville

About the Author

Robert Tenison was born of Spanish parents in the UK and spent fifteen years as a commercial and investment banker, including a spell in the Cayman Islands. On leaving banking, he worked as a freelance business consultant and authored two Financial Times Management Reports until founding an online recruitment company which was eventually sold to a leading newspaper publisher.

For the last seven years he has been living in Southern Spain, working in the property and financial services sector. As a result, he has had numerous dealings with estate agents, property developers and banks and has an in-depth knowledge of the subject matter of Deadly Secrets. At the same time, he was advised by a number of professionals, such as lawyers and policemen, regarding some of the technicalities covered in the book.

Acknowledgements

The author wishes to thank the friends and family who read and commented on various drafts including, but not limited to: Tony Tanner, Mike Goggs, Peter Sire, Miriam Nugent, Viv Moore, Graham Tennant and Nicholas Le Seelleur, as well as the three lawyers who advised him on certain legal aspects of Spanish and UK Wills, Spanish taxation and money laundering and extradition treaties, and not forgetting the Spanish Police Inspector who gave invaluable advice on procedures following deaths in Spain.

He also owes a debt of gratitude to numerous fellow writers on YouWriteOn.com for their constructive criticism, comments and advice, especially Avery Mathers, as well as to Yvonne Koot for her guidance and assistance in the publishing and cover design process. Finally, Katie Holland deserves a special mention for her invaluable support in printing, binding and sending out many versions of the manuscript to a host of different people.

At the end of the day, this is a work of fiction, so any errors or omissions regarding any of the legal or taxation aspects are purely those of the author. Likewise, any resemblance of any character to any real person, living or dead, is entirely accidental and wholly unintentional.

Late September

Andy Montalvo threw his suit carrier onto the bed and walked through to the living room. It had been a busy but productive trip, and he was looking forward to a nice glass of wine to help him unwind.

As he tried to decide whether to open an Australian Cabernet Sauvignon or a Ribera del Duero, the phone rang. From the display he saw it was Mike Cameron, so he picked the handset up.

"Andy, great you're there – I thought you said you'd be back tonight."

"Hi Mike, I've literally just walked in. I'm knackered and I was about to have a glass of wine before hitting the sack, can it wait until tomorrow?"

"Err… yes… well actually… no."

Andy couldn't help laughing. "You sound confused, make your mind up!"

"Ok, listen, I've got some exciting news – I've been approached to see if I can find buyers for over three million square metres of rustic land which is going to be reclassified to allow a golf course with five thousand residential properties, a commercial centre and a hotel. The price is two hundred and fifty million euros and I can probably get an exclusive – Andy, this could be our first big deal!"

Andy was suddenly all ears. After more than twenty years in the City, and having broken up with his long-term girlfriend earlier that year, he had decided he was ready for a complete change of direction and lifestyle. He was not rich by any stretch of the imagination, no million pound bonuses for him; but with no mortgage on his flat in Kensington, no family commitments, some savings and the villa in

Spain, he could afford to look at other options. Mike was an old friend, and in August, Andy had agreed to buy a stake in his estate agency and move to Los Cipreses as soon as possible – it would be a return to his Spanish roots, although his father had emigrated to the UK in the 50s and Andy had never lived in Spain before.

The town and its surrounding area were still relatively unspoilt compared to the rest of the Spanish costas, but things were about to change. The imminent completion of the new coastal motorway, along with the growth in low-cost flights into Malaga and Granada, was making the town and its surrounding area increasingly accessible, and hence very attractive to large property developers.

As a result, a new urban development plan, commonly known in Spain as a PGOU, proposed the reclassification of millions of square metres of land for residential, commercial and leisure use. If approved by the Junta de Andalucia, the autonomous regional government, it would mean a step change in the development of the area, so he and Mike had discussed how to re-position Mike's business in light of these probable changes.

During their discussions it had become clear that a partnership would play to their respective strengths, with Mike's local knowledge and contacts, and Andy's City experience and connections, enabling them to take Mike's business to another level – hence Andy's decision to buy into Mike's business.

This transaction was a perfect example of the type of deal they hoped to get involved in.

"Ok, slow down Mike. That's a potentially big deal – what makes you think it's for real?"

"Well, the person who's approached me is a businessman who's already been involved in a number of successful developments in the area."

"Fair enough, but what makes this project special? I thought there were proposals for eight golf courses in the area, four in Los Cipreses and another four in El Castillo."

"There was, but earlier this week the Junta announced that it's only going to allow one golf course in the area."

"Really? Why?"

"Oh, mainly pressure from environmentalists, but also to prevent excessive development of the coast. The problem is they've not announced which of the eight sites will get the nod, but my contact is very confident that his site is the one which will be approved."

"What makes you think he's a horse worth backing?"

"He's successful and well connected, at local and regional level."

"Normal Spanish practices then!" exclaimed Andy, who knew that in Spain it was who you knew not what you knew that got things done. "Who is he? Do I know him?"

Mike hesitated for several seconds. "I'm sorry Andy but I've been sworn to secrecy. I'll give you the low down when you're officially on board but for now why don't we call him Mr. Brown – after all Reservoir Dogs is one of your favourite films."

"It all sounds very mysterious but I guess it's understandable with such a potentially lucrative transaction. But why has this Mr. Brown approached you – surely he knows plenty of developers who'd be interested in such a project?"

"He knows I've got connections with major foreign investors via my property management clients."

"And why does he want foreign investors?"

"Because he says they have much higher design and construction standards than local developers, as well as better access to foreign buyers, who, at the end of the day, are the main target market."

"There's certainly logic in that. Do you know which of the eight sites we're talking about?"

"No, he's not willing to disclose which site it is until he's got acceptable references, a signed Confidentiality Agreement and a five-million euro reservation deposit's been paid. Also, the deal needs to be agreed before the new PGOU is approved, which leaves us three months at most."

Andy thought about this. "It's not going to be easy to find investors for such a big deal so quickly."

"I know, but it's a unique opportunity, so there should be significant interest. Also, with completion being conditional on the land being reclassified, it's relatively low risk."

"That's true – apart from the five-million euro deposit, of course.

So, have you made contact with any potential investors yet?"

"Not yet, I wanted to tell you first, but I'm going to approach one of my clients whose villa I look after – he's got excellent connections with leading international property developers and investors."

"Sounds promising. What commission has this mysterious Mr. Brown offered you?"

"One percent of the total purchase price. What do you think?"

"Not bad! Two and a half million euros, even after tax, means you could quite happily retire."

"Yes it would be great, but I'm not quite ready to retire and go walking in the hills just yet. What I really want to do is to slow down a bit and spend more time with Sonya and the kids."

Andy knew that when Mike had split with Ann earlier that year he had begun to see Sonya, a divorced expat with two children. He was happy that Mike had found solace in a new relationship instead of going off the rails, but was also a little concerned about the speed with which it had happened. In his experience rebound relationships tended not to last.

"Good. I'm looking forward to getting to know Sonya better, she's obviously very special. So what's next as far as this deal's concerned?"

"I'll contact my client tomorrow to see if he has anybody who might be interested and who can provide acceptable references – then we can start the real negotiations. We've also got to get the paperwork sorted regarding your investment in the business."

"Quite, but the problem is, as you know, my notice period doesn't end until mid-November and I've got a couple of major cases that need to be tied up before I leave, so I'm not going to be able to come out for at least a month."

"Don't worry, it'll wait. We'll stick to the terms we agreed last month, whether this deal comes off or not. My word is my bond, as you City boys say!"

"I'm not worried. I'd trust you with my life Mike, you know that."

Late October

Mike and Johan had been propping up the bar for over three hours. Aside from them and the owner Pepe, the Cutty Sark was empty.

"One more for the road?"

"Why not," replied Johan. "I'll have plenty of time to sleep my hangover off before my weekly visit to the kids. What are you doing?"

"I've got to go and see my lawyer about my divorce – it's becoming a bit messy."

"Why? Is she trying to screw you?"

"Yep."

"So what are you going to do?"

"Unless she sees sense, the lawyers will have to sort it out. Thank God she doesn't know about the big property transaction I'm working on, or she'd want a share of that too."

Mike slipped off his chair and walked uncertainly in the direction of the gents. Johan sobered up quickly on hearing Mike's reference to the deal he was working on. Unbeknown to Mike, he knew all about it and wondered how many other people Mike had discussed it with; hopefully none.

"So what's this property deal you're working on?" Johan asked when Mike returned.

"Oh, that's top secret," Mike replied, tapping his nose with his forefinger, "but, anyway, it's not about the money."

"If it's not about the money what is it about then? Surely money is what it's all about!"

Mike glanced around the bar. It was still empty, but he could hear Pepe clearing up in the kitchen. He leant forward and lowered his voice:

"Listen Johan, I can't say anything about the deal except that if it goes ahead I'll get a very nice fee, but what I really want is to bring one of the parties involved to justice. The problem is that I still haven't got enough information to go to the authorities – but I should have soon."

"Sounds intriguing – what do you mean bringing one of the parties involved to justice?"

"Oh, forget I said that, I've drunk and said too much already, so no more questions – let's finish up and be on our way," said Mike staggering to his feet, the effects of the night's drinking now all too apparent.

"Ok, but who else knows about this deal?" said Johan rising from the bar stool and towering over Mike, his dark expressionless eyes carefully regarding Mike as he fumbled to put his three-quarter length padded jacket on.

"As far as I know, no one except me and the owner of the land. Now, come on, point me in the direction of my car."

Mike's keys slipped through his fingers and fell with a dull thud onto the beach as he approached his jeep, which was parked on the beach directly in front of the Cutty Sark. Fortunately, using the light of the moon he was able to find them. "Sonya's going to kill me," he said to himself, as he clambered into the driver's seat "but at least she's a lot more understanding than Ann ever was."

He started the jeep, reversed on to the road and drove along the beachfront towards Cerro Grande for a few hundred metres and then turned down a dirt track on the right. This was the shortcut to Sonya's house; however, it did mean that he had to drive past his own house in Los Romeros.

Johan sat in his car and watched Mike drive off. As soon as Mike's jeep disappeared from sight, he took a mobile phone from the glove compartment – it was a popular flip-lid model which had been bought anonymously on a pre-paid basis – and punched in a nine-digit number.

As Mike drove unsteadily, but slowly, along the bumpy track, he recalled how he and Ann had acquired the house for a song from a distressed seller during the property slump of the early 1990s. They had subsequently lavished much care and attention on it and, following the recent boom in property prices in Los Cipreses and the surrounding area, he reckoned that the house was now worth about one million euros.

There was no mortgage on the property, and he thought his offer to Ann of a cash payment of six hundred thousand euros and to see Emily through university was more than fair. In fact, it was more than she was entitled to under Spanish law. Unfortunately, now she wanted a share of the proceeds from Andy's investment in the business as well as some of his offshore "pension fund."

As he approached the house, he saw that the lights were on and could just about make out the figures of Carlos and Ann standing in the living room, talking in what appeared to be an agitated manner. "Nothing new there then," he muttered to himself, driving past the house.

Initially, it had been a shock to be supplanted by a younger man, especially one who appeared to be clinging to the fast-disappearing stereotypical image of the macho Andalusian male, but, now he had Sonya, he realised it was the best thing that had happened to him.

Carlos was tall for a Spaniard, with classic dark hair and smouldering eyes. He was in his late twenties and Ann, like many other women, had been attracted by his Antonio Banderas-type looks and his Latin charm.

Ann's relationship with Mike had fallen into routine and complacency a number of years ago. Emily's departure to university a couple of years ago had left her with even less to do, while Mike devoted more and more time to his business. It was a dangerous combination, and Carlos had blown away the remaining vestiges of her relationship with Mike like a category-four hurricane hitting a beach hut.

As she listened to him, she remembered the first time she had seen him in El Boqueron, one of the most popular restaurant-bars on Los Cipreses beach. He was dressed in the classic black waiter's trousers with a white shirt and a black waistcoat. He walked upright, head held high and without shuffling his feet, which, along with his looks and easy smile, distinguished him from his fellow waiters. She was smitten and had asked her friend Carmen if she knew who he was.

"Oh, he's new in town. Rumour has it that he comes from Marbella but had to leave in a bit of a hurry because of some woman trouble. Hot but dangerous apparently!"

"Very hot!" Ann had replied, making a mental note to return to El Boqueron in the next day or two more appropriately attired. One thing had led to another and a few months later she and Mike separated, although it was Mike who had left the family home and who had recently decided to formalise their divorce.

She was jolted back to reality by his raised voice. "Sweetheart, I know six hundred thousand euros is a lot of money but it won't buy us a half decent villa with a garden and pool – more like a two- or three-bedroom apartment in one of those non-descript blocks on the beachfront. Surely you're entitled to more?"

"Carlos, my lawyer says all I'm legally entitled to is fifty percent of the value of the house – which is five hundred thousand, give or take. When I talked to Mike earlier this week he told me that he's going to pay me from his offshore account, which means it won't be subject to tax either."

Carlos paced agitatedly round the Jali coffee table. "You've been married to him for twenty years, had his child and supported him through thick and thin, forget the law – don't you think you deserve more?

"You told me Mike's got over a million euros in his offshore account and I bet he's about to get a nice sum for selling a share in his business to Andy Montalvo – I tell you, he can afford to pay you more!"

"Carlos, calm down, Mike started the business before we were married so under Spanish law I'm not entitled to any proceeds from its sale. The offshore account is in his sole name and if we bring that up in court it would open a can of worms with the tax authorities. Remember, he's also setting aside some of that money for Emily's education so I don't think it is fair to ask for more."

She looked at him imploringly. She hated confrontation with Carlos, something which seemed to be occurring with increasing frequency. "Listen darling, we don't need a villa with a pool overlooking the sea. There're only two of us and I fancy buying a finca inland to do up. I'm fed up of the beach and the in-crowd on the Punta de Palermo and Cerro Grande, and it's only going to get worse as the area becomes more popular."

Carlos stopped pacing and turned to face Ann. "Sweetheart, that'd be very nice when I'm in my forties – like you, or as a weekend hideaway, but there's going to be plenty of opportunities to make money here over the next few years and I want us to be part of that. Actually, I've recently been offered an interesting business so the more money we can get from Mike the better."

"Alright, alright – I'll try and talk to him one more time before he starts formal proceedings."

"Now you're talking," said Carlos, sitting down on the sofa opposite Ann "but I don't think asking politely is going to get you anywhere. He needs to feel that it's in his best interests to pay you more than he's currently offering."

"What do you mean?"

"Well, imagine if the tax authorities were to find out about his offshore bank account. They're getting very hot on all this black money and tax evasion stuff. Mike could lose all of that money and more, not to mention potentially spending some time inside Alhuarin gaol. Wouldn't be in his best interests to give you more money from the offshore account in return for the authorities not finding out about it?"

Ann stood up and moved over to the bar. "Actually, that's not a bad idea," she said turning to face Carlos, "but I wouldn't want to resort to overt blackmail. It'll have to be done subtly because, if he feels threatened, Mike is quite capable of making the money in that account disappear."

"Ok, so be subtle," said Carlos in a quieter voice. "By the way, does Mike have a Will?"

"Yes, actually we both have Spanish and English Wills."

"And what are the provisions of these Wills?"

"Each of us inherits the other's assets inside and outside of Spain. Mike's also made a provision for Emily to receive a lump sum of four hundred thousand euros from his offshore account. Why do you ask?"

Carlos ran his fingers through his hair. He had calmed down and looked more pensive.

"Sweetheart, forgive me for thinking out loud but if Mike were to die you would inherit all of his assets. This would presumably include the house, the offshore account and the shares in the business, less Emily's four hundred thousand euros of course."

"And since when were you an expert on UK and Spanish Wills?"

"Ah, my love, in my relatively short life I have met a lot of people and discussed many things, including the consequences of death."

"Anyway, it's immaterial, I can't imagine Mike dying. He's not as fit as he used to be and he's still drinking too much, but his last annual checkup gave no cause for concern."

Neither of them noticed the lights of Mike's car as he drove past the house on his way back to Sonya's from the Cutty Sark.

Wednesday, 14th November

The night air was still; the smell of the sea lingered in the air as Johan Gaards retraced his steps back to the office.

A metal security blind covered the large, single-pane window from top to bottom. To its right, a second security blind hung, half-mast, over the frosted glass door, leaving just enough room for most adults to enter without stooping. The door was closed but a soft glow emanated from inside, so Johan turned the handle and pushed. The door remained closed. He knocked on the glass. "Mike open up, it's me. I've been waiting for you at Luque's for more than half an hour."

He waited a few seconds, knocked again, and, when there was still no response, he stepped sideways and pressed his face against the security blind. As he peered through a small chink in the blind, he thought he caught a glimpse of flames flickering in the corner of the office. He immediately started kicking at the door, but to no avail – the reinforced frame and five-lever lock Mike had recently installed held firm. Giving up after a few kicks, he turned, ran the five hundred metres back to Café Luque, and rushed over to the bar.

"Luque, quick, call 112, it looks like there's a fire in Mike's office. The door's locked so I can't get in and I don't know if he's in there or not, but that's where I left him more than thirty minutes ago."

A couple of minutes later, just as Luque and Johan were about to try and break the door down, a Guardia Civil Nissan Patrol screeched to halt outside the office. Two burly officers exited the vehicle. "Stand back," one of them shouted at Luque and Johan and the small crowd that had gathered, as they began to batter the door, one using his feet and the other his shoulder. After a few hefty blows, the door gave way, violently swinging inwards and allowing a cloud of acrid smoke to escape the enclosed space.

The bystanders shuffled forward, led by Luque and Johan, trying to peer inside the office. Smoke was now billowing out of the door into the night and orangey-yellow flames could be seen dancing and leaping ever higher at the back of the smoke-filled room. One of the officers turned to face the crowd, stretching his arms wide and forcing them back. His companion crouched on the pavement close to the entrance, covering his nose and mouth with a cloth, scouring the room for any signs of Mike Cameron.

He was momentarily distracted by the sound of the fire engine's alarm, as it hurtled towards them down the beachfront road, but then he saw a body slumped on the floor under the solitary desk in the left-hand corner of the office. The sofa next to the desk was being engulfed by flames, which were growing fiercer by the second, but he dashed in, grabbed the inert body under the arms, and dragged it into the street.

Johan Gaards stood to one side, watching dispassionately as the Guardia tried to resuscitate Mike Cameron. After a few minutes, when the officer finally gave up his attempts, Johan walked across the road to the beach, took out his mobile, and made a brief phone call before returning to join Luque and the growing crowd of onlookers.

Friday, 16th November

Ordinarily he looked forward to driving the last few kilometres to Los Cipreses. This stretch of coastline, with its cliffs and promontories, pine-filled valleys and hidden coves, always left him awestruck. Looking along the ragged coastline he could see a few white houses in the distance clinging to the side of the cliffs, desperately resisting the pull of gravity which sought to send them tumbling into the sea far below.

But today was no ordinary day. The news of Mike Cameron's death had come like a bolt out of the blue and, given recent events, Andy approached Los Cipreses with a sense of trepidation, wondering what secrets lay waiting to be discovered.

Only a few days ago, Mike had told Andy that he had finally received references from the potential property investors, and had passed them on to the mysterious Mr. Brown.

"They're great references so he should respond favourably – but we've only got a few weeks to complete the deal. Get down here as soon as possible so you can help me with the negotiations."

The timing could not have been better for Andy. He was finishing his three-month notice period that very week and had been planning to fly down to Spain the following week to finalise his acquisition of fifty percent of Mike's business.

"By the way, just so you know, I'm officially initiating divorce proceedings next week."

"About time too," Andy had replied. He'd never been terribly fond of Ann, who had rather a sharp tongue and aggressive manner, and he had often wondered why Mike had stayed with her so long. He assumed it was because of their daughter, but Andy didn't believe that a couple should stay together for the sake of the children. Nevertheless, Emily had not appeared to suffer too much from her parents' constant bickering and Ann's difficult personality, so maybe it had been the right decision. Anyway, who was he to judge, with several failed relationships and no children in tow, he had thought to himself.

"I suppose so, but now she's putting pressure on me to give her more money than I'm offering her."

"What do you mean, putting pressure on you?"

"She's threatening to tell the Spanish tax authorities about my offshore account unless I give her at least a million euros plus a share of the proceeds from the sale of the business to you."

"That's outrageous," Andy exclaimed. In truth, given the nature of his job, Andy felt a little uncomfortable about Mike's offshore account. Nevertheless, he was sure that Mike had earned the funds legitimately and, so, in the end it was a personal matter in which he didn't want to get involved.

"Tell me about it. Personally, I put it down to Carlos, he's out for all he can get and she's totally besotted by him."

"So what are you going to do?"

"It's very complicated and I'll tell you all about it when you're here, but don't worry, I'm not concerned about the Spanish tax authorities and you can be sure that there's no way she's going to get what she's asking for."

"Good, you've offered her a fair deal so stick to your guns. Listen, let me know as soon as Mr. Brown gets back to you, but I'll book a flight for next week anyway."

Little had he known that was to be the last conversation he would have with Mike; his sudden death not only meant the loss of a very good friend but also a rethink of his plans.

Andy had been a regular visitor to Los Cipreses since childhood, when his parents had bought a villa on the Cerro Grande headland, and its charm and beauty had attracted an eclectic mix of both Spanish and non-Spanish residents. He had many friends in the area, including Mike Cameron, who he'd first met over twenty years ago during the long summer following Andy's finals. Mike himself had stumbled across Los Cipreses earlier that summer, as he travelled around the Mediterranean searching for a purpose in life.

There was only a year between them and they bonded immediately, enjoying a wild summer, partying late into the night and then recovering lazily by Andy's parents' pool or on the beach during the day.

Those were the heady days when Spain had just joined the then European Community and was moving full steam ahead to catch up with its Northern neighbours. Optimism abounded and Mike had decided to stay, believing that Los Cipreses would provide him with opportunities for a relaxed but profitable life. It had been a very good choice as his estate agency, the first in the town, had grown steadily, providing Mike with regular income from property sales, rentals and management.

At the same time, Andy's career in investment banking had thrived as he became a leading expert on international financings, from mergers and acquisitions to major infrastructure projects.

However, Andy had become increasingly disillusioned with the money-is-king, greed-is-good, attitude that pervaded the City. So a couple of years ago he had accepted the role to head up the City of London Police serious fraud squad; Andy's experience in international finance had proved invaluable in successfully achieving a number of high-profile prosecutions.

He and Mike had maintained contact, predominantly through Andy's flying visits for the occasional long weekend, which had continued after his parents passed away and he inherited their villa. Andy's desire for a change and their discussions that summer had convinced him that the new PGOU presented many opportunities, hence his decision to buy into Mike's business and move to Los Cipreses.

But Mike's unexpected death changed everything and Andy needed more time to gather his thoughts before his meeting with Ann, so, as he approached the Cerro Grande tunnel, he took the sharp right turn onto the old coast road which climbed over and round the Cerro, offering even more stunning views of the coastline.

As Andy drove along the old coast road, Vicente Maldonado was sitting at his desk in Granada looking at his computer screen. He moved the mouse with his right hand, placed the cursor over the green Skype button and clicked on it. It was their preferred way of talking, since Skype calls were impossible to trace. A few seconds later Javier Urquiza answered.

"Don Javier, what's the latest news?"

"My source within the Policia Nacional says Mr. Cameron's death is being treated as an accident."

"No surprise there. Does he know whether UDYCO are investigating Project Pulpo or any of your other activities?"

"No, but he's spotted nothing unusual in internal communications and there are no rumours of any investigation, so it looks as if Project Pulpo is still on track."

"That's good news. We can go ahead with tomorrow's meeting. How do you want to handle it?"

"We'll tell them that in light of Mr. Cameron's death, you're taking over the negotiations with the investors. Then we'll confirm how the deal's going to be structured as well as the financial arrangements."

"Ok, let's meet down at the marina tomorrow at twelve and go over the paperwork before the meeting."

Andy pulled over just after the derelict Moorish watch tower, which stood where the furthermost part of the Cerro jutted into the sea, and got out. His body felt taut after the flight and car drive, and he stretched his limbs to loosen up. He was just under six foot in height and of medium build, with a full head of shortish brown hair, tempered by flecks of grey, hazel eyes and well-defined lips. He was a regular gym goer and so was in good shape, despite a love of food and wine.

It was a glorious day – the sea was calm, the sky clear and blue, and as he stood surveying the sweeping horseshoe bay of Los Cipreses, a slight breeze brought the faint, but familiar, smell of the sea to his nostrils. Above him, seagulls glided and swooped on the currents and eddies rising above the Cerro. Directly in front of him, at the far end of the bay, was the Punta de Palermo. This wooded headland, with its fabulous views back across the bay and out to the Mediterranean, was where the elite lived in the villas which were dotted all over the Punta.

He turned his head slightly to the left to view Los Cipreses itself. Like many towns and villages along the coast, the majority of the houses were located on a hill approximately one kilometre inland from the beach. In the old days this afforded residents some security from the constant raids of the Barbary pirates. This was known as the Casco Antiguo, or Old Town, and was mainly the preserve of older generation Spaniards and a few foreigners who were buying up old town houses to renovate.

In front of the Old Town, clustered in the lee of the Punta de Palermo, close to the beachfront, was what appeared to be a separate village which comprised, at most, a hundred traditional Andalusian white houses. This was La Caleta de Los Cipreses, or La Caleta for short, and was where the fishermen had lived and plied their trade for generations until competition, pollution and tourism had finally made their efforts uneconomic. A few hardy souls still went out at night in their boats to catch whatever fish they could, but it was a very difficult way to make a living and they were a rapidly dying breed.

As he took one last look at Los Cipreses, the sunlight suddenly faded as a solitary cloud passed directly in front of the sun, casting a deep shadow over the town. It only lasted a few seconds, but he wondered whether it was an omen. With this thought fresh in his mind, he climbed back into the car to complete the short drive to his villa.

When he arrived at his villa Ann was sitting in Mike's old pick-up waiting for him. He parked, got out of his car and gave Ann a quick hug. He stepped back and looked at her. Her hair had been permed and highlighted with blond streaks since Andy had last seen her, but he wasn't sure it suited her. She was not an unattractive lady but it was clear that too many years in the sun and too many long lunches were beginning to take their toll. Her face was fleshier and weather worn, making her small eyes appear more sunken. Nevertheless, her snub nose, which Mike had considered "cute," continued to be a redeeming feature.

"How are you doing?" he asked her.

"I'm bearing up but I am beginning to feel rather tired – it's been a long couple of days."

"I can imagine. I'll fix us a drink and then you can tell me exactly what happened."

He unlocked the front door and ushered Ann through the hall and into the living room. The house was full of sunlight as all the external window blinds had been raised, at very short notice, by Alejandra, his regular cleaner for the last four years, in preparation for his arrival. She was his life saver and he was very grateful for the economic crisis in Argentina that had brought her and her family to Spain in search of work.

"Tea or something stronger?"

"Tea is fine. I think anything stronger will knock me out."

Once the kettle had boiled, Andy carried the two mugs of tea through to the terrace. The house had been one of the very first built on the Cerro Grande headland nearly forty years ago and, although it was now surrounded by other properties, none blocked the view from the terrace across the bay to the Punta de Palermo.

Ann was standing with her back to Andy admiring the view and turned to face him as she heard him approach. "Sit down and tell me all about it when you're ready," Andy said, pulling out two chairs from under the round teak table which occupied the centre of the terrace.

"Actually, there's not much more to tell you. Mike was out drinking with Johan Gaards at the Cutty Sark and by all accounts they were pretty smashed by midnight. According to Johan, they decided to go on to Luque's but on the way Mike stopped off at the office to check for an email he was expecting from a client."

"Why would he want to check an email in the middle of the night?"

"Apparently, the client was arriving later that morning and the email was meant to give him the flight details so he could collect him from the airport."

"Typical Mike, still doing the airport pick-ups himself," remarked Andy.

"Yes, he's always liked to provide a personal touch. Anyway, Johan left Mike at the office and went straight to Luque's but when

Mike failed to turn up a bit later he went back to look for him. The rest is what I told you on the phone."

"And you said he was already dead when they pulled him out?"

"Yes."

"What was the cause of death?"

"They think it was suffocation from the smoke."

"And how did the fire start?"

"The Guardia Civil and fire department think that an electrical fire started under the desk and that Mike probably panicked while trying to put it out, banging his head in the process and knocking him out for long enough for the smoke to overcome him."

Andy thought about this. "If crime novels and CSI programmes are to be believed, it takes a lot of smoke to overcome a relatively healthy adult. Surely there wasn't sufficient time for that to happen?"

"They think the waste paper bin under the desk caught fire and that the old sofa he kept for clients, which was next to it, went up in flames pretty quickly, releasing all sorts of toxic fumes.

"Mike didn't have a chance. The fact that he'd locked the door from the inside hampered the rescue attempts. That's it really, but we're still waiting for them to do the autopsy to confirm the cause of death."

As Ann took a sip of her tea, Andy asked: "And when are they expecting to carry out the autopsy?"

"Early next week."

"Why so long? They're usually pretty quick with these things."

"Oh, the investigating judge wants the senior pathologist from the Institute of Legal Medicine in Granada to do it. He's away on a conference in the US and returns over the weekend."

"Well, the sooner the better, then at least you can bury Mike. By the way, do you happen to have the name and phone number of the Guardia Civil officer in charge of the investigation?"

Andy knew there should be no particular reason why the Guardia Civil would want to talk with him, but he felt he ought to tell them about his agreement to buy into Mike's business and about the golf course transaction Mike had been working on so that they were fully in the picture.

"Actually, although the Civiles would normally be given the case, the investigating judge has allocated the case to the Policia Nacional. A Chief Inspector Diaz is in charge and he's based in El Castillo.

Andy looked perplexed. "That's a bit odd. Do you know why?"

"No, but I think it's probably because the Chief Inspector speaks English," Ann said, rising from the chair. "I need to go; Carlos is expecting me for lunch. I'll call you later with his number."

Andy accompanied her to the front door. "By the way, how's Emily? Is she flying out?"

Mike and Ann's daughter was in her second year of university in England and he had known her since she was born, although, as she had grown older and developed her own social circle, Andy had seen less of her during his occasional visits to Los Cipreses. Nevertheless, Mike had kept him up to date with her exploits, from her first serious boyfriend to gaining entry to university.

"As you can imagine, she's very upset. She was closer to Mike than to me. She's due to arrive tonight on the last flight in, so I'll leave for Malaga at about nine-thirty to pick her up."

"Give her my love and tell her I'll call her tomorrow."

When Ann had driven off Andy took a beer from the fridge, went back to the terrace, sat down on the swing seat and pondered over what she had told him.

She was not looking forward to lunch as she was expecting Carlos to continue to pressurise her for the money to buy Bar Salamander, especially as Mike's death meant she would now inherit the house, the business and the offshore funds.

She had seen enough bars open and close in Los Cipreses to know this was probably not a good investment. Carlos was a waiter, and a good one when he put his mind to it, but running a successful bar was a totally different ball game which required hard work, late nights, a personal touch and a fair amount of luck. He might have the charm but she doubted he was ready to make the necessary commitment. More likely, after an initial splash, he'd hire a manager and it would become a drinking den for him and his friends.

Maybe I'm being a bit harsh, she thought, and perhaps I should give him the benefit of the doubt, as well as the opportunity he deserves. After all, it was only one hundred and fifty thousand euros and she had discovered that morning that Mike's offshore account actually contained close to two million euros. Of course, Carlos didn't need to know that, but it brought home the fact that Mike had been trying to short change her with his offer of six hundred thousand euros.

She pulled up outside the house. Carlos opened the front door before she could put her key in the lock, his tan and dark complexion perfectly setting off the orange floral-pattern swimming shorts and stone-washed Billabong T-shirt that she had recently bought him. He does look dead sexy she thought and couldn't resist reaching up and giving him a quick kiss while squeezing his left buttock.

"Careful sweetie, or lunch will be served late. How was Mr. Montalvo? Is he amenable to buying the business?" Carlos asked, as Ann edged past him into the living room.

"You don't waste any time do you? All he wanted to know were the circumstances surrounding Mike's death. It wasn't appropriate to mention the possibility of him buying the business."

"So what did you tell him about Mike's death?"

"The truth of course."

"And what did he say?"

"Nothing really. Just that he wanted to call Chief Inspector Diaz in case he needed to talk with him about anything."

Carlos looked pensive. "At the end of the day, him buying the business is not that important anymore; Mike's death means you inherit everything and, from what you say, there's over one million euros in his offshore account."

"True, but you know that legally I can't touch that money until probate is granted on his English Will, even if it's held in an offshore account."

Carlos approached Ann from behind and put his arms round her waist, squeezing her close to him. "As ever, you're right cielo, but I might need that money next week. Jorge says that someone else is seriously interested in the bar and so I have to confirm by this afternoon that I can go ahead. You've got the online login details so you could transfer some funds to your account in Gibraltar and then go and withdraw the cash next week. Nobody will be any the wiser and, anyway, the money does belong to you," he said, nuzzling her neck and moving his lips up to nibble her ear lobe.

Ann sighed and turned to face Carlos as he relaxed her grip. "It's something I'd rather not do but if Jorge is serious and you're prepared to put the effort in to make a go of it then tell him you can go ahead. Now leave me alone for a second while I call Andy with Chief Inspector Diaz's phone number. Then maybe we can skip lunch and have a siesta," she said, looking into his eyes with a knowing smile.

Carlos smiled back. This woman will do anything I want, he thought to himself, so long as I keep her happy; and that really isn't too difficult.

As Andy finished his beer the phone rang. "Hi Andy, here's Chief Inspector Diaz's number. He said he was going to Granada for the weekend so it's probably best to call him first thing Monday morning."

"Great, thanks Ann. I'll do that. Do you happen to have Johan Gaards' number handy? He was the last person to see Mike alive and I'd like to talk with him too."

"Yes, hang on a second – here it is." She gave Andy the number and then continued, "I don't think he can tell you anything I haven't told you but, if he does, let me know."

"I will."

"Oh, by the way, I almost forgot. I understand Mike was in the process of selling fifty percent of his business to you. Since I'll inherit the business, I was wondering whether you'd be interested in buying it lock, stock and barrel from me. I don't need to work and Carlos doesn't think estate agency and property management are his thing."

Andy was taken aback at the insensitivity of the request so soon after Mike's death. He knew Mike had intended to exclude the business from the divorce settlement, despite Ann's attempts to pressurise him into giving her a share of the sale proceeds, but, since the divorce had not been formalised, presumably Ann would now inherit everything.

"I don't know Ann. You're right, I had agreed to but into the business, but nothing's been signed and now I'm not sure it would make any sense for me to buy a business whose principal asset is no longer alive," he responded, managing to maintain an even tone.

"Well, give it some thought over the next few days and let me know."

"Will do Ann, but let's bury Mike first before you start selling his assets," Andy said hanging up.

Later that evening, Andy drove down the hill and almost the entire length of the beach to Casa Luque, which was located in La Caleta. He had known Luque since the summer he had met Mike and Luque had established the bar at the end of that summer in a beachfront unit which belonged to his father. Over the years it had evolved from a simple beer and tapas bar to a more sophisticated café-cum-restaurant serving brasserie-style food. As a result, it was very popular with the resident expats and out-of-town holidaymakers. However, eating was not compulsory and Andy had spent many a late night there knocking back the beers.

"Hombre, que tal?" said Luque, spotting Andy immediately as he walked in. "I haven't seen you since the summer and I guess you're here for all the wrong reasons."

"I'm afraid so. I was meant to be coming out next week but Ann called me yesterday with the news and here I am. I see you're busy," he said, surveying the restaurant. "Have you got a table for me and perhaps a little later we can catch up over a beer."

"Yes, the good weather has brought the usual crowd down from Granada and Jaen for the weekend but things will calm down in an hour or two. There's a table in the corner by the kitchen – not a great spot but, unless you want to wait a while, it's all I've got."

"No problem, at least it should be quiet – aside from the kitchen door flapping in my face every few seconds," replied Andy, smiling.

After ordering a Caesar salad and French omelette, Andy looked around the restaurant. The restaurant and outside terrace overlooking the beach were full with about twenty-five clients – Luque had space to handle more but didn't want or need the aggro.

The bar was semi-circular and was at the far end of the dining room. It was usually busy early evening and after eleven, when the diners had finished and the late-night drinking crowd moved in, but tonight Andy could see a group of four men at the bar talking animatedly. From where he was sitting he couldn't see them properly and could only catch snippets of the conversation when they raised their voices above the general din of the restaurant, but he thought he recognised Carlos as being one of the party. He'd never met him, but Mike had pointed him out once and he was sure it was him. By the looks and sound of him he was quite drunk.

An hour later, as the restaurant slowly began to empty, Luque pulled up a chair at Andy's table. "Finally, some breathing space! So, tell me Andy, what have you heard about Mike's death?"

Andy proceeded to tell Luque what Ann had told him that afternoon.

"Yes, that's the chain of events but until the autopsy is carried out we won't know for certain how drunk Mike was and whether he actually knocked himself out."

"You sound dubious, why?"

"Well, let's be honest, it's quite difficult to knock yourself out."

"I agree, but he was drunk and found under the table close to the source of the fire. Also, the door was locked from the inside so he must have been alone."

Luque cast a glance over his shoulder to ensure no one was within earshot and then, lowering his voice, said: "You probably don't know, but there is another door in the back office which Mike used as a storeroom and which is accessed via the garage at the rear of the building."

Andy looked at Luque in surprise, "You mean there's another way in and out of Mike's office? Ann didn't mention that to me."

"As I said, the door is in the storeroom and, to my knowledge, Mike never used it but I am sure he would have had a key to that door and to the garage."

"I assume the police are aware of this?"

"Yes, I mentioned it to Chief Inspector Diaz."

"And who owns the garage?"

"The family that owns El Boqueron. They use it as a storeroom and the youngest son, who is over there at the bar with that Carlos, sometimes stores his motorbike there," Luque said, turning his head in the direction of the bar.

Andy was perplexed. Why had Ann not mentioned the rear office door to him? Did she think it was not relevant? Of course, it was conceivable that she knew nothing about it. On the other hand, surely she had been in the storeroom at some point in the last few years and would have seen, or even used, the door. It was probably not important but he made a mental note to ask Chief Inspector Diaz whether it had any relevance, if he agreed to meet with him.

"Also, don't you think it's a little odd that the Policia Nacional have been given the case instead of the Guardia Civil? After all, the Civiles have jurisdiction in Los Cipreses and were first on the scene."

"Ann thinks it's because the Chief Inspector in charge speaks English but who knows, maybe there are some local rivalries involved or favours to be repaid – you know better than me what it's like here."

As the restaurant began to empty, the noise from the bar increased; it now looked as if Carlos and his friends were drinking vodka shots or something similar.

"Don't worry Miguel, I'm a rich man now and I've promised you that there'll be room for a man of your capabilities in my new venture. It's going to be the hottest bar in town, full of pussy and THE place to be seen," Carlos was shouting.

"Charming isn't he?" Luque said to Andy.

"I thought he was a waiter, so why is he saying he's rich and is going to open a bar?"

"It appears that he has suddenly come into some money but I bet he's sponging off Ann. Anyway, I'm going to ask him and his friends to leave before they get too carried away."

Before Luque could get up to ask Carlos to leave, Andy saw a smartly dressed woman, followed closely by two men, enter the restaurant. They stopped inside the doorway and began to talk. From their demeanour it was clear that she was controlling the conversation but she did so in a self-confident, rather than haughty or arrogant manner.

She was probably in her mid-thirties, of above average height, with shoulder-length ash blond hair and a slightly angular face. The black skirt of her well-tailored two-piece suit finished just above the knee and Andy could see that her calves and ankles were slim and she had what looked like an athletic figure under her suit. They finished their brief conversation and began walking towards the bar, steering away from the side where Carlos and his friends were standing. Luque got up and approached her.

"Good evening Cristina, can I help you?" asked Luque.

"Hello Luque, we were wondering whether you are still serving food," replied the woman in a firm and slightly husky voice.

"I'm afraid the kitchen closed ten minutes ago but I think El Boqueron may still be open. More traditional food I'm afraid, but food nonetheless."

"Yes darling, try El Boqueron. I'm well connected there so if you leave Tweedle Dee and Tweedle Dum behind and come with me I'll make sure you are well looked after – if you know what I mean," interrupted Carlos, lurching towards her.

"Thank you, but we don't need any help finding somewhere to eat and it seems to me that you're the one that needs looking after before you fall down and do yourself an injury."

"We've already had one of those accidents here earlier this week. Bit unfortunate really, but he probably had it coming. But don't you worry about me darling, I can look after myself. It's you that needs looking after."

"Ok Carlos, that's enough. You are very drunk, hassling my customers and insulting Mike Cameron, so please leave before, as the lady says, you find yourself in need of assistance. And don't bother to come back – you're not welcome here."

"Suit yourself Luque, this place is a shit-hole anyway – full of old fogies and snotty bitches like madam here. My new bar will be the place for the in-crowd to hang out, just you wait and see."

On that note, Carlos and his three cronies staggered off. One of them, a small wiry man with a pock-marked face, turned to Luque, "He's a bit boisterous tonight but it was a bit over the top to ban him, Luque. I'm sure you'll change your mind."

"Not a chance Miguel and, while I'm at it, the rest of you are banned as well. Good night."

Luque turned to Cristina, "I'm sorry about that. They're the unsavoury side of Los Cipreses but fortunately there aren't too many of them here, yet."

"Don't worry, I can look after myself. Thanks for the recommendation but I don't fancy beach-restaurant food so we'll pop up to the Old Town to see if La Cantinetta is still open."

As they turned and left the restaurant, Andy cast her an admiring glance. He hadn't managed to catch her eye during her exchanges with Carlos and Luque but he wished he hadn't eaten so he could go up to La Cantinetta, order a veal escalope and find an excuse to talk with her.

"Well, well, that was quite a little fracas. Tell me all about the beautiful Cristina."

"You don't miss a trick, do you? Yes, she is a bit special is our Cristina and you won't be the first, or the last, to fall for her."

"Ok, Ok, let's not get carried away. She's attractive and has a certain air about her, which is very unusual down here, so I assume she's from the city and down for the long weekend?"

"One out of two. Her name is Cristina Ibañez and she's from Madrid, but she arrived here a few weeks ago. She's the area manager for Samesa, one of Spain's biggest property developers. Her role is to buy land for development under the new PGOU."

Interesting, thought Andy to himself, I wonder if she's aware of the golf-course site; maybe we'll end up being competitors and, as they say, you should always keep close to your enemies and your competitors.

"Is she married?"

"Apparently she's recently divorced from some hot-shot lawyer in Madrid and is in no mood for dalliances. Believe me, a number of people have been making a bee line for her office on the pretext of having land for sale and most have been shown the door rather rapidly."

"What about her two companions?"

"They work for her. Samesa already have approval for a two hundred and fifty unit development the other side of Cerro Grande, overlooking the protected nature reserve. Jose Luis is the Project Manager and Paco the Sales Manager for that development."

"Well, she's a very attractive lady and I'm sure that she is used to being pestered, including by lowlifes like Carlos. Tell me, is he always so obnoxious?" asked Andy, as he took a sip from the Lepanto brandy Luque had poured him a little earlier.

"As far as I can tell, aside from his supposedly classic Andalusian looks, there is nothing remotely appealing or attractive about him and I don't know what Ann sees in him – youth and energy I assume," he said with a shrug. "He's been in Los Cipreses for about a year and has already broken up Mike's marriage and fallen in with a bad crowd."

"You mean the three musketeers?"

"Yes. Miguel's a nasty piece of work and I have it on good authority that he's mixed up in drugs. The other two are never far from him. As I said, one of the others, Alvaro, is the youngest son of the owner of El Boqueron and he has a fancy Harley Davidson, while Miguel and Paco drive smart cars. None of them have any visible means of support other than working in El Boqueron from time to time."

It was now half-past eleven and Andy was feeling tired after a very long day which had started at four o'clock in the morning in London. He had a lot to think about before trying to arrange a meeting with Chief Inspector Diaz. As for Ms. Ibañez, he was sorely tempted to pop up to La Cantinetta for a night cap, but it was late and hopefully he'd have plenty of time to get to know her better.

"Things certainly seem to be getting more interesting in Los Cipreses these days; I'd like to know where Carlos is getting his new-found wealth from. Anyway, I must be off, it's been a long day and I can't handle hangovers like I used to! I'll catch you again in the next day or two," and he left, just as a few late-night revellers walked into the bar.

Saturday, 17th November

The next day Andy awoke at ten. After showering and dressing, he called Maria Salcedo. He hoped that her mobile number had not changed and that she would agree to meet him for lunch.

"Diga?" said a woman's voice.

"Hi Maria, this is Andy Montalvo, remember me?"

"Hmm, let me think. Are you the Andy Montalvo who works for a major investment bank, lives in London and occasionally spends long weekends in Los Cipreses?"

"Spot on, as usual, but no longer working for a bank and planning on spending a lot longer in Los Cipreses. Actually, I'm here at the moment and I was hoping that you're free for lunch."

"That's a bit forward for someone I haven't seen or spoken to for over three years, but I suppose I might be able to find a slot sometime next week," she replied teasingly.

"Ah, ever the tease and I can't wait that long to see you. I was thinking of tomorrow, say at El Asador?" El Asador was run by an Argentinean immigrant who sourced the beef from his home country. As such, the quality of the meat was fantastic and the wine list comprehensive, and it had been one of their favourite restaurants when they'd been dating.

"You know that El Asador is one of my favourite restaurants so that's very tempting. Ok, let me see, today I'm having a lazy day on the beach followed by some late night shopping, so a long lunch tomorrow afternoon sounds like the perfect way to end the weekend."

"Great, you've made my weekend. I'll see you there at half past two. It's been too long and I look forward to catching up."

"Me too. You'd better book though as it may be busy."

She's a character, thought Andy. Feisty and fiery, but with a sharp intelligence and a warm heart under what appeared to be a haughty exterior. It could have been a serious relationship, but long distances and long periods of time apart always made things difficult and, in the end, it had petered out, both of them wanting more but realising it was a no-win situation.

They had not been in touch for over two years but the old rapport still seemed to be there, at least on the phone. Nevertheless, he wasn't seriously thinking of reinitiating a relationship with her, assuming of course she was available and interested. In fact, he rather hoped that he might get an opportunity to get to know Cristina Ibañez better. However, right now, his priority was to see if Maria could give him any information about the ownership of plots on the potential golf course sites.

He then called Emily to see how she was. She sounded tired and upset so they agreed to have lunch at his place on Monday. Next he dialled Johan Gaards' number and left a message asking Johan to call him.

Ann had driven down to the town at half past nine leaving Carlos in bed to catch up on his sleep after another late night in El Boqueron. The fine weather had attracted large numbers of weekend visitors and, as a result, she eventually got home at eleven.

To her surprise, Carlos was sitting on one of the wicker chairs on the terrace smoking a cigarette with a cup of coffee on the table at his side. The rising sun shone directly on to the terrace and Carlos was wearing nothing but the figure hugging boxers he had gone to bed in.

"Buenos dias cariño. I see you've been for the newspapers. Did you bring Ideal?"

"Of course. You can read it while you finish your coffee, but why don't you make yourself decent in case Emily wakes up while I go and make breakfast."

"That sounds good, I'm starving," said Carlos, rising from the chair and putting out his cigarette in the ashtray. "Can you make me some bacon and eggs? It's one of the few English meals I love."

"Actually, you're not working until this evening and Emily is going to Granada today, so we're having a steak and a salad for lunch. Why don't you have a bowl of cereal or a tostada instead?"

"Cereal is for wimps so it'll have to be a tostada – with olive oil and tomato."

"Alright, but go and put on a pair of swimming trunks and a T-shirt before Emily makes an appearance."

"You don't think she actually cares what I look like or even what I do, do you?"

"Don't be silly, darling. Emily may not be too happy about my leaving her father for you but in her heart of hearts she knows the relationship was over. I'm sure she'll come to accept you in due course; it just may take a little time, and Mike's death will not be helping."

Carlos shrugged his shoulders. "I don't think she'll ever accept me."

As Carlos walked off towards the bedroom Ann placed the Daily Mail and Ideal on the table and then went to make breakfast.

A few minutes later they were seated at the table eating their breakfast when Carlos read the headline on the front page of Ideal: "Guardia Civil break up major drug-smuggling ring" The article went on to describe how the special UCO unit of the Civil Guard had dismantled a leading cocaine smuggling ring based in Andalucia. The drugs were dropped off the Spanish coast by fishing boats which in turn had been supplied out at sea by fast motor launches based in Morocco, although the drugs originated from South America. Apparently they had seized over four tonnes of cocaine in Malaga and Seville and prevented further drops of eighteen tonnes.

That should help take the pressure off us tonight, he thought to himself.

Emily finally emerged from her room at half-past twelve, giving a polite good morning to her mother but studiously ignoring Carlos. She left for Granada forty-five minutes later, taking Ann's car. "I'm not sure what time I'll be back but I might just stay at Jaime's if we have a few drinks or it gets late. I'll call you later and let you know my plans," she said, disappearing through the front door.

With the controversial Los Cipreses PGOU being so close to approval, Javier Urquiza knew full well that he could not be seen in public with Vicente, Enrique and Fernando. Neither could he afford for Enrique or Fernando to be seen entering or leaving his villa, which was why the meeting was taking place on his Rodman 41 motor yacht.

He had bought her last year and she was a beauty. At forty feet with three cabins, a large lounge area below decks, a good size bathing platform and a range of just over two hundred miles cruising at thirty knots, she was perfect for day cruises along the coast as well as longer trips across to Africa or even the Balearics.

He left the marina with Vicente Maldonado and Johan Gaards on board, and drove the Rodman across Los Cipreses bay, round the Cerro Grande headland to Tesoro beach, where they anchored two hundred metres offshore. It was a small but busy beach with three restaurants, the most famous of which was Las Maravillas, and Javier Urquiza was a regular visitor. At one-thirty Johan collected two people from the beach in the tender. They all gathered in the main cabin where Javier Urquiza addressed them:

"Gentlemen, welcome aboard and thank you for coming at such short notice. I realise that you're looking forward to a long, lazy lunch so I'll try to be brief.

As you know, Mike Cameron recently provided me with references on the potential investors. These are acceptable but, unfortunately, he died in an accident two days ago – before he could arrange a meeting with them to discuss the terms of the deal in more detail.

The silver lining is that, as we have the references, we now know who the lawyer representing the investors is and Vicente is meeting him in London on Tuesday to see if they'll agree to pay a five million euro deposit in return for exclusive negotiating rights."

Johan regarded Vicente Maldonado, who was standing to the right of, and slightly behind, Javier Urquiza, with a gin and tonic in one hand. He was in his late forties, tall and slim. His hair was a little long for a lawyer and, combined with his tan and neatly trimmed beard, gave him the appearance of a fading Latin rock star.

He then looked across at Enrique Gonzalez and Fernando Echevaria. Both were seated on the main sofa directly in front of the wet bar and were listening to Don Javier attentively. Johan was familiar with Enrique since, as the Urban Planning Officer for Los

Cipreses he was often out and about in the municipality. In addition, in recent months he had, together with the Mayor, been appearing much more frequently in newspapers and on television, as the proposed new PGOU was debated.

Fernando Echevaria was based in Seville and, aside from the traditional holiday month in August and the odd bank holiday weekend, rarely came to Los Cipreses. But, as chairman of the Junta's Environmental Planning Committee, and a member of the Urban Planning Committee, he was a vital key to the reclassification of the land for use as a golf course and residential housing project.

Johan felt no loyalty or true friendship towards any of them, or anyone else for that matter. He had realised many years ago that he was a loner with poor social skills and no interest in developing close relationships with anyone, except where money was involved. Nevertheless, he had come to respect Vicente Maldonado as he'd seen how he had helped Don Javier develop his business interests and manage his finances. He'd come to respect him even more when Vicente had suggested a way in which he could benefit substantially if Project Pulpo went ahead.

Fernando cleared his throat. "Don Javier, are you satisfied that there is no risk of both us, and the site in question, being identified?"

Javier Urquiza took a draw from the Monte Cristo No. 4 cigar in his right hand. He was stocky and slightly overweight, but powerfully built. He was wearing a short-sleeved pale yellow linen shirt with navy blue shorts and deck shoes – very much the picture of a successful businessman relaxing on his yacht, but his jovial manner belied the sense of power his presence gave.

"Yes, Vicente's already agreed the terms of a confidentiality agreement and, as far as the investors are concerned, he's acting as the legal representative of the unnamed principals, not as one of the principals.

Also, as you know, the options over the land are owned via companies registered in Belize and the Seychelles, which guarantees anonymity. That's right, isn't it Vicente?"

Vicente Maldonado had been listening to this exchange with interest. Through a combination of hard work, ruthlessness and cultivating the right relationships, he had finally reached the position where, if all went according to plan, he would become very, very rich – to the tune of twelve and a half million euros, or significantly more, if his discussions with Fernando and Johan came to fruition.

It was therefore in his interests to make Project Pulpo happen and to keep the identity of the principals involved secret. He stepped forward and drew level with Javier Urquiza.

"Yes, the way we're going to sell the options makes it virtually impossible for these people to identify any of us as the principals behind the transaction. Our main problem is timing – as you know, we must complete the deal before the first of January when the new legislation requiring Notaries to advise the authorities of any transactions done by companies in offshore jurisdictions comes into effect.

We also need to pay our friends on the Environmental Planning and Urban Planning Committees their fees, so the reservation deposit must be paid as soon as possible."

"On what basis are you asking them to pay the five million euros?"

"The same as we discussed last month, Enrique. The deposit will be held in an escrow account controlled by an independent trustee agreed between the parties. The funds will be released to us in three stages:

One million euros if, after reviewing the option agreements, the underlying title deeds and the feasibility and environmental studies, the investors wish to proceed to the next stage.

Another two million against a copy the Environmental Planning Committee's recommendation of the site to the Urban Planning Committee and the final two million upon approval of the PGOU by the Urban Planning Committee."

"The Environmental Planning Committee meeting is scheduled for the tenth of December so we'll need the first million to be released to us a few days before then," Fernando interjected.

"I know, and that's easily achievable, but clearly my meeting on Tuesday is vital and if they agree to our terms I have drafts of all the relevant agreements drawn up ready to give them."

Fernando reached over to the table in front of him and took a bottle of mineral water. "Don Javier, is the asking price the same as we discussed in September?"

"Yes, there's no change as far as I am concerned, it's still two hundred and fifty million euros."

"And the percentages for each us?"

Javier Urquiza took another puff of his Monte Cristo cigar. "The same as we agreed in August, that is to say: eighty-five percent for me and five percent each for the three of you. Given the risks involved and that I've funded the entire project, I think this is a more than fair distribution of the proceeds. Wouldn't you agree?"

Enrique Gonzalez was finding it hard to keep the smile from his face at the thought of a twelve and a half million euros payout. He knew that he would have to share two and a half million of this with the Mayor once the deal had gone through, but ten million euros was more than enough to retire on in Argentina, he thought.

"I think the returns justify the risks," Enrique replied, with a broad smile on his face.

"Well, some of us are taking more risks than others but I suppose I can't complain," said Fernando, glancing sideways at Enrique, whom he considered to be a country bumpkin who happened to be in the right place at the right time. Still, he thought, if his own discussions with Vicente came to fruition then he'd be getting a much larger slice of the pie.

"Good, it looks as if we are in agreement; let's hope Vicente can persuade the investors to go to the next stage. Thank you Fernando and Enrique, we'll be in touch via the usual channel as soon as we have some news. In the meantime, go and enjoy your lunch."

He turned to Johan Gaards. "Johan, please drop Señor Gonzalez and Señor Echevaria on the beach and then join me below."

After Emily left, Ann began to prepare lunch. Carlos was sitting by the pool on a sun lounger listening to music on the iPod which Ann had bought him.

"Carlos, put a T-shirt on and come to lunch," Ann shouted. Carlos continued with his eyes closed and tapping his feet.

Ann marched over and prodded him. "Come on. Lunch is almost ready."

Carlos jumped up startled. "Ok, Ok, but you nearly gave me a heart attack."

"Don't exaggerate. I wish I'd never bought you that thing, you spend more time with it than with me when we are alone."

"That's not true sweetheart and if you have any complaints about my attention to you then please make them at the appropriate time and in the appropriate location," said Carlos with a wink.

As he tucked into his rare steak, Carlos looked at Ann. "Cielo, Jorge wants me to sign the deeds for the bar this week so can you transfer the money to your Gibraltar account this weekend? In fact, if you make it one hundred and seventy-five thousand that will cover taxes and notary fees and leave a little for some minor reforms and publicity before reopening."

"Carlos, you know I'd rather not do that until probate is granted and we don't even have Mike's Will yet or his death certificate. Do you need to complete the purchase this week? Can't it wait a week or two?"

"I'm afraid not. Jorge is adamant that if I don't complete by Friday he'll sell it to someone else that same day. In fact, he's already booked the notary for Friday midday."

"Alright, but we have a slight problem."

"What do you mean a problem?" asked Carlos, a look of concern on his face.

"Well firstly, we had agreed one hundred and fifty thousand not one hundred and seventy-five, but in any case the maximum that can be transferred out of the account in any thirty-day period is one hundred and twenty-five thousand euros, so this is all I can withdraw at the moment."

For Ann, it was an unexpected restriction which limited her ability to access all of Mike's funds instantly and one she intended to renegotiate with the bank as soon as probate had been granted. Not that Carlos needed to know that.

"Can't you raise the fifty thousand from somewhere else? I mean don't you have cash or savings in a bank account in Spain?"

"No Carlos, I can't get my hands on that sort of money. Maybe five or ten thousand at most if I use my credit cards and talk with my bank manager."

Carlos stood up and started pacing agitatedly. The frown on his face created deep furrows around his forehead and nose, giving him a dark and sinister look.

"If you can raise ten thousand euros I can probably raise another thirty thousand from friends, which should just about cover the purchase price and the costs. I'll have to make a few calls but in the meantime transfer the hundred and twenty-five thousand to your account. I'll confirm to Jorge that we can sign on Thursday just to keep him sweet, and I'll take Wednesday off so we can go to Gibraltar and collect the cash."

Ann sighed resignedly. "Yes, I suppose so but I hope you know what you are doing."

"Don't worry my love. This is going to be the hottest bar in town." As well as a cover for my new activities, he thought to himself. "By the way, I'm going for a dive first thing tomorrow morning with Johan."

"Oh, you know how much I love our Sunday lie-ins," said Ann, with a disappointed look on her face "but I suppose we could make up for it now with a little siesta," she continued, taking Carlos' hand and leading him towards the bedroom.

"What did you make of that, Vicente?" Javier Urquiza said as the tender with Enrique and Fernando headed for the beach.

"Everything went as planned. In reality, Mr. Cameron's unfortunate accident is what allows us to progress the transaction but there was no need for them to know that."

"Precisely, and they're already committed. Anyway, they both stand to make very tidy sums so why bother them with details that no longer matter. Talking of which, are the three million euros ready to be transferred to the Galician if the goods are delivered tonight?"

"Yes. Just let me know when you want me to make the transfer."

Ten minutes later, Johan returned and clambered down into the cabin after tying up the tender.

"They're back on dry land, safe and sound," he said. "Do you want me to take us back to the marina?"

"No, that won't be necessary. Vicente is driving us back while you and I go through the details of tonight's operation."

Andy had arranged to meet Sonya at four at the Isla de Ibiza café on the La Caleta beachfront. The Isla comprised a small indoor unit where the coffee and food were prepared and a large exterior terrace which ran parallel to the beach road. Sonya was sitting at one of the round plastic tables in a corner of the terrace furthest from the entrance.

She looked up and saw him approaching. "Hi Sonya, sorry I'm late but I had to park a bit further away than normal."

"Yes, it's busy this weekend but by four o'clock tomorrow it will be like a ghost town."

"So how are you?" asked Andy giving her a kiss on both cheeks. She was petite, with short blond hair, blue eyes and a kind, uncomplicated face. He had seen her around over the years, but he had only met her twice since she and Mike had become an item. Nevertheless, she struck him as being a sincere and down-to-earth person.

"I'm Ok, thanks Andy. It's been a terrible shock and I miss Mike dreadfully already. I'm still not sure what it all means and as soon as the funeral's out of the way I think I'll disappear to the States for a while. You know I have family there."

"I understand and I'm sure everything will work out for the best."

Maria, one of the regular waitresses, hovered around the table pad in hand with a bored look on her face. Some things don't change, thought Andy.

"A peppermint tea, please Maria," said Sonya. "I'll have a fresh orange juice," added Andy. Maria nodded, scribbled on her pad and wandered off nonchalantly towards the counter.

"Sonya, Ann and Luque have told me what happened. I know it may be a strange question, but do you think there was anything suspicious about Mike's death? I mean, to your knowledge did he have any enemies, was he involved in anything unusual, had he mentioned anything to you that was worrying him?"

"No, I don't think his death was suspicious. Of course, there were people that he didn't get on with, but not that many, and certainly no one that he considered an enemy in the true sense of the word. He was involved in a number of projects, after all it was part of his job, but the only thing of any significance that I knew he was working on was selling some of the business to you. He was quite excited about that and said that you already had a potential deal in the pipeline."

"It was Mike's deal really," said Andy "but yes, we were trying to put something together. Did he tell you anything about it?"

"No, just a passing reference. He was very discreet about his work, except of course where some of his property management clients were involved. He thought most of them were tight-fisted whingers who expected him to jump to it at the drop of a hat."

Andy thought about this for a moment. Mike had only been with Sonya for a few months and had told Andy that he was sworn to secrecy about the identity of Mr. Brown, so it was highly unlikely that he would have disclosed anything of relevance about the potential transaction to her.

"What about his relationship with Ann and Carlos?"

Sonya considered this for a moment. "His relationship with Ann was reasonably amicable until she started asking for more money as part of the divorce settlement. Then they had a few heated discussions, but he put it all down to Carlos."

"And did he and Carlos argue or threaten each other?"

"Not that I am aware of. They tried to steer clear of each other but it's a small town and it's more than likely they crossed paths. If they did, I'd be surprised if Mike didn't have a go at Carlos, he couldn't stand him, but he never mentioned anything to me."

Andy nodded. "Don't you think it was unusual that Mike had locked the door from the inside? "In my experience, when Mike worked late or returned to the office after a few drinks, he always left the door open, as people were in the habit of popping in if they saw him in the office. He couldn't stand having to get up and open the door."

"That's true. I often put my head round the door to drag him away from the office but he had been getting more security conscious in recent months. In fact, he recently had the door and lock replaced with much stronger versions, and maybe that contributed to his death – if Johan had been able to open the door sooner then Mike might still be alive."

Her voice began to break up and Sonya took a tissue from her bag and wiped the tears from her eyes. "I'll be alright, just give me a minute," she replied, as Maria placed their drinks on the table and sauntered off.

They sat in silence for few minutes sipping their drinks and watching the beach slowly empty of people as the temperature dropped and the light began to fade.

"So what are your plans now Andy?" she asked, her voice back to normal.

"I'm going to stay in Los Cipreses for the autopsy result and Mike's funeral. Then I'll decide whether I want to take over Mike's business – I'm not sure if I can, or even want to do it without him. In the meantime, I know Mike was extremely fond of you so if there is anything I can do then let me know."

"That's very kind of you. Mike had a tremendous respect for you so don't worry I'll be knocking at your door the minute I need your help."

"Good, promise me you'll do that," said Andy covering her hand with his and squeezing it. After a few minutes, Andy caught Maria's attention and signalled for the bill. "That should take at least ten minutes," he joked, trying to lighten Sonya's mood.

When Maria arrived with the bill, Andy handed her a ten-euro note before she could wander off, then rose to leave. "Don't forget to call me if you need anything," he said, giving Sonya another hug.

Back home, Andy put on his Young Chet CD and settled down on the sofa with *A Short History of Nearly Everything* by Bill Bryson. Bryson was one of his favourite authors, combining astute observations with a wry, and sometimes hilarious, sense of humour. Later that evening, after cooking himself supper he showered, put on some jeans and a jumper and by eleven he was in Casa Luque enjoying a beer and chatting to a couple of acquaintances.

It was busy but by half past midnight the restaurant was virtually empty while the crowd in the bar area had thinned. "Fancy a beer at La Cabaña? The Free Soul Band are playing and they were great in the summer," Luque asked Andy.

On a Saturday night, for those aged over twenty-five, there was really only one place to go: La Cabaña, down on the beach front close to the Cutty Sark. It was a long-established feature of Los Cipreses and was renowned for its funky style, mixed crowd and variety of live music acts at the weekends. Nevertheless, this being southern Spain, the action started after midnight and really only got going after one. It was not uncommon for the place still to be buzzing at three-thirty in the morning, and even later in the summer months.

"Good idea, I caught them one night in August and they're certainly one of the better bands."

"Great. I'll leave Diana and Pepe to close up."

The main bar area of La Cabaña was crowded and Andy struggled to the bar and ordered a rum and coke for Luque and a beer for himself. The club consisted of an L-shaped bar with a large garden terrace at the back. The Free Soul Band were warming up in the corner close to the entrance and the expectant crowd forced Andy and Luque to stand at the top end of the bar, close to the garden terrace.

"At least we won't get jostled so much here," remarked Andy "and we'll still be able to hear the band."

"We'd be able to hear them from the Punta de Palermo," Luque shouted, as they launched into their first number. As the band worked through their repertoire, some covers and some original songs, the crowd became livelier, dancing and singing along.

Andy and Luque stood watching and listening, receiving the odd push and shove as the crowd swayed and moved with the music or as people made their way to and from the garden terrace.

Suddenly Carlos, Miguel and Alvaro emerged from the crowd and stood against the bar a few feet in front of them. They did not appear to see Andy and Luque and had their backs turned to them as they watched the band. About five minutes later the Free Soul Band wound up their first session and the loud music was replaced by the hubbub of the crowd.

"Thank God for that," said Carlos to his mates "give me decent flamenco anytime."

"But it seems to be popular," said pock-faced Miguel.

"You're right, but look at the people it attracts. My bar is going to be for the younger, trendy crowd who want to see and be seen, just wait and see."

"So when are you signing the deeds?" asked Alvaro.

"On Thursday, although I need to ask our friend Mr. Gaards for a little extra cash to cover taxes and expenses. I think he has plenty and, anyway, I'll be able to repay him in a month. I'll have a word with him tomorrow after we finish moving the goods."

Andy looked at Luque inquisitively and then gestured in the direction of the door. Luque nodded in agreement and they managed to leave without attracting the attention of Carlos and his friends. "So our friend is a little short of cash after all and is going to approach Johan Gaards," Andy said once they were outside. "Did you know that Carlos knew Johan and that he is doing some work for him?"

"No I didn't, but it is a small town and it appears that they have some mutual friends so it's not surprising."

"I suppose not. I wonder what goods they are moving tomorrow; after all it is a Sunday."

"Best left alone," said Luque as he got into his car. "Pop in for lunch tomorrow if you fancy – my treat."

"Thanks, but actually I'm having lunch with Maria Salcedo."

"You don't waste any time do you. Not sure if her new boyfriend will be impressed though, apparently he's the jealous type."

"Maria was never bothered by jealousy, that's one of the things I liked about her," replied Andy.

Johan Gaards' apartment was located in a quiet part of the Las Gaviotas urbanization on Cerro Grande and was surrounded by mature landscaped gardens. Being on the top floor, it had excellent views across the bay of Los Cipreses and was not overlooked. In short, it was secluded, well located and with a clear line of sight across the bay to the Punta de Palermo and out to sea and, as such, was ideal for his work for Don Javier.

As Andy and Luque left La Cabaña, he surveyed the bay from his terrace using his powerful 10 X 15 binoculars. His Mac sat open on the table by his side, connected, via WiFi, to the Internet.

He rued the fact that it was clear night with not a cloud in the sky. Both visibility and ambient light were very good, too good, so if anyone else was monitoring the bay they would see exactly what he saw, provided, of course, they looked in the right place at the right time.

They preferred to make the drops on nights with a new moon and, ideally, with cloud cover – although the latter was down to luck.

Unfortunately, this drop had been forced on them prematurely by the Guardia's recent successful operation against the cocaine smuggling ring as Don Javier and his suppliers thought they would not be expecting another major drop so soon after that operation.

At three he looked at the far end of the bay through his binoculars and focused on the three fishing boats just inside the lee of the Punta de Palermo. They were about fifty metres apart and, along with their navigation lights, each had a series of bright lights focused on the sea to attract fish. He could make out the chugging of their engines as two of them moved virtually imperceptibly towards him.

Johan focused on the stationary fishing boat nearest the Punta de Palermo. He saw the flare of a match and then a cigarette being lit. This was rapidly extinguished as it was thrown overboard but another cigarette was re-lit almost immediately. Again the cigarette was thrown overboard and then another one a minute later. They were in position and ready.

Johan turned to the Mac, placed the cursor over the green Skype button and clicked on it to dial a pre-selected Spanish mobile number. "All systems go," he said when the call was answered, and then hung up, although no one at the other end had spoken.

Almost immediately, there was the roar of a large, powerful engine from Johan's right. He swung round almost one hundred and eighty degrees and trained his binoculars just beyond the headland of Cerro Grande and caught sight of a fast-moving, low-slung shape in the water. It was a sleek power launch of the type used by drug smugglers. The power launch raced around the tip of Cerro Grande into the bay and headed directly towards the beach, staying parallel to the headland. Perfect, thought Johan, that will attract the attention of the Guardia if they're watching.

He turned his binoculars back to the fishing boat which had been the subject of his attention moments earlier. On the boat he could make out two or three people moving on the deck and manhandling a number of large objects towards the edge of the deck. As the power launch on the other side of the bay slowed down to a crawl they began to throw the objects overboard.

After a couple of minutes the power launch suddenly accelerated, did a sharp U-turn, and roared out back towards the open sea. If the Guardia stopped it in one of their high powered ribs they would find some well-to-do gents from El Castillo entertaining a couple of impressionable young ladies with champagne and speed.

As the launch disappeared round the Cerro Grande headland Johan could see that the men on the fishing boat had finished throwing the objects overboard. The rhythm and volume of the chugging of the engine increased as the boat slowly moved away from the spot where it had been for the last few minutes.

"It's going to be another long night but it'll be worth it," Johan said to himself, as he thought of the hundred thousand euros he would make from this drop alone – fifty percent payable once they had moved the hashish from its current location to the secret compartments in his catamaran and fifty percent once the distributors had taken delivery. Miguel would be rewarded with a total of twenty five grand but Carlos would only receive five thousand as this was his first operation.

He zipped up his polar fleece and settled into his chair to monitor the drop site until daylight just in case any boats approached it. Assuming the coast was clear, at nine o'clock in the morning he, Miguel and Carlos would take out a rib dive boat to the site and recover the packages under the cover of an early morning dive. They would hang the packages from cables attached to the bottom of the rib and then slowly make their way across the bay close to where his catamaran was moored. Then, while ostensibly undertaking a second, shallow water dive in the lee of Cerro Grande, they would transfer the packages to the secret compartments in the twin hulls of the catamaran.

At the merest sign of trouble or of another genuine early morning diving expedition coming close, they would jettison the packages knowing that, unless they were caught red-handed with them, the Guardia Civil could do nothing. It would put an end to future drops, but then as far as he was concerned these would be unnecessary if Project Pulpo went through and his agreement with Vicente and Fernando came to fruition.

In truth, the biggest risk was if the packages were found in the catamaran, but they should all have been dispersed by the middle of the week. In any event, he could always activate the remote-controlled ejection system at any hint of a raid from the Civiles.

Sunday, 18th November

It took Johan Gaards, Miguel and Carlos over three hours to complete the transfer of the waterproof packages containing the hashish to the catamaran. The transfer had gone without incident and now they were propping up the bar in El Burro celebrating.

El Burro was tucked away in a side street in the Old Town and was a haunt of locals. Enrique, the owner, was a large, scruffy-looking individual with permanent dark stubble which refused to develop into a full beard. He had a toothpick permanently in his mouth that he moved constantly from one side to the other, somehow managing to avoid the large gap in the middle of his bottom row of teeth.

Enrique was a local and had been running El Burro for over thirty-five years. Very little local business escaped his notice and he was well aware of Johan Gaards' activities. He had very strong suspicions about who was the brain behind the operation but, even if he could prove it, as far as he was concerned it was none of his business.

"Well, how was it for you, Carlos?" Johan asked, taking a swig from his bottle of Alhambra 1925 Special.

"The first time is always special and I'm looking forward to many more. By the way, when do I get paid?"

"Don't worry. You'll get what we agreed before you leave this bar, with the balance by the end of the week."

"I appreciate that Johan but I was wondering if I could ask you for a favour. Can we have a chat in private?" Carlos said, inclining his head towards the door.

"Are you sure you don't want to ask him into the gents instead," said Enrique in a voice so loud everyone in the bar could hear.

Carlos gave Enrique a withering look. "I thought that was reserved for you and your boys."

"Now, now, children, let's not squabble," Johan said, as he led Carlos outside. The street was empty and they stopped on the pavement a few yards from El Burro.

"Carlos, it's best not to cross Enrique; be careful what you say to him. He was only joking."

"Ok, Ok, but I don't like his sense of humour."

"You'd better get used to it if you are going to frequent his bar. So what's this favour?"

"I don't know if you know, but I've agreed to buy Bar Salamander from Jorge. I'm meant to be completing on Thursday and, although I've got most of the money, I need an extra forty thousand euros. I'll have this in thirty days so I was wondering if you could lend me the money until then."

"That's not an insignificant sum of money. I assume you want it in cash?"

"Yes, you know how it works here and, given what we've done today, I'm sure this won't be a problem for you."

Johan's eyes narrowed and he barely concealed his anger as he fixed his gaze on Carlos. "Listen Carlos, let me make one thing clear. Today's business has nothing to do with any other business that we may or may not do together and I don't want it mentioned again," he said in a low voice and hard tone. "Now, going back to your cashflow problem. Assuming I'm willing to do this, what's in it for me?"

"It is only for a month so I was thinking that I'd pay you back forty-two and a half thousand. That's a healthy return for a thirty-day loan."

Johan considered this. "Let's call it forty five thousand. How does that sound?"

"A bit expensive to me, especially as I know I can get the money in thirty days," Carlos responded.

"Fine. Take it or leave it."

Carlos bit his lip, a look of concentration on his face. "Ok, I'll take it."

"Good. Let's meet here tomorrow afternoon and I'll bring the money."

"Ok, thanks. Now I must get back to Ann's for lunch. Please give my apologies to Enrique."

"I think you can do that yourself the next time you see him. See you tomorrow," said Johan as he turned and walked back into El Burro.

When Carlos arrived home he found Ann curled up on the sofa reading the Sunday Express. Emily was nowhere in sight and Carlos assumed that she had not returned from Granada. He was relieved; the last thing he needed was the stuck-up little bitch souring the atmosphere, especially as he needed to remind Ann to transfer the balance of the money he needed to her account in Gibraltar, if she hadn't done so already.

"Hola, I'm sorry I'm late but I went for a beer and tapas with the boys after the dive."

"Well, I hope you're not expecting any lunch," retorted Ann, without looking up from the newspaper.

"Don't worry, we had some tapas so I'm not hungry. I'll have a sandwich later. How was your morning?"

"Lazy. I got up late, popped into town for the paper and, after tidying up a bit, I haven't really moved from the sofa."

Carlos sat down at the end of the sofa and started to stroke Ann's bare feet. "Well I've got some good news. I've borrowed forty thousand euros from a friend, but on the condition that I pay forty-five thousand back in thirty days."

"Some friend," said Ann "five thousand euros interest for a thirty-day loan."

"Ok, Ok, but it's difficult to get your hands on that sort of money at such short notice. Since you'll be transferring more money to your account in thirty days, it seemed like the best thing to do. Talking of which, have you transferred the one hundred and twenty-five thousand to your Gibraltar account?"

"No, I'll do it later this afternoon. I also need to make an appointment to see Jonathan Westwood of Fernandez & Fernandez in Marbella to discuss Mike's Wills. Mike used them for personal matters so they should have his Wills."

Carlos' hands moved slowly up Ann's legs, gently rubbing and stroking her calves and thighs. Ann closed her eyes "You can keep doing that all day," she moaned.

"I will, but not here," Carlos whispered in her ear, taking her by the hand and leading her towards the bedroom.

Andy arrived at El Asador at twenty past two. It was a large open-plan restaurant but divided into two distinct dining areas, one a large rectangular room, whose longest side ran along the beach front pavement, and the other, a smaller room directly behind it. The front room was enclosed by large windows with access via sliding glass doors which opened directly on to the pavement. Andy entered the rear room by a wooden door in the side street.

Maria's job at the notary meant she might be able to shed light on which of the golf course sites Mike had been dealing with and who Mr. Brown was so he asked the owner to swap the table he'd been allocated for one in the corner where they could talk with less danger of being overheard.

Andy ordered a mineral water, as well as a bottle of wine from the extensive Argentinean wine list, asking the waiter to open the bottle and leave it on the table. Although Maria had said half past two, based on past experience, he really didn't expect her to turn up before quarter to three at the earliest so, as he waited, he surveyed the restaurant.

From his vantage point he could see that most of the tables in the front dining area were laid out for groups of six or more, while those in the rear room were set up for foursomes or couples. The large windows flooded the front room with natural light but being set further back the rear room had a few strategically placed wall lamps to provide additional lighting.

A few of the tables in the front room were already occupied by groups of families and friends, and over the next few minutes several more groups arrived, noisily taking their places after the usual discussion and debate as to who should sit where. In the rear dining area Andy was alone until two young couples arrived and were seated at separate tables in front of him. As the restaurant came to life, the smell of grilled meats slowly began to permeate from the kitchen.

After twenty minutes he resisted the temptation to try the wine and ordered another mineral water instead. He knew that by three o'clock El Asador would be virtually full and very noisy, which suited him perfectly. At ten to three, he saw Maria enter via the sliding glass doors. He got up, raising a hand to attract her attention. After a few seconds she saw him and made her way over to the table, turning a few heads as she passed through the restaurant.

Her long black hair hung loose over a charcoal grey pashmina, under which she was wearing a three-quarter length sleeveless black wool dress. Her high cheek bones and olive skin set off her dark almond-shaped eyes perfectly, while her sensuous lips were accentuated by crimson lipstick.

"You look as stunning as ever," he greeted her, kissing her on both cheeks.

"Ever the charmer, Señor Montalvo. Actually, I'm three years older and five kilos heavier."

"You could have fooled me. You look exactly the same as the last time I saw you."

"Oh, shut up and order me the usual," she said, laughing.

They sat down and Andy beckoned the waitress over and ordered a red Martini. They chatted for a while, briefly filling each other in on their respective lives over the last two years. Andy explained that he had just left the City of London Police serious fraud squad and had been planning on buying into Mike's business.

"So I'd probably have been yet another estate agent hassling you for special treatment at the notary," he said smiling. "Unfortunately, Mike's death is making me reassess my plans."

"Yes, it's terrible what happened to Mike. I only knew him professionally but he was highly respected. He was always a pleasure to deal with and it's a shame there aren't more people around here with the same degree of professionalism. I'm afraid it's only been getting worse – the proposed new PGOU means that every Tom, Dick and Harry is trying to get a piece of the action."

"Actually, that's something I wanted to talk to you about, but let's order first."

They decided to skip starters and for her main course Maria chose grilled fillet steak while Andy went for the sirloin steak. As an accompaniment they agreed to share the ubiquitous "tropical" salad which was served in most restaurants in the area and included avocado, sweet corn and pineapple.

"I hope you don't mind but I've taken the liberty of ordering a bottle of Familigia Bianchi San Rafael 2004, Cabernet Sauvignon. I'm sure you'll like it, unless your taste in wine has changed."

"Sounds perfect, and my taste in wine has not changed, so pour me a glass quick."

Andy poured out two glasses, and raised his glass to Maria's: "Salud, dinero y amor y el tiempo para disfutarlos."

"I'm healthy – touch wood – earn good money and my love life is looking up, it's the time to enjoy all three that I need," she laughed.

They savoured the wine, swilling it around their glasses and smelling it before tasting a small amount.

"Wow, good choice Señor Montalvo and perfect for the fillet."

"I thought you'd like it," he replied. "Anyway, you can tell me about your love life later but first I'd like to talk business if that's alright with you."

Maria raised her eyebrows. "So this is not a social lunch?"

Andy looked embarrassed. "Actually, it's a bit of both. I hope you don't mind?"

"Same old Andy. Fire away, let's get the business out of the way."

"Thanks. Now, I understand from Mike that the Junta is only going to allow one golf course for the whole region, including El Castillo, which means that the chosen site is going to be hot property. Was he right?"

"Yes. It's been common knowledge since September that they're only going to allow one golf course in the area so I'm not letting you in on any secrets there."

"Do you know which site it will be?"

"That's the million-euro question. No one outside the Junta knows and they have until the end of the year to choose the site and approve the PGOU."

"Ok, so if I told you that Mike had been approached by someone claiming to own the site which will be chosen to see if he could find a buyer, what would you say?"

"I'd have no reason to disbelieve him, but if it was a serious approach or not depends on who it was who approached him. This is Spain, and you know as well as I do that it's conceivable that someone has an inside track on this, and other, projects. For example, see that man sitting at that table over there, the one wearing the green checked shirt and smoking a cigarette?"

"Yes, I don't know why but he looks vaguely familiar. Who is he?"

"That is Enrique Gonzalez, the Urban Planning Officer for Los Cipreses. He's been in that job for a long time, knows a lot of people and, rumour has it, has done a few deals over the years, if you know what I mean. All talk and not a shred of evidence of course, but it would be amazing if he and his cronies had not found a way to benefit from the new PGOU. Now, whether that would extend to the proposed golf course is another matter, since the final decision is in the hands of the Junta."

Andy looked at Enrique Gonzalez with renewed interest. There was nothing particularly unusual about him. He was probably in his mid-fifties, with short-cropped grey hair and a chubby face. His eyes were small and inset and his face had that ruddy complexion that came from too much eating and drinking.

"But why is this of interest to you?"

"To be honest, I'm not totally convinced that Mike's death was an accident and I'd like to tell the police about this deal just in case there is any connection. The problem is that I don't know who it was who approached Mike. He wouldn't tell me. All he said that it was a very successful businessman who is well connected at all levels, up to and including the Junta."

"That could describe at least ten people in Los Cipreses alone, forgetting El Castillo. Anyway, what makes you think Mike's death was not an accident?"

"Nothing specific, just a niggling feeling. I'm probably making a mountain out of a molehill but if I could find out which site was involved and who the owner is then at least I could give this information to the police and they could investigate, if they think it's relevant of course."

"Andy, I'd love to help you but neither us, nor the local authority, nor the Land Registry are allowed to release any information concerning current ownership, or recent changes of ownership, of any land that might be included in the PGOU. Unless, that is, there is something unusual, suspicious or downright illegal about a change of ownership transaction, and then I'd go directly myself to the authorities."

"I understand your position Maria, but can you give me any idea of whether there might be something unusual going on – off the record, of course."

Maria looked at Andy for a few seconds and then leant forwards towards him. "What I can say without compromising myself is that I have not reported any suspicious transactions to the authorities. But remember, I've only been working at the notary's office for eighteen months and I don't get to see every transaction – it's a busy office, so that's not to say something has not been going on."

Andy topped up both their glasses and looked at Maria. He had expected this response from her. She was, after all, a professional, but at least he had established that there were no change-of-ownership transactions currently being investigated, and that made him feel a little better. However, he knew that deals could be structured in many ways or that the land could have been steadily acquired by Mr. Brown over a period of years. Also, as Maria had admitted, she didn't get to see every transaction that went through the notary's office.

Andy held her gaze. "I appreciate your position and thanks for sharing that information with me but, for Mike's sake, do you think you could look into any transactions related to the potential golf course sites over the last few years?" he asked.

"I suppose I could, but there are probably hundreds of plots involved. Also, remember that transactions can be completed at any notary office in Spain, regardless of where the property is located. It's only the when the change of title is officially registered that the authorities know a transaction has taken place."

"What do you mean?"

"In Spain property-related transactions typically involve three stages. Firstly, there is usually a private purchase contract which states the terms of the purchase, sets a completion date and which normally entails payment of a deposit. These contracts are private in the sense they are not signed in front of a Notary but they have full legal validity. Completion usually happens at the Notary's office via an escritura de compraventa. The third stage, where the title deeds are registered at the local Land Registry in the name of the new owner, is the one that some parties do not take in order to avoid making the change of ownership public."

"So, if I've understood this correctly – you can sign an escritura of compraventa at any Notary in Spain and this is not a public document BUT officially registering the change of ownership must be done at the local land registry office which is when the change of ownership becomes a matter of public record."

"You've got it."

"Wow, that's quite a large loophole as far as the tax authorities are concerned."

"Yes it is, but from next year a new centralised database of property transactions signed at all notaries throughout Spain will be put in place. At the same time, notaries will be obliged to inform the relevant Land Registry of any change of ownership."

"Ok, but that's next year. Right now, if something unusual has been going on then it may be difficult to pick up."

"Yes, but I'm sure that if anything unusual was happening with the plots in question someone in the office would have noticed. "So will you do me a favour and look to see if there's been any unusual activity related to these plots? You don't have to tell me, but if you find anything unusual you could go to the authorities."

"Let me give it some thought, but now lighten up and enjoy the food and, of course, the company."

They managed to finish another bottle of the Familigia Bianchi by which time Maria had told him all about the new love of her life – a tall, blond Norwegian who had recently moved to Los Cipreses. Apparently, he had an Internet hotel-booking business which was growing nicely and, being based in Southern Spain, provided him with better access to his suppliers than from Norway. It was early days yet but she seemed very happy and Andy was delighted for her.

By the time they finally finished their meal it was nearly half past five. The service had been slow and they had talked a lot, but since Tord was not arriving back from a business trip until later that evening they had been in no hurry.

Andy walked Maria to her car, which was parked on the edge of the beach opposite El Asador. "Maria, it's been great seeing you and I'd love to meet Tord; give me a ring and we'll go for a drink. In the meantime, please think about what we discussed about looking into any transactions over the last couple of years, it would take a weight off my mind. Now drive carefully – even with your connections I don't think you could avoid losing three penalty points."

When he got home, Andy dozed for over an hour on the sofa and woke with a fuzzy head. He knew that, if he wanted to, he could catch the early crowd in Casa Luque for a beer or two and a Sunday night La Liga football game.

Instead, he decided on a takeaway pizza and a movie. It was still too early to eat so he put on his DVD of the Last Seduction, one of his favourite neo-noir movies, and made himself comfortable on the sofa, ordering the pizza just as Linda Fiorentino's femme fatale character discovers she is being watched by a private investigator. It arrived when she killed him by driving into a tree, resulting in him flying through the windscreen while her seatbelt and airbag saved her.

Monday, 19th November

Despite a relatively early night, the last few days had finally caught up with him, and Andy struggled out of bed at eleven. He showered, dressed and then made himself a strong cup of coffee to kick-start the day.

Switching on his laptop, he wondered if Maria would check to see if there were any suspicious transactions relating to any of the proposed golf course sites. His inbox was empty, apart from the usual spam emails offering him various products to enhance certain parts of his anatomy, which he deleted. He switched the laptop off, finished his coffee and called Chief Inspector Diaz, who picked up the phone almost immediately.

"Hello, Chief Inspector Diaz?"

"Speaking," said a gravelly voice.

Andy explained who he was and his connection with Mike Cameron. "I think it would be worth meeting so I can tell you what I know about Mr. Cameron's business activities," he suggested.

"Of course, any information relating to Mr. Cameron's business activities is of interest. I'm in Granada all day today so shall we say tomorrow at twelve o'clock at the Police Station in El Castillo?" responded Chief Inspector Diaz in excellent English. Andy agreed and hung up.

Emily arrived at Andy's villa at one o'clock. He had planned a simple lunch, starting with a salad followed by barbecued chicken. There were also a couple of bottles of wine in the fridge, which somehow he knew they would get through.

The Weber was all primed and ready to go and when Emily arrived

Andy lit the charcoals and opened a bottle of Rueda. They sat at the round teak table under the shaded pergola, with a stunning view across the bay to Punta de Palermo. The sun was high in the sky and the air was warm, but there were virtually no craft in the bay, as most of the weekend visitors had returned to their city homes the previous evening.

"It's very nice of you to cook me lunch, but we could have gone to one of the beach restaurants."

"Don't mention it. I can imagine how you must be feeling right now and I thought a quiet lunch out of the public eye, so to speak, would be best."

"You're right, and getting away from Mum and that awful Carlos for a couple of hours is a relief. He's a creep but Mum is besotted with him, and it makes me sick to see how she behaves despite what happened to Dad."

Andy studied Emily as she spoke. He knew she had a strong character and he could see that she was angry.

"Yes. From what I hear and see he is not very pleasant, but then love knows no limits as they say."

"Love!" Emily snorted angrily. "Lust more like and now it looks as if Mum is lending him some money to buy a bar."

Andy looked pensive. "Hmm. I wondered if that's where he's getting the money from. I hope your mother knows what she is doing."

"I doubt it very much and by the time she sees sense it'll probably be too late."

Andy checked the barbecue coals and announced that the chicken could now be safely placed on the grill without danger of being burnt. He poured them each another glass of wine and told Emily briefly about his negotiations with her father to buy into the business, but was careful to avoid mentioning the property transaction and any of his suspicions about Mike's death. Emily asked few questions and seemed more concerned about her mother's relationship with Carlos than with the death of her father, which she saw as an unfortunate accident.

As they ate lunch, Andy asked Emily about how her studies were going and what her plans were. She told him that once she completed her course she would look for a job in the UK, as she no longer had strong ties to Los Cipreses, or for that matter to Spain. She had made a lot of friends at university and thought that there were greater opportunities in graphic design in the UK than in Spain.

"So when are you going back?" he asked her, as they finished their meal.

"Well, of course, I'll stay for Dad's funeral but then I want to get back as soon as possible. There is nothing for me to do here and I really want to get away from my mother and Carlos."

She left at half past four to meet a friend for a tea at La Cabaña. "I think I'll stay with Elena tonight," she said to Andy as she left. "It just makes me angry having Carlos in the house."

"Well, just make sure your mother knows where you are as otherwise she'll worry about you; you know where I am if you need me," he said, kissing her on the cheek.

Vicente Maldonado looked across the city towards the Sierra Nevada mountains from his penthouse apartment. As he watched the sun set, spreading a pink and purple glow over the Sierra Nevada, he reflected how much Granada had changed in recent years.

Its major claim to fame was the Alhambra, the fabulous 14th Century Moorish palace nestling in the foothills of the Sierra Nevada mountains. This monument attracted hundreds of thousands of tourists each year and was what put Granada on the map internationally.

However, its relatively isolated location and a lack of investment in transport infrastructure meant that the city had remained largely a provincial backwater during the boom years of the 1980s and 90s, as Spain became the single largest recipient of EU grants. For the same reasons, its coast, which lay adjacent to the Costa del Sol, had never attracted large numbers of foreign tourists and had therefore not been subject to excessive development.

Well, our day has come, he thought – Granada was playing catch-up, and fast. The airport was now being used as a hub by several low-cost airlines flying to and from various European cities; motorways were being built from Granada to the coast and along the province's coastline. A high -speed train link with Madrid was also in the pipeline.

As a result there had been a significant increase in property developments, both in the city itself and along its coast, with much more to come. He was already a rich man, but Project Pulpo would be the crowning glory and put him in a different league altogether, one where he knew he belonged.

As the pink and purple glow faded from the sky and darkness descended, the floodlit Alhambra stood out in all its glory. Vicente turned away from the view and went to his study to double check that he had all the necessary documents for his meeting in London.

Tuesday, 20th November

It was still dark when Vicente got up, and the drive to the airport only took him twenty minutes. With no luggage to check in and having paid extra to pre-book his seat online, he had timed his journey to arrive a few minutes before the check-in desk closed, thus avoiding having to stand in a long queue. Being the first flight out of the airport that morning there were no delays, and shortly after the scheduled departure time they were airborne.

He closed his eyes and catnapped as the plane flew almost due north over Madrid and then the Bay of Biscay before turning east to approach Gatwick airport. Of the four airports serving London, it was his favourite since, outside of the peak holiday season, it was usually not too busy and had excellent rail connections to the West End and the City.

Passport control was a mere formality and as a European national, Vicente only had to show his Spanish national identity card. Maybe one day the British will accept the advantages of having identity cards, he thought to himself but somehow he doubted it. By 9.40 (he had already turned his watch back one hour – another British idiosyncrasy he didn't understand) he was at London Bridge station. His meeting with Peter Roberts of Moore, Moore & Blackthorn was at eleven so he had plenty of time for a tall latte before catching the tube to Blackfriars.

As Vicente Maldonado was entering Moore, Moore & Blackthorn's offices, Andy Montalvo was being shown into Chief Inspector Diaz's office at the police station in El Castillo.

He knew that the Policia Nacional were responsible for policing all provincial capitals and any other towns designated to them by the Ministry of the Interior while the Guardia Civil, a military corps, was responsible for policing smaller towns and villages and rural areas, such as Los Cipreses. Both forces had special units responsible for investigating corruption, organised crime and drug trafficking and he was aware that there was fierce rivalry between them as much of their work overlapped.

In truth, Andy had been a little surprised that the Chief Inspector had agreed to see him; after all, Mike's death seemed fairly clear-cut, but at least it presented him with an opportunity to try and dispel some of his niggling doubts.

He entered a sparsely furnished office which contained a metal desk, a large filing cabinet in the far right-hand corner of the room and two rather battered steel-framed, plastic chairs placed immediately in front of the desk. There was a window in the far left wall and a picture of the King on the wall behind the desk. The man behind the desk rose and extended his hand to Andy. He was over six feet tall, well built and about forty-five years old. He was bald, with piercing blue eyes that seemed to drill into Andy as they settled on him.

"Chief Inspector Diaz," he said, shaking Andy's hand with a bear-like grip. "Please take a seat, Señor Montalvo."

"Thank you seeing me, Chief Inspector. As I mentioned when we spoke, I've known Mike Cameron for over twenty years and was in the process of buying into his business. His death came as a complete shock and I wanted to tell you about our discussions just to make sure you're fully in the picture."

"I appreciate that; any information about Mr. Cameron's business activities is of interest and may even help us with our investigation."

So there is an investigation, thought Andy, as he proceeded to tell the Chief Inspector about his relationship with Mike, his negotiations with him to buy into the business and details of the property deal Mike had been working on.

Chief Inspector Diaz listened attentively, without interrupting, and now and again jotted some notes in a pad on his desk. When Andy had finished, Chief Inspector Diaz looked at Andy and said, "Thank you Señor Montalvo. May I ask you a couple of questions?"

"Of course, fire away."

"Who else was aware that you were negotiating to buy a stake in Mr. Cameron's business?"

"To my knowledge no one, although Mike's wife did mention the fact to me the other day."

"I see. And was anyone else aware of the potential property deal Mr. Cameron was working on?"

"Mike had been sworn to secrecy so, aside from myself, as far as I know, he'd only discussed it with this client of his who had contacts with potential investors."

"You said that Mr. Cameron didn't tell you the name of the person who had approached him about selling this piece of land. Do you have any idea who this is?"

"No. All Mike said was that he was a successful businessman who was very well connected."

"And do you happen to know who the client Mr. Cameron was in touch with is?"

"No, Mike would only give me all the relevant details once I'd joined the business."

"Ok, thank you, Señor Montalvo. You have been most helpful."

"My pleasure, and I realise you may not be in a position to do so, but there are some aspects of Mike's death that I wonder if you could clarify for me."

"I'll do my best, but there really is very little I can say until the case is closed."

"I appreciate that, but any feedback you can give me would be most welcome. Firstly, I understand that the front door to Mike's office was locked from the inside but that there is also access to the office via a door in the back storeroom. Is there a possibility that someone gained access to the office via this rear door?"

"As you say, the front door was locked from the inside and in fact Mr. Cameron's keys were in the lock. We are aware of the existence of an alternative entry point but this was locked too, more than that I cannot say."

"Thank you. Secondly, I'm intrigued as to why the Policia Nacional were given this case although the Guardia Civil were first on the scene and have jurisdiction in Los Cipreses."

"Well Señor Montalvo, unlike in your country, in Spain a judge is usually appointed to investigate deaths from unusual circumstances, and it is they who decide which police force will be given jurisdiction over the case. Nine times out of ten the case is given to the force that arrives at the scene first but Judge Bustamente has passed the case to us because it involves the expatriate community and I speak English."

"And excellent English if I may say so."

"Thank you, that's very kind. I'm fortunate enough to have an American wife, which helps tremendously."

"One last question, if you don't mind. Is there any particular reason why the autopsy is being undertaken in Granada and not by the local pathologist?"

"Again, this is a decision made by Judge Bustamente. The local pathologist retired recently and it appears that the judge feels that his replacement is not sufficiently experienced to handle this case and so he's decided to use a senior forensic pathologist in Granada. Unfortunately, this man has been at a conference in the United States so we have been waiting for him to return."

"And when might that be?"

"Actually, he got back last night and so, jet-lag permitting, he'll be performing the autopsy as we speak or a little later today," Chief Inspector Diaz said, standing up and indicating that the interview was over. "Thank you for coming to see me, Señor Montalvo and hopefully this matter will be resolved satisfactorily in the near future."

He doesn't give much away, thought Andy as he shook Chief Inspector Diaz's hand again, this time bracing himself for the firm grip. "My pleasure and I hope that what I've told you helps."

The policeman watched him leave and then walked over to the window and looked through it pensively. After a minute or two he returned to his desk, picked up the phone and dialled a number in Seville.

As Andy walked back to his car he thought about his meeting with the Chief Inspector. He had been polite and professional and had listened with interest to what Andy had told him, but he had also been non-committal and had given Andy very little information.

However, the fact that Mike's keys were found in the lock of the office door was new information to Andy and indicated that if there had been anyone else with Mike they would have needed keys for both the rear door and the garage.

The reason why the investigating judge had allocated the case to the Policia Nacional seemed plausible, while the appointment of a senior forensic pathologist might be justified if the new boy in town was still a little wet behind the ears.

Still, his use of the word "investigation" and his interest in the people behind the golf course deal seemed odd, and Andy couldn't help feeling that something was not quite right.

Moore, Moore & Blackthorn's offices occupied five upper floors of a tall, rectangular-shaped building which, like so many modern office blocks, appeared to be made primarily of glass and held together by a few thin strips of steel. It was, in truth, rather nondescript, unlike the famous Swiss Re "gherkin," which was a few hundred yards away and dominated much of the City skyline.

After signing in at the main reception on the ground floor, Vicente Maldonado caught one of the lifts to Moore, Moore & Blackthorn's reception and told the smartly dressed lady behind the desk that he had an appointment with Peter Roberts. "You must be Mr. Maldonado," she said, smiling and passing him a clear plastic lapel badge with his name printed on the label inside. "Please take a seat and I'll tell Mr. Roberts' secretary that you are here."

How efficient and professional compared to the one-man band "law firms" like his that operated in Granada and all along the coast he thought. But then this was the City and an entirely different league to almost anywhere in the world, let alone Granada and the Spanish costas. He would never be able to operate in such a formal, not to mention structured, environment and, although senior partners at these City law firms earned millions, he too would soon be very rich – all he had to do was convince Peter Roberts and his clients to proceed with the purchase of the land.

At three minutes past eleven, a woman wearing black trousers and a crimson red blouse got out of the lift, approached him and introduced herself as Joanne, Mr. Roberts' secretary. "The meeting is in one of the conference rooms on the fifteenth floor. It's only one floor but unfortunately the stairs are out of bounds except in the case of emergencies so we have to take the lift."

On getting out of the lift, Joanne used her electronic security card to open a glass-frosted door and led Vicente Maldonado through an open plan office to a conference room at the far end of the office. "Please help yourself to coffee, tea or water," she said pointing to a collection of catering size thermos flasks and an array of bottles on a sideboard at the far end of the conference room. "If you prefer a soft drink I can arrange for one to be brought to you."

"That's alright, I'll have a coffee, thank you," he said, moving towards the cups and saucers which were in the middle of a long rectangular dark wood table running almost the entire length of the room.

"I'll tell Mr. Roberts and Ms. Nuñez that you are here," she said, leaving him alone in the room.

Vicente Maldonado sat down at the far end of the table, which could comfortably seat eight people down each of its sides, and took a file from his briefcase. Just as he was going through the documents for the fourth time that morning, there was a knock at the door and a man, followed by a woman, walked into the room.

"Hello, I'm Peter Roberts and this is Elena Nuñez," as they walked the length of the room towards Vicente Maldonado who stood up to shake Peter Roberts' and Elena Nuñez's outstretched hands.

"Ms. Nuñez usually works on any transactions involving Spain or which require Spanish to be spoken as I don't speak much Spanish at all – can't teach an old dog new tricks, as they say," he laughed. "Anyway, we find it helps to avoid any misunderstandings and usually speeds things up. Aside from that, she's a damn fine lawyer."

He looked young, probably late thirties/early forties, and was wearing a classic navy blue pin stripe suit with bright red braces, a white shirt and yellow polka dot tie. Although of above average height, his girth gave away the fact that he was fond of his food and this, combined with his receding hairline and jovial manner, gave him an almost Bunter-like appearance.

On the other hand, Ms. Nuñez was small, very slim and conservatively dressed in a two-piece business suit and a plain white blouse.

Her hair was fine, straight and cut short, giving her an elfin appearance. They were like chalk and cheese.

"Thank you for seeing me at such short notice, Mr. Roberts, and under such unfortunate circumstances. I realise you must be busy so I'll get straight to the point."

"Before we get down to the nitty-gritty, can you tell me exactly what happened to Mike Cameron," interrupted Peter Roberts. "He'd looked after my villa for a number of years and I considered him a good friend."

"From what I have been told, he had been out with a friend and was, how do you say in English, "a little the worse for wear"? It was late but he decided to go to his office to check for an email he was expecting before going on to Luque's for a nightcap. It appears that an electrical fire started and in attempting to put it out he panicked and knocked himself out. He was subsequently overcome by fumes from an old sofa which had caught fire. By the time they got to him it was too late."

"Surely somebody would have seen the fire and got him out sooner?" Peter Roberts said.

"Had it been a busier time of the year, then yes, there is a good chance that would have been the case but, being mid-week in November, there was nobody in the street at that time of night. Also, it didn't help that he had locked the office door from the inside."

"Poor sod, but if he was already unconscious I guess he didn't suffer. Let's sit down and then you can tell me what I can do for you. Elena, I'd love a cup of white coffee. Thanks."

Elena rose and walked over to the sideboard while Vicente addressed Peter Roberts. "As I explained on the phone, I represent the principals behind the transaction that Mr. Cameron had approached you about."

"Yes, and I was wondering why you approached us via Mike instead of directly?"

"Because of his good reputation, knowledge of the Los Cipreses area and contacts with potential investors."

Peter Roberts nodded as Vicente continued. "As you know, Mr. Cameron had passed on the references provided by your firm to my clients and now they would like to establish the extent of your clients' interest.

If we have sufficient common ground then we would like to try and get a reservation deposit in place as soon as possible and a definitive agreement by the middle of December."

Peter Roberts took the cup and saucer from Elena Nuñez's outstretched hand and beckoned her to sit down opposite him. He turned to Vicente Maldonado, "I must say the little that Mike Cameron told me was enough to get my clients' attention, but there are a number of questions that need answering before we can even think about paying a reservation deposit."

"That's perfectly understandable, so what would you like to know?"

"Clearly our first question is; who are your clients?"

"Unfortunately, I am not at liberty to disclose that. My clients wish to receive any proceeds of the sale offshore and would prefer to remain anonymous. We are therefore proposing a structure which will achieve both these objectives."

"Tax avoidance we can live with but tax evasion we cannot. It sounds like what you are proposing is the latter and not the former," said Peter Roberts, looking Vicente Maldonado directly in the eyes.

Vicente held his gaze. "The structure we propose does not involve the sale, or the passing of title, of any assets located in Spain, but rather the purchase of shares in an offshore company whose only assets are a series of options over land based in Spain.

"Title to the underlying land will only pass when the options are exercised and it is at that point that tax will be due in Spain by the sellers of the land and not the company that exercises the options."

As Vicente Maldonado spoke, Peter Roberts made notes in a Black n'Red ruled notebook which he had placed at his side on top of the table. He stopped writing, turned his Montblanc pen upside down and tapped the notepad with the white-capped top.

"Hmm, that sounds like a clever solution but of course we'll need to check the relevant Spanish legislation. The transaction will also have to be undertaken in an offshore jurisdiction which is not on the OECD blacklist."

"Of course, that goes without saying and these things have already been taken care of. For example, we are using a Cayman

Island company. As you know the Cayman Islands is not on the OECD blacklist of tax havens."

"Assuming we go ahead on that basis, we would still need assurances from the Cayman authorities that the principals involved are not subject to any investigation with regard to tax evasion or money laundering."

"Of course, and we would provide a Certificate of Non-Investigation from the Cayman Islands Monetary Authority."

"Looks like you have that covered so why the rush to get the deal done? Wouldn't it be easier for everybody if we were to wait until the new urban development plan is approved and then buy the land if it is reclassified as your clients expect?" asked Peter Roberts.

Vicente was well prepared for this question. "Two reasons. Firstly, my clients are very confident that their site will be the winner. However, they have incurred considerable expense to date in acquiring the options and also undertaking environmental impact and feasibility studies for presentation to the Junta de Andalucia. They also have some final payments to make with regard to the option premiums on some of the bigger plots. So, while they are reasonably wealthy, shall we say that, from a liquidity perspective, it would suit them if they could find a way to fund these final payments before the land is reclassified."

"And the second reason?"

"Under the revised urban development plan, only one golf course will be allowed in the whole area. This means the winning site will attract considerable interest from developers and will be worth a lot more than if several golf courses were to be permitted.

"So, in return for some cash up front, my clients are willing to enter into exclusive negotiations, but only for a limited period given the attraction of the site once it is reclassified."

"I see, but there are no guarantees that the land will be reclassified," Peter Roberts said. "Nevertheless, your clients want some money up front – an option for an option, so to speak. Is that a fair synopsis?"

"Yes it is. In effect, a reservation deposit would give your clients the exclusive right to buy the options at a pre-agreed price in the event the land is reclassified for golf course use. The deposit would be held in escrow with agreed amounts being released to my clients when certain milestones are met.

"This will ensure that my clients only get the agreed amounts when they deliver certain things and your clients are protected in the event the agreed milestones are not met. I think you call it a win-win situation in England," Vicente Maldonado said, looking first at Peter Roberts and then Elena Nuñez.

"In principle yes, but it depends on the size of payment we are talking about and the milestones involved, Mr. Maldonado. Can you tell me what you have in mind?"

Vicente Maldonado nodded and proceeded to describe how the investors would be given access to the key documents via a secure data room and what amounts would be released from the escrow account at each stage in the process.

"Well I must say this has been well thought out but you'll understand that we have to satisfy ourselves that there are no laws being broken. This may take a few days, but assuming we get the all-clear from the experts then I'll recommend to my clients that we initiate negotiations along the lines you have suggested."

Vicente Maldonado smiled, "Of course I fully understand but, as you'll appreciate from what I have told you, time is of the essence so we would certainly welcome a response at your earliest convenience."

"We will get back to you as soon as we can Señor Maldonado. More than that I cannot promise," replied Peter Roberts. "My secretary will take you down to reception. It's been a pleasure and I hope that we can do business together."

All three stood up and Vicente Maldonado extended his hand first to Peter Roberts and then to Elena Nuñez. "Thank you for your time and I look forward to hearing from you," he said, leaving the conference room and rejoining Joanne, who had remained seated at a desk close by.

Peter Roberts and Elena Nuñez sat down again at the table. "What do you make of that?" he asked Elena.

"Very interesting. The structure might work but the insistence on offshore payments and anonymity concerns me."

"My thoughts exactly; you had better start looking into the

relevant Spanish legislation regarding the structure he is proposing – and tax implications, Elena."

"I'll start right away; it's probably a good idea to bring in Pelayo y Parra's Madrid office, as they are the foremost experts on Spanish legislation in this area."

"Agreed. I'll leave it with you and get back to me with an opinion as soon as you can."

Wednesday, 21st November

Carlos and Ann set off early for the bank in Gibraltar to collect the cash, as the drive from Los Cipreses could take anywhere from two and a half to three and a half hours, depending on the rush-hour traffic around Malaga and Marbella.

"If we arrive early I can always pop into Marks and Spencer for a little retail therapy," Ann said, as they joined the A7 coastal motorway. "I won't have much time afterwards as I've got lunch with Jonathan Westwood at Da Bruno's."

"I wish you hadn't agreed to meet him there," Carlos said in a disgruntled voice. "I'm persona non grata and I'll have to go and find somewhere else to eat."

"Oh, don't be so miserable. I didn't have much choice. It's close to his office and he suggested it since we'll have limited time. In any case, no offence, but I'd rather have my conversation with him alone. After all, it's a sensitive subject which does not directly concern you."

"I suppose so and I'm sure I'll find somewhere to eat, something to do or someone to see in Puerto Banus," replied Carlos, looking at Ann with a mischievous glint in his eye.

As expected, they got caught up in the morning rush-hour traffic around the Malaga ring road, which was compounded by an accident at one of the main junctions; they arrived at La Linea at a quarter to eleven. There was a long queue of cars at the border, so they decided to park by the Maritime Club and enter the Rock on foot.

Ann was uncomfortable about carrying a large amount of cash back across the border, but Carlos reassured her that she was safe with him. "Anyway, one hundred and twenty-five thousand euros in five-hundred euro notes is not actually very bulky," he said knowingly. "If you put them in your shopping bag no one will be any the wiser."

Both had dressed smart casual so as not to attract too much attention. The walk from the spot where they had parked to the border took five minutes and they were waved through after a cursory glance at Ann's passport and Carlos' Spanish identity card. "Well at least they are getting less officious about letting people cross the border," Ann said once they were on British soil.

"Maybe they are learning to live with a little bit of Britain being part of the Spanish mainland after nearly thirty years in the EU," replied Carlos. "But I wouldn't count on it. More like just busy with bigger fish to fry than us. Spain will never give up its claim to sovereignty over Gibraltar – the Pope is more likely to turn Protestant first!"

"Never mind that, Ceuta and Melilla form part of Morocco's land mass but Spain will never cede these to Morocco and they weren't even obtained by treaty. I suppose if Spain ever gets Gibraltar then Portugal and Andorra will be next on their list. Anyway let's leave the politicians to sort all that out," retorted Ann, as they approached the bank entrance.

Mr. Evans, the bank manager, greeted Ann warmly and Ann introduced Carlos as a business associate of her husband. Mr. Evans showed them to a private room where he offered them coffee or tea while he completed the paperwork. Ann chose tea while Carlos elected to have a black coffee. Mr. Evans explained that it was relatively unusual to withdraw such a large sum in cash and warned that, if stopped, they would be asked to prove its provenance.

"As it stands, I do not have to advise the Spanish authorities of this cash withdrawal. All I have to do is confirm the source of the funds and, since they were transferred from your husband's account with our Jersey branch, I have prepared a certificate to that effect."

"I understand and thank you for organising the withdrawal at such short notice."

Once Ann had signed the relevant forms, Mr. Evans passed over an A4 brown envelope which appeared to be padded. On closer inspection Ann saw that the envelope contained bundles of five-hundred euro notes.

"I'll leave you alone for a few minutes so you can count them. You can do it manually or, alternatively, you can use that automatic note-counting machine in the middle of the table. Just put the notes in the feeder tray and push the 'count' button on the front. The electronic display will tell you how many notes it has counted," said Mr. Evans, getting up from his chair and moving towards the door.

A few minutes later, after Ann and Carlos had manually counted two hundred and fifty notes, Mr. Evans returned, asked Ann to sign the final release paper and then escorted them to the front door.

Ann had placed the envelope with the notes at the bottom of a Marks and Spencer carrier bag and covered it with two lamb's wool jumpers they had brought with them. She and Carlos walked side by side, with the carrier bag in her left hand so that it hung between them. They passed through the border and customs control without incident.

"That's a relief. I was worried that the customs guards were going to stop us and ask to see inside the bag."

"I'm sure hundreds of people pass through with Marks and Spencer bags every day and you look very respectable; so I can't see why they would choose to stop you."

"I thought the fact that I was with a good-looking Spaniard who is not my husband might raise few eyebrows," Ann joked as she took the car key from her handbag and opened the door of the car. "Its half past twelve and I had better put my foot down if we're going to get to Marbella by two."

Vicente Maldonado's flight back to Granada the previous evening had been delayed an hour due to French military manoeuvres over the Bay of Biscay, and he had eventually got back to his apartment just after midnight. When he arrived he found that his ADSL line was down and so decided to wait until the morning in order to update Don Javier on his meeting with Peter Roberts, rather than call him on his mobile.

The next morning, the ADSL line was still down, so Vicente made his way to his office to call Don Javier. His office was a converted first-floor apartment just off Calle Recogidas in the centre of Granada and, although it was only a ten minute walk, Vicente liked to drive his Porsche Cayenne through the heavy traffic. In recent years, the number of top end BMWs, Mercedes and Audis had increased significantly in Granada as the city prospered, but Porsche Cayennes were still relatively rare and it gave him a sense of power to sit in the car, cocooned from, but highly visible to, the outside world.

He arrived at ten-thirty, just as Carlos and Ann were driving through Algeciras. Belen, his secretary-cum girl Friday, greeted him and asked how his trip to London had been.

"Good, thank you, but I don't want to be disturbed for an hour; why don't you put the answering machine on and go and grab yourself a coffee and some breakfast?" he said briskly.

Belen was accustomed to these instructions and had given up questioning them or telling her boss that she had only had breakfast an hour ago. Instead, she used these opportunities mainly for visiting the shops and boutiques located along Calle Recogidas and its immediate vicinity, since most tended to be closed during her long lunch break. So she just nodded at Vicente Maldonado as he disappeared into his private office and closed the door behind him.

Vicente turned on his desktop computer. While he was not a great fan of computers, he greatly appreciated the importance of the Internet in enabling him and Javier Urquiza to carry out and develop their activities, in a fast, efficient and anonymous manner, via services such as Skype or Web-based email services.

Vicente typed in his password and the computer proceeded to load Windows. He had been careful to ensure that neither his Skype nor web-based email accounts were automatically loaded on start up. He started Skype, logged in to his account and saw that Javier Urquiza was online. He placed his Bluetooth headset in his ear, selected Don Javier's pseudonym and then clicked on the large bright green dial button at the bottom of the Skype pop-up window.

Javier Urquiza answered almost immediately. "Vicente, I was expecting your call last night. I was getting worried. Has anything happened?"

"No, don't worry. I didn't get in until late and my ADSL line at home was down, both last night and this morning, so I'm calling you from the office."

"But you could have sent me an email from London before you caught the plane," Javier Urquiza said in an admonishing tone.

"I'm sorry but the Internet café I found was full of backpackers and the only Internet access at Gatwick was WiFi; I couldn't access it since I didn't have my laptop with me thanks to all these hand luggage restrictions."

In truth, he'd had time to find another Internet café after his meeting with Peter Roberts but instead had spent some time buying shirts from Turnbull and Asser in Jermyn Street before catching the train back to Gatwick. In any event, whenever possible, he preferred to speak with Javier Urquiza to avoid leaving an email trail, albeit an anonymous one.

"Ok, I understand. So how did it go?" asked Don Javier in a more relaxed voice.

"Pretty much as I expected," and Vicente went on to describe his meeting and discussion with Peter Roberts and Elena Nuñez.

"And when do you think they'll get back to you?"

"Hopefully by the end of the week."

"Let's hope so and that they want to go ahead – we'll need the reservation deposit in order to pay our friends on the Environmental Planning Committee before their meeting on the tenth. In the meantime, can you arrange to transfer the funds to the Galician via the usual channel.

"Of course, consider it done."

That morning Andy went for a bike ride, as much for the exercise as to try and clear his head of thoughts about Mike's death.

As he cycled along the beachfront towards the Punta de Palermo, he noted how devoid it was of cars. Despite the sub-tropical climate, the absence of the soon-to-be completed coastal motorway and appropriate tourist infrastructure, such as golf courses, to attract winter tourists, meant that the next time Los Cipreses was likely to experience an influx of visitors would be the long weekend in early December to coincide with Spain's Constitution Day.

Fifteen minutes later, after a brief stop to catch his breath and drink some water, Andy reached the top of the Punta de Palermo. On the way up, he had passed many villas, most of them hidden behind whitewashed walls or natural fences made of bougainvillea or Cypress trees, and he now surveyed the bay from the opposite direction to which he was accustomed.

The view was equally stunning, with the majestic sweep of the bay ending at the Cerro Grande headland which was, in fact, slightly bigger than its sister. Jutting out behind Cerro Grande and into the distance stretched the Spanish coast all the way to Malaga and beyond.

After a couple of minutes Andy set off again, descending via a very steep tarmaced single lane track to the Old Town. By ten to eleven he was back at his villa; before showering he checked his mobile phone and saw that he had missed a call from a withheld number. He also had a voicemail, presumably from the same caller. To his great surprise the voicemail message was from Chief Inspector Diaz, asking him to call him back as soon as possible.

Andy dialled Chief Inspector Diaz's number and the phone was answered almost immediately.

"Ah, Señor Montalvo, thank you for getting back to me so quickly."

"No problem. How can I help you, Chief Inspector?"

"Well, following our meeting yesterday morning, I have been discussing our conversation with some of my colleagues and we feel it would be helpful if you were to meet one of them to discuss Mr. Cameron's business activities in more detail."

"Really. I was under the impression that the investigation into Mike's death was very much under control. In fact, that it was almost wrapped up," said Andy, surprised.

"Let's just say that there are still a number of loose ends that need tidying up and that maybe you can help us," replied Chief Inspector Diaz, in a warmer tone than he had used with Andy until now.

"As I said yesterday, if I can be of any assistance then please count me in. So when would you like to meet?"

"Good. My colleague would like to meet you tomorrow lunchtime at the La Bobadilla hotel in Loja. Do you know it?"

"Yes I do, but it's been a while since I was there. It's probably at least an hour's drive from Los Cipreses. Can't we meet at your office or at my house?"

"I realise it is an unusual request but, for security reasons, we would rather the meeting took place away from Los Cipreses or El Castillo."

"This all sounds very mysterious. And who am I meeting?"

"I'm afraid I am not in a position to disclose that either. It will only be the two of you and my colleague will approach you. If you are still willing to go then please be at the La Finca restaurant at La Bobadilla at two o'clock tomorrow."

"Ok, I'll be there."

"Thank you, I'll let my colleague know to expect you. By the way, please don't mention this meeting to anyone, not even Mr. Cameron's immediate family," Chief Inspector Diaz said before hanging up.

Andy was intrigued and at the same time concerned. The Chief Inspector had specifically said they wanted to discuss Mike's business activities in more detail, but Andy had already told him all he knew – so why a meeting with an unidentified colleague, and why the need for secrecy?

The traffic back to Marbella was light but road works for the new underpass at San Pedro de Alcantara just west of Marbella meant that Ann arrived at Da Bruno's at a quarter past two.

"Let's see if he has Mike's Wills, or at least knows where they are," she said to Carlos before he sulked off in the direction of Puerto Banus.

The restaurant was located on Avenida Ricardo Soriano, in the heart of Marbella's commercial district, with at least three notaries and innumerable lawyers' offices within a five-hundred metre radius. The food was traditional Italian, the service efficient and the ambiance business like. It was therefore a popular lunch-time venue for lawyers and their clients and was almost full when Ann arrived.

Ann asked for Jonathan Westwood; she didn't know him by sight as he had only joined Fernandez & Fernandez a few months earlier. She was shown to a table in the far corner of the restaurant, at a discreet distance from the surrounding tables. A tall slim man, with sandy-coloured wavy hair, who was probably no more than thirty-five years old, stood up and shook Ann's hand.

"Jonathan Westwood. Pleased to meet you Mrs. Cameron and I'm sorry that we are meeting for the first time under such unfortunate circumstances. Please accept my condolences. I must say I was shocked to hear of Mike's death; it sounds like a horrible accident."

"It was and, despite the fact we were getting divorced, it's all been a bit of shock. Frankly my daughter and I would like to put his affairs in order and then move on."

"I quite understand; how can I help?"

"Well as a UK national but resident of Spain I know Mike made two Wills – an English one and a Spanish one, and I need these in order to sort out his estate. Since your firm handled all of his personal affairs, I thought you would be able to help me locate them."

As Ann finished, looking at Jonathan Westwood expectantly, a smartly dressed waiter approached the table, notepad at the ready.

"I see. First let's order our lunch while we have his attention and then I'll explain the procedures involved in locating and executing Spanish and English Wills."

After they had placed their orders, Jonathan turned to Ann. "You're right, we did act for Mike with regard to his personal affairs. As far as a Spanish Will is concerned, these are registered with the official Wills Registry. Once you have the death certificate, the Wills Registry will provide you with a certificate showing you which Notary the original Will is lodged with. Then, any beneficiary under the Will can apply to the relevant Notary for an authorised copy."

He stopped and took a sip of water.

"That sounds relatively straightforward; where is the Wills Registry?"

"There is one in every major city in Spain; the nearest one to you is in Malaga. Do you have the death certificate yet?"

"No, but we are expecting the autopsy result any day now; apparently the pathologist has been away at a conference, and I assume the death certificate will come with the autopsy result."

"Yes, normally if an autopsy is held the death certificate is made available to the next-of-kin at the same time as the result of the autopsy. Since you are not officially divorced you'll receive the death certificate. Just remember that the Will can only be released to a beneficiary, or a lawyer with a Power of Attorney from one of the beneficiaries," Jonathan said, as the waiter placed a large mixed salad in the centre of the table.

"Now, as far as an English Will is concerned, as you probably know, there is no such thing as a Wills Registry and usually people lodge their Wills with their solicitors or in a safe place where it'll be found on their death, for example, a bank safety deposit box.

An original Will can be read by anyone as soon as it is found but only the executors can apply for Grant of Probate from the Probate Registry of England and Wales. They must apply in person with the death certificate. However, a UK solicitor can apply by mail for Grant of Probate without a death certificate, provided they have written authority from the executors."

"So the important thing here is to find the original Will?"

"That's correct."

"And do you have Mike's English Will in safekeeping?"

"I'm afraid not. Whilst we've always helped Mike to prepare his Wills, we have never retained originals. Of course, his Spanish Will is lodged with a Notary."

"I see. So I guess I'm going to have to try and find it amongst his papers or perhaps at the bank."

"That would be as good a place as any to start. Now let's have some salad before they bring our main courses."

Ann filled Jonathan in on the details of Mike's death over lunch, but refused dessert and coffee. Jonathan insisted on paying the bill and, once the waiter had taken away the signed credit card slip, he turned to Ann, "Unfortunately, because Mike was our client and had initiated divorce proceedings, even if you do locate his Wills, we cannot help you any further as it would be a conflict of interest."

"That's fair enough, I suppose. Thank you for letting me know what the correct procedures are. At least I can make a start."

"My pleasure; drive carefully. The early evening rush-hour traffic on the Malaga ring road can be like driving in the Indianapolis 500," he said, shaking Ann's hand and heading off in the direction of his office.

Ann walked in the opposite direction towards the car park while calling Carlos' mobile. Five minutes later, she picked him up at the entrance to Puerto Banus and told him about her conversation with Jonathan Westwood as they headed back to Los Cipreses. They agreed that Ann would go through the papers that Mike had left in the house to see if his English Will was there. If not, she would go to the bank and ask to see the contents of Mike's safety deposit box. In theory, the bank should not allow her access to the safety deposit box, since it was solely in his name but she was certain that Antonio, the long standing bank manager, would indulge her.

"Getting the Spanish Will should be easy enough once we have the death certificate," she said. "Now let's change the subject. Why don't you tell me about your plans for the bar – tomorrow will be a big day for you."

As Ann drove, Carlos described the refurbishment he was planning and his ideas for turning the bar into the "in" place for the young and trendy. It sounded fantastic but Ann could not help but harbour doubts about Carlos' ambitious plans for an area which was not an all-year-round tourist destination like the Costa del Sol. However, she knew better than to question some of his ideas or a major row could follow.

Although the traffic around Malaga was heavy it was flowing freely, and they managed to get back to Los Cipreses in time for Carlos to shower, change and head off to El Boqueron. "This is going to be my last night working for someone else and tomorrow a whole new world of opportunity begins," he said to Ann, giving her a short but firm kiss on the lips before disappearing out of the front door.

Thursday, 22nd November

As Andy approached La Bobadilla, the digital clock in the hire car indicated the time was quarter to two. Perfect timing, he thought. It had been a few years since he had stayed at the hotel, which in the past had entertained the King of Spain, Hollywood film stars and sports personalities amongst other celebrities. Now he thought the exterior of the Moorish-style building looked tired and jaded, rather like an ageing madam in need of a little tender loving care.

He parked in the virtually empty car park at the side of reception and made his way to the La Finca restaurant through the courtyard beyond reception, not knowing what to expect.

As he walked through the large rustic wooden door of the restaurant, to his amazement, Cristina Ibañez appeared as from nowhere and approached him. "Good afternoon Mr. Montalvo. My name is Cristina Ibañez and I believe that we're having lunch together," she said, in the slightly husky voice which had made such an impression on Andy nearly a week ago in Casa Luque.

"Well, to be honest, I didn't know lunch was with you Ms Ibañez – but I'm not complaining," Andy replied, smiling.

In keeping with the smart but rustic surroundings, Cristina Ibañez was wearing crisp denim jeans with a white linen blouse and a pink tweed Chanel jacket. Her shoulder-length ash-blonde hair was pinned back with a black velvet brooch. Being this close to her Andy could not fail to notice her green eyes and the light splattering of freckles on her nose and upper cheeks.

The combination of looks, dress and voice was stunning and he could imagine this woman driving men crazy. Nevertheless, her demeanour was cool and professional and he decided that any overt attempt to flirt with her would be pointless, as well as inappropriate.

"I've reserved a table in a dining room just off the main restaurant; why don't we go there? We can talk in private."

"I'm all ears," said Andy, following her as she walked towards the back of the dining room.

In the middle of the private dining room was a table set for two. It was of a size which would facilitate private conversation without encouraging intimacy. On the top of the table, next to the place setting furthest from the door, was a small plastic box with a red button protruding from its centre.

Cristina Ibañez sat down at the place setting with the plastic box and indicated to Andy to sit down on the remaining chair. "Would you like an aperitif?" she asked.

"I'll have a manzanilla please."

"I think I'll join you," she said, pushing the red button.

Almost immediately a waiter entered the room and Cristina Ibañez asked him to bring two manzanillas. On leaving the room she turned to Andy. "Why don't we order and then I can tell you why we asked you to this meeting."

After reviewing the menu, they placed their orders when the waiter brought the manzanillas. They were both driving so they ordered a bottle of still water to accompany their meal.

"Good, that's the fun part over with, now let's get down to business. I work for the Drugs and Organised Crime unit, or UDYCO as we call it, of the Policia Nacional, which is charged with investigating organised crime and money laundering."

Andy was stunned, but at least it explained the cloak-and-dagger antics. "I've heard of UDYCO."

"Given your background, I'd be surprised if you hadn't."

"So you know about my role at the serious fraud squad?" Andy asked, looking at her intently.

"Yes."

"And you know that I've just left?"

"Yes."

"So what interest has UDYCO got in Mike Cameron, and why do you want to talk with me?"

"Well, I am currently working undercover on an investigation in which Mr. Cameron was involved; we think that you may be able to assist us with this investigation."

Cristina paused and Andy remained silent, his mind racing. "Does this have something to do with the golf course deal Mike was working on?" he asked eventually.

"Before I tell you more, I must stress that Chief Inspector Diaz does not know my identity – this meeting was actually set up via our regional HQ. He is aware that there is an ongoing UDYCO investigation in Los Cipreses, but not of the precise nature of that investigation or, as yet, its principal focus. Therefore, regardless of whether you agree to help us or not, I must insist that you do not disclose my identity or role to Chief Inspector Diaz, or anyone else for that matter. Do you agree?"

"Absolutely. It's clear something important is going on so I'll do everything I can to help you get to the bottom of whatever it is you are investigating – if only for Mike's sake and that of his daughter."

"Good. We had our doubts about revealing anything to you but hopefully it will prove to be mutually beneficial."

Right on cue, the waiter appeared with a tray containing the starters they had chosen. When he had placed the plates on the table and left the room, Cristina Ibañez continued.

"The subject of our investigation is a businessman based in Los Cipreses who we suspect of bringing large quantities of hashish into Spain via North Africa. We have been investigating him for some time but, until recently, have been unable to gather any evidence of his involvement in the drugs trade. He's very careful about using open lines of communication and, to date, we've not been able to trace the movement of any illegal funds. Nevertheless, our sources indicate that he is a major player in the drugs trade in this part of Spain."

"But I'd swear on my mother's grave that Mike would never knowingly get involved with the drugs trade," interrupted Andy, looking surprised.

"I'm sure you're right Mr. Montalvo, but Mr. Cameron's involvement was not entirely voluntary. Let me explain. As you know, in September this businessman approached Mr. Cameron for assistance in finding foreign investors who might be interested in buying a golf course site in Los Cipreses. Fortunately for us, the call to Mr. Cameron was made on an open telephone line which we were monitoring and, even though the mooted transaction appeared to have nothing to do with drugs, we felt sure it was a front for a money laundering and tax evasion exercise. Thus we were able to identify Mr. Cameron as being of potential use to us."

"I see. So this has got something to do with Mr. Brown, as Mike referred to him, and the golf course site. But how did you persuade Mike to cooperate with you – if he suspected there were criminals and/or drugs involved he would have run a mile."

"You're right. Initially, Mr. Cameron didn't want to become involved in helping us but, how can I put this," she said, hesitating for a moment before carrying on "we became aware of some offshore funds held by Mr. Cameron which he had not declared to the Spanish tax authorities. So, in return for a tax amnesty, Mr. Cameron agreed to continue to cultivate his relationship with Mr. Brown, as you call him, and keep us informed of any developments with regard to the proposed land sale."

"So essentially you coerced him into working for you," Andy said, with a hint of anger in his voice.

"You could put it like that, but we prefer to think that Mr. Cameron agreed to do his citizen's duty in bringing a criminal to justice while at the same time retaining all of his hard-earned income."

Andy was shocked but not surprised at what Cristina Ibañez had just told him; it explained the comment Mike had made to him a couple of days before his death about not being concerned about the Spanish tax authorities. Given the same situation he would probably have done the same, so he could not blame Mike, but now he wondered whether his death had anything to do with Mr. Brown and the undercover investigation into his activities. Had Cristina Ibañez and UDYCO put his friend's life at risk? If so, what was expected of him, and was he prepared to do the same?

Back in El Castillo's Notary office, Carlos was leaning over the desk leering at Maria. "Darling, we've been waiting two hours already – when are we going to be able to sign the purchase deed? My friend Jorge is an important man and is getting impatient and I'm hungry. If you can speed this up I'll treat you to lunch. How does that sound?"

Maria stood up, picked up some papers from her desk and looked directly at Carlos, "I am not your "Darling" and would appreciate it if you could sit down in the waiting area and stop making a fool of yourself. The deed is being checked to ensure that the amended payment terms are correctly reflected and then you and Señor Haro will be able to sign it – probably in about five or ten minutes. I can assure you that we would all like to get this transaction completed and close the office. You can also rest assured that I have no intention of joining you for lunch."

"Suit yourself, it's your loss," replied Carlos, sauntering over to the waiting area. "The smug bitch says five to ten minutes so I am just popping outside to make a phone call," he said to Jorge.

Ann answered her mobile as she was driving back to the house. "Hi sweetheart, have you signed the purchase deed yet?"

"No, but they say it'll be ready in a few minutes."

"And how about you, how was your morning?"

"Very successful. Antonio had no problem giving me access to Mike's safety deposit box but I had to go back at one o'clock because the secure area is on a timer. Anyway, I used the security code Mike had told me and, bingo, the box opened no problem."

"That's great," interrupted Carlos in an excited tone "and what did you find?"

"Maybe I should wait until you're back to tell you, after all, you're not working tonight, but it looks as if we both have something to celebrate."

"Don't tease me. There will be plenty of time for celebration – come on, tell me what you found."

"Ok. Well firstly there was ten thousand euros in cash which will come in handy and, along with some insurance policies, an envelope containing Mike's English Will."

"And...?"

"It's the same one that he updated about a year ago so, aside from Emily's four hundred thousand Euros, I inherit all of Mike's assets."

"Fantastic, so no more financial worries."

"It seems that way. Once we have the death certificate I can contact the executors and ask them to apply for Grant of Probate."

"These are just formalities; at least you know everything is yours."

"Actually, Mike's UK Will specifically excludes his Spanish assets, so we still have to locate the Spanish Will to see if I inherit the house and the business, but if he didn't change his UK Will then he's unlikely to have changed his Spanish one."

"Cariño, that's fantastic news. I'm going back into the Notary's office now to see if we can sign the paperwork and then I'll come straight home and we can spend the rest of the day celebrating with French champagne – none of that Catalan Cava!"

"Sounds like heaven – don't be long, I'll be ready and waiting."

Once the waiter had removed the empty starter plates and brought their main courses, Andy looked at Cristina Ibañez. "So did Mike's death have anything to do with Mr. Brown and your investigation, or was it merely an unfortunately timed accident?"

Cristina Ibañez paused before replying. "Mr. Montalvo, I must stress that whatever we discuss must stay within these four walls. You agree?"

Andy nodded, so she continued, "We have reasons to believe that Mr. Cameron's death was not an accident. However, we have nothing to connect his death to Mr. Brown – although we suspect he may be involved."

Andy put down his cutlery. "Why do you think Mike's death was not an accident?"

"Well, the autopsy results show that there was no smoke in his lungs, while a broken hyoid bone, along with bruises inside the neck tissues and at the base of the tongue, indicates he was strangled."

"Which means he was already dead by the time the fire started," Andy continued.

"Exactly. There are also indications that the door in the rear storeroom has been opened recently."

"That sounds like compelling forensic evidence for murder; what makes you think Mr. Brown might be involved?"

"It's a long shot, but Mr. Cameron had been drinking with Johan Gaards most of the evening of his death and we suspect that Johan Gaards is Mr. Brown's main fixer. It seems strange that he left Mr. Cameron at the office, and also that he took more than thirty minutes to go back for him when he failed to turn up at Casa Luque."

"So you think Mike could have been set up?"

"It's a definite possibility. We're trying to establish at what time Mr. Cameron got to the office and whether Johan Gaards had sufficient time to strangle him, start a fire, leave by the rear door and then go to Casa Luque to ostensibly wait for Mr. Cameron."

"According to Ann, they left the Cutty Sark one or two minutes after Pepe closed the bar at midnight and the office is a five-minute walk away, so they should have got there just before ten past twelve."

"Yes, that's what we're assuming for the time being, but what we haven't been able to confirm yet is the time Johan Gaards arrived at Casa Luque without Mr. Cameron."

Andy considered this carefully. "But if Mr. Brown was behind this why would he do it? Especially as Mike was just about to introduce the investors to him. Surely if Mr. Brown wanted Mike out of the way he would at least have waited until he was in direct contact with the investors?"

"That's the problem. We cannot see why Mr. Brown would want, or need, to get rid of Mr. Cameron, particularly at this delicate stage of the transaction."

"Then, assuming Mike's death had nothing to do with Mr. Brown, who would want to kill him and why?"

"We have no idea, but when we have all the results of the forensic tests these may yield some extra clues. We also want to establish what emails Mr. Cameron received that evening, as they may have a bearing on the case. Unfortunately, the fire destroyed all of Mr. Cameron's paperwork and damaged his computer and so far we have been unable to recover data from the hard drive. We are also going to check details of any calls or SMSs he made or received that evening, but this will take a few days. So at the moment we have no other lines of enquiry."

"And when do you intend to make the fact that Mike was murdered public?"

"We only got the autopsy results yesterday afternoon and, in accordance with Spanish law, the investigating judge, Judge Bustamente, has to formally open a murder enquiry. Given the evidence, this will not be a problem and we expect to receive the instruction today. However, we would rather wait a little longer before publicly confirming this is a murder enquiry, in order to give us time to try and identify the murderer before they become aware of our investigation."

"Actually, opening a murder investigation might help flush out the murderer or murderers," responded Andy.

"That's true, but at this stage we would prefer to keep the investigation low profile. Even if Mr. Brown has nothing to do with Mr. Cameron's murder, any investigation into Mr. Cameron's affairs is likely to scare him off from pursuing the property transaction.

So, Mr. Montalvo, given all that I have told you, are you still willing to help us?" Cristina Ibanez asked, holding Andy's gaze.

"Please call me Andy. This is certainly a more complicated and dangerous situation than I'd imagined. Although I agreed to help you, dead is not something I'm planning on being for some time and I still don't know what it is you want me to do."

"I fully understand; if you decide to withdraw your offer of assistance once I've told you how we would like you to help us then that's fair enough. However, we would then require you to absent yourself, at our expense of course, from Los Cipreses until we complete our investigation."

"Sounds reasonable, a few weeks in the Caribbean wouldn't go amiss," said Andy with a smile.

"Mr. Brown's arm is long; we were thinking more of Russia or Northern Scandinavia – not particularly pleasant this time of the year," replied Cristina Ibañez with the faintest hint of a smile.

When they finished their main courses Cristina Ibañez pushed the red button to summon the waiter. They skipped dessert and ordered coffee. When they were alone again, Andy asked Cristina how he could help them.

"Our objectives are now twofold. Firstly, to find Mr. Cameron's murderer and, secondly, to bring Mr. Brown and his associates to justice. As we have discussed, these matters may, or may not, be related, but we think you can help us find out."

"And how can I do that? I don't know who this Mr. Brown is and have no reason to become involved in the proposed property transaction now that Mike is dead. I don't even know who the potential investors are."

"As I mentioned, so far we have been unable to access the hard drive of Mr. Cameron's office computer to check for any files or emails. We would like you to try and gain access to his laptop, his web-based email accounts and any other paperwork he has at home to see if there are any clues or information concerning the golf course deal and/or his murder before our murder enquiry becomes official."

"Why can't you wait until your investigation is official?"

"Because requesting access to any of Mr. Cameron's effects now may raise Mr. Brown's suspicions, and he may decide to pull out of the negotiations with the investors."

Andy put down his coffee cup and reached out to pick up a petit four from the plate in the middle of the table. "I see, but how do I get access to his laptop and papers?" he said with a puzzled expression.

"Since you were in the process of buying into Mr. Cameron's business we think it would be reasonable if you were to continue to try and do this, despite his death. This would give you a perfect excuse, as a legitimate part of the due diligence process, to ask his widow for access to any paperwork or other material she might have relating to the business."

Andy thought about this. "In fact Mike's wife has asked me if I would be interested in buying the business; she expects to inherit it and is not interested in keeping it. The laptop and paperwork will probably be at Sonya's house, so Ann will have to ask Sonya for access. I can't see that it will be a problem; they actually get on reasonably well."

"Excellent. So can I assume you are willing to help us? If so, you must act quickly. We cannot delay informing his wife and daughter of the results of the autopsy much longer. Once they are aware of the results it won't be long before everyone in Los Cipreses knows that Mr. Cameron was murdered – that's the nature of small towns."

"Yes, I'll try to help you, but I'll need his passwords to access Mike's web-based email accounts or any files on his computer. Anyway, it's worth a try; maybe Ann or Sonya knows the passwords."

"Good, thank you. Will you be able to do it tomorrow?"

"Yes mi Capitan," said Andy, giving Cristina a mock salute "but how do I contact you? Do you have a business card?"

"Maintaining my cover is paramount and, given your closeness to Mr. Cameron, I don't want to bring any undue attention to myself, so the best thing to do is to set up an anonymous Gmail account and then email me at this address," Cristina Ibañez said as she passed over a piece of paper with a hand-written email address on it.

I check it regularly throughout the day and it is also monitored by some of our people in Seville on a 24/7 basis so you can be assured anything urgent will receive immediate attention. Of course, I'm assuming that you have regular access to the Internet?"

"I do. In fact I have an ADSL line at the villa and I suppose I can take my Blackberry out of retirement."

"No, please don't use a POP3 mail account, either on your laptop or Blackberry, just stick to web-based mail. If you don't have access to email and need to contact me then call this mobile number and leave a voicemail," she said, writing down a nine-digit number on another piece of paper and handing it to Andy.

"Please memorise the email address and phone number and destroy the papers before you leave here. In an emergency you can call me at the office or on the mobile number on my card. Jose Luis and Paco in the office don't know my real identity so make sure it's a business-related call by asking for more information on one of the penthouse apartments in phase two of our proposed new development."

"I've worked on a few sensitive deals in my time but I have never had quite so much cloak-and-dagger stuff – James Bond would be proud of me," said Andy with a wry smile.

"I think that just about covers everything. Do you have any more questions?"

"No, I can't think of any right now. I'll set up a Gmail account when I get back home and send you an email from the new address. I'll also talk with Ann tonight about getting access to Mike's laptop and business papers as soon as possible. It will appear a little insensitive to some, especially Sonya and Emily, but Ann should cooperate; after all, she herself asked me whether I would be prepared to buy the business."

"Good. Thank you for your time and for agreeing to help us; I hope you have some positive news for us very soon," said Cristina, standing up and offering Andy her hand.

As Andy and Cristina Ibañez were having lunch, Carlos arrived at the villa to find Ann sitting by the side of the pool in a skimpy black bikini, drinking a glass of champagne.

"I couldn't wait any longer darling. Come over here and join me – and since Emily is not here you can take your shirt and trousers off – your boxers can stay on, for now at least," she said giggling.

Carlos made his way from the terrace, across the grass to the pool. As he got closer, Ann's body looked decidedly less glamorous, as the stretch marks and excess flab around her stomach came clearly into view. It was not that she was fat, but a combination of a lack of exercise, and excess alcohol, meant that her muscle tone was fast disappearing; she had gained nearly a stone in the last twelve months. Still, he thought, she's not a bad lay and has money, which is what I need right now.

He kicked off his shoes and began to undo his shirt buttons. Ann rose from the sun lounger and reached for his belt buckle.

"Not so fast sweetheart. I can manage. Just pour me a glass of champagne; I can do the rest," he said, taking a step away from her.

Within a minute they were both sipping champagne, with Carlos down to his boxers, his taut, lithe body contrasting with Ann's less than firm flesh.

"So, you have Mike's English Will and all we need now is the death certificate in order to apply for Grant of Probate and to locate his Spanish Will," said Carlos, caressing Ann's back with his finger tips.

"Yes, and I'm going to call Chief Inspector Diaz tomorrow to find out when we can expect the autopsy result – for this afternoon I have other plans for my hot Spanish lover," she said, putting her arms around his neck and pulling Carlos towards her.

"I can see that, but don't you want to hear about my purchase of the bar?"

"What's to hear? Hang around for a few hours to get the paperwork in order because it never is, sign a few papers in front of the Notary, hand over the money and Bob's your uncle. Now let's forget all this Will and bar business and have a little fun!"

On leaving La Bobadilla, Andy took the scenic route back to Los Cipreses. It was a spectacular alternative to the main road, passing first through arid, flatish terrain, then a pine forest, followed by a tortuous but stunning mountain section, leading in turn to a lush sub-tropical valley before reaching the coast close to Los Cipreses.

Andy loved the drive, but the mountainous section was not for the faint hearted and required extra concentration. Nevertheless, he usually found it a peaceful and relaxing drive. Unfortunately, his lunch with Cristina Ibañez had unsettled him, and as he began the descent down the mountainous section he realised that perhaps it had not been such a good idea to return via this road.

He concentrated fully on driving until reaching the outskirts of the sub-tropical valley. He had descended over eight hundred metres in altitude to virtually sea level in less than ten kilometres; now sharp bends became gently sweeping curves as the road unwound. As he approached the coast, avocado and custard apple trees in full leaf filled the right-hand side of the valley.

He began thinking again about his lunch with Cristina Ibañez and the implications of what she had told him. Although Mike had been murdered, given the delicate stage, the negotiations with Mike's clients were at it seemed unlikely that Mr. Brown would want to get rid of him. So if not Mr. Brown, then who and why? Would Mike's laptop and papers be able to provide the answer?

The first thing he did when he got home was to power up his laptop and open an anonymous Gmail account. He sent an email to the address that Cristina Ibañez had given him, thanking her for the lunch and confirming he would call Ann to ask for permission to access Mike's laptop and any business papers he had at Sonya's.

After making a peppermint tea he called Ann on her home number. After four rings a slightly groggy Ann answered.

"Hi Ann, Andy here. Sorry to disturb you, it sounds as if you were having a siesta."

"Yes, sort of, but now you've got me on the phone what can I do for you?"

"I've been thinking about your offer to buy Mike's business and I'd like to look into that in more detail. Mike and I were going to go through the accounts and client list in detail next week. I need this information to decide what the business is worth, so I was wondering if I could have a look at his computer and business files to see what I can find."

"I see, but as far as I know, his computer and files were all destroyed in the fire."

"Yes, but he also had a laptop, which is probably at Sonya's, along with his papers. If he did then, as his widow, I need your permission to gain access to them."

"You're right; he definitely had a laptop and it must be at Sonya's. I'll ring her and ask. If she's got it I'll ask her to give it to you along with any business papers he may have left at her house."

"That would be great, thanks. Will you call me back when you have spoken with her? I'd like to try and make a decision about buying the business as soon as possible."

"Of course, it's in both our interests. I'm a bit tied up right now but I'll call her as soon as I can and get back to you."

Andy hung up, drank his tea and then logged in to his new Gmail account to see if the enigmatic Cristina Ibañez had responded to his earlier email. He doubted she would be that quick but, just to confound this thinking, his inbox contained an email from the email address she had given him earlier that day. He clicked to open it. The text was short and to the point:

Diaz will advise family of autopsy results and murder investigation on Saturday morning. Please let me know if you make any progress with Mr. Cameron's files tomorrow.

Very efficient. That was not a great surprise having seen how she handled Carlos in Casa Luque the other evening, and having had the experience of a closer encounter with her himself earlier. She's one sexy lady, but probably not someone you would want to cross, he thought to himself.

Ann's conversation with Sonya was brief. They were not rivals or enemies but had little in common other than Mike Cameron.

Sonya confirmed that Mike had a laptop at the house along with a desk and that she was happy to give Andy access to these.

"Thanks. I'll let him know and no doubt he will call you to agree when he can come round. I think he wants to make a decision quickly about buying the business so he may want to see them tomorrow."

"That's fine Ann, I've got nothing special planned."

"By the way Sonya, do you happen to know if Mike had any personal papers in his desk?"

"I've never looked in the drawers but I thought he kept anything of importance, work or personal related, in the office, especially since he'd had the office door and locks changed."

"That makes sense and sounds like Mike. Anyway, I'm sure if Andy finds anything of importance he'll let me know. Once Andy has finished with Mike's laptop and papers I'll pop round to collect them."

Ann immediately called Andy and told him Sonya was expecting his call. "I think most of his papers related to the business were in the office, but if you find anything of interest let me know. Hopefully we can discuss your purchase of the business over the weekend."

"Thanks Ann, I'll call Sonya in a minute. As you say, it's unlikely I'll find too much but it's worth a try. Just a thought, do you happen to know the password and usernames for Mike's laptop?"

"Not a clue. Mike was very particular about people accessing his computer; you'd think he had the secret coca-cola formula or some state secrets on it."

"Oh well, if I can't find the passwords there is no way I am going to be able to access his computer so it might be a short due diligence process. In any case, I'll let you know how I get on."

Andy pondered the computer password issue for a couple of minutes and then called Sonya.

"Hi Sonya, Andy here. I think you're expecting my call?"

"Yes, I only got off the phone with Ann a few minutes ago."

"And how are you doing?"

"Tired of waiting, to be honest. I just wish they would give us the autopsy result and let us bury him in peace."

"I'm sure it won't be long now and then we can all move on. I also need to decide whether to get involved in Mike's business so I was wondering if it would be convenient to come round tomorrow morning and have a look at his laptop and any papers he has over there."

"I've got aerobics first thing; why don't you come over any time after ten-thirty."

"That's fine, I'll see you then."

It had been a long day and tomorrow he would need to be fully alert to try and crack the password on Mike's laptop. So after rustling up a spaghetti a la pomodoro, washed down with a glass of Casa de La Ermita from the up and coming Jumilla region, he retired to bed to read a bit more of Bill Bryson's A Short History of Nearly Everything. At eleven he switched off the lights and soon fell into a deep sleep.

Friday, 23rd November

In London, Peter Roberts was listening attentively as Elena Nuñez summarised Pelayo y Parra's opinion about the structure proposed by Vicente Maldonado. Unless they were satisfied no laws were being broken they could not proceed with the transaction.

"Mr. Maldonado is correct that the responsibility to pay tax will fall on the sellers of the land once the options are exercised. At the same time, if we obtain a Certificate of Non-Investigation from the Cayman authorities, then we don't need to know the identity of the principals involved. However, if the owners of the Cayman Island company are Spanish residents, under Spanish law they must declare any income they obtain from that company."

"But if we are satisfied that they are not under investigation, do we have an obligation to inform the Spanish authorities about the transaction?"

"Only if we have reasonable cause to believe that Spanish residents are involved and money laundering or tax evasion is going on."

Peter Roberts considered this. "In all likelihood tax evasion is the objective, but if we get a Certificate of Non-Investigation and also put a rep and warranty in the agreement that the beneficial owners of the Cayman Island company are in compliance with the tax legislation in their countries of residence, then we would be in the clear."

"Technically that's correct, but wouldn't we also want a financial indemnity just in case Spanish residents and tax evasion are involved?"

"Yes, you're right. Let's call Sr. Maldonado now and see if he wants to proceed on that basis."

It was just after ten o'clock in the morning in Granada, and, since his ADSL line at home was still down, Vicente Maldonado had been in the office since eight making payments to various offshore accounts on behalf of his clients.

Belen had not arrived yet and he was just about to leave the office to grab a coffee at a bar around the corner when his mobile rang. From the 44 prefix he saw it was a call from the UK.

He flipped the phone open and placed it to his right ear. "Vicente Maldonado."

"Good morning Sr. Maldonado, Peter Roberts and Elena Nuñez here. Is it convenient to talk?"

"Good morning. Yes I can talk. I was just on my way out for a coffee."

"Well Mr. Maldonado, we have some good news for you. Our Spanish lawyers have confirmed that the structure you propose is legal, albeit with some provisos which we would like to discuss with you before proceeding."

"Are these provisos deal breakers?"

"I couldn't say. That's for you and your clients to decide."

"Ok, tell me what they are so I can consult my clients and get back to you as soon as possible."

"Well, we're happy with the proposed structure in terms of reservation deposit, stage payments against milestones and ultimately acquiring shares in a Cayman Island company.

We are also prepared to accept your clients' need for anonymity provided that, in addition to the Certificate of Non-Investigation, we include a representation and warranty in the Share Purchase Agreement to the effect that the bona fide owners of the Cayman Island company are in compliance with the tax legislation in their country of residence and also that ten percent of the proceeds are held back in an escrow account as an indemnity against any claims against us in respect of any tax that may be due on the transaction."

There was a long silence at the other end of the phone. "I understand where you're coming from but obviously I need to discuss this with my clients. Are there any other conditions?"

"No. That's it."

"And if my clients agree to these new conditions how quickly could we proceed?"

"That's up to you, but the quickest way forward would be for you to email us a draft of the proposed deposit agreement. If that is acceptable then we can meet in Madrid next week to finalise it and also work on the Share Purchase Agreement."

"Very well, thank you and I'll get back to you later today," said Vicente, closing his phone.

Accepting this proposal would mean that they would probably never see the twenty-five million euros again. On the other hand, losing ten percent was a hell of a lot better than paying fifty-six percent in tax, and what alternative did they have? The deal had to be done before the thirty-first of December if they were to avoid falling under the new notary disclosure laws, and there were no other investors on the horizon.

Javier Urquiza was not happy but reluctantly agreed with Vicente that the twenty-five-million reduction be allocated on a pro-rata basis between all four of them.

"But I hope Enrique and Fernando appreciate it means that I'm taking the biggest hit, even though I've funded this deal to the tune of three million euros already."

"Javier, at the end of the day you're still going to come out with over a hundred and ninety million euros and we still need their cooperation; reducing their take further might jeopardise that."

"Ok, Ok, but there is no need to tell them about the reduction until both agreements have been finalised and the PGOU is approved. In the meantime, call Mr. Roberts and tell him we accept but, please, no more surprises Vicente; let's get the deposit paid as soon as possible so we can pay our friends on the Environmental and Urban Planning Committees. What does the timing look like?"

"I'm confident that we can wrap up the deposit agreement by the end of next week. The Share Purchase Agreement will take longer but, as you say, the priority is to get the five million euros paid into the escrow account."

"Absolutely, so move it along as quickly as you can. By the way, you are sure that they will not be able to identify any of us, even when we sell the shares in the Cayman company to them?"

"Yes, I'm certain. The Cayman authorities will only disclose the names of the shareholders if the requesting authority can demonstrate they have reasonable cause to believe the company and the individuals concerned are involved in criminal activities. Since the transaction itself will not occur until after we ask for the Certificate of Non-Investigation there is no reasonable cause."

"So our anonymity is guaranteed?"

"Yes. Also, remember the transaction per se is not illegal until such time that we fail to notify the Spanish authorities of our interest in the proceeds, by which time the funds and us will be long gone."

"Excellent, good work as usual Vicente. By the way, did you transfer the funds to the Galician?"

"Yes, I did it earlier this morning."

"Mr. Roberts, my clients are prepared to proceed on the basis you outlined earlier but they don't expect any further material changes."

"Splendid. Please send the draft deposit agreement and any other drafts you have by email to Elena, with a copy to my secretary, as I still haven't figured out how to use my new fangled Blueberry or Blackberry thing, whatever it's called.

In any event, Elena will be handling most of the negotiations – I just want to go to Madrid for the seafood and the Prado! Seriously, Elena will review your draft to ensure there are no major issues with it and then she or my secretary will get back to you later today with some times and dates for a meeting in Madrid next week."

"Very well, I'll email the drafts in a few minutes and look forward to hearing from Elena."

Andy had set the alarm on his mobile phone for nine. Nevertheless, he awoke earlier, thus avoiding being abruptly awoken by its shrill tone. He got out of bed, padded down the corridor to the living room in his boxers and went over to the stereo. He plugged in his MP4 player and selected J.J. Cale's Special Edition album from the on-screen menu. I wonder how many people realise this man is responsible for Cocaine, I Shot the Sheriff, Cajun Moon and They Call Me the Breeze, he thought to himself.

After showering he made himself some scrambled eggs with smoked salmon and sat on the terrace watching the sun rise ever higher above the Punta, its rays gradually warming his face. As he ate his breakfast, he thought about today's task and hoped his luck would be in, and that Mike's papers and laptop would have clues as to who had murdered him – provided, of course, he could access the laptop and emails.

When he'd finished his breakfast, he checked his emails, both personal and also the new anonymous Gmail account he'd set up to communicate with Cristina Ibañez. As expected, both inboxes were empty so, after quickly checking the latest business and financial news he logged off and put his laptop in its carry case. At half past ten, he picked up the carry case, grabbed an A4 pad and went out to his car and drove to Sonya's, taking the shortcut through Los Romeros.

Sonya made him his second cup of coffee of the day and then left him alone in Mike's study, which was actually a small outhouse at the rear of the main house. It had probably been built as a tool shed or storage room but Mike had converted it for office use, installing proper electrics, a phone line, painting the walls and re-tiling the floor. He had also made the south-facing window larger to let in more natural light and his desk, on which sat a laptop, was directly underneath the window.

It was a proper office desk with cut away holes for computer and telephone cables and a set of drawers on either side of the chair, which was tucked under its centre.

Andy pulled out the chair and sat down. The laptop was closed but appeared to be plugged in to the mains, along with a router which blinked away in the top right-hand corner of the desk. He opened the laptop, hoping that Mike had left it in sleep mode and without password protection.

No such luck. When he pushed the power button the Windows XP booting up screen appeared and then, after a minute or two, the login screen blipped its welcome. Before continuing with the laptop, Andy decided to open the drawers to see if Mike had written down the password somewhere, but both were locked and there were no keys in the locks. Sonya didn't have the keys and agreed to let Andy force the locks with a screwdriver, which proved easier than he expected.

Aside from the two sets of drawers with hanging files, there was a shallow drawer which was full of the usual paraphernalia, including a diary, pens, pencils, staples, loose invoices, mobile phone charger and various cables and connectors for phones and computers.

Andy carefully emptied the contents of this drawer onto the desk. The most obvious place to look for any passwords was the diary, but this appeared to have been a gift from a bank and had not been used. The invoices and receipts were for petrol and groceries and Andy could find nothing which resembled a password for the laptop. He put all the items back into the drawer and then began looking at the hanging files.

There were about eight hanging files in the right-hand drawer and ten in the left-hand drawer. The right-hand drawer tabs included credit cards, bank statements, utilities, insurance, pensions, ancestry and divorce and these were obviously Mike's personal papers. The left-hand drawer tabs had names such as Marysol and Acacia and a quick glance revealed them to be properties Mike had on his books.

There was nothing to indicate that either set of files would contain the password for the computer but Andy decided to look at the credit card and bank statement files – which in fact was all they contained. He noticed that there were recent statements from a bank account in Jersey showing a balance of a little under two million euros. Not bad, thought Andy, that must be the offshore "pension fund" that Mike mentioned to me a couple of times and that the Spanish authorities had discovered.

It was now half past twelve and he went back to the house to ask Sonya again if she had any idea what the computer password might be or where it might be found before he sat down for what was likely to be a long afternoon at the keyboard.

"I'm sorry Andy, I've racked my brains and I can't think what the password might be apart from the obvious like house name, Emily, phone number, date of birth, etc."

"Oh well, I suppose I'll have to try guessing a few combinations once I've finished going through his business papers."

A couple of hours later Sonya called to Andy to ask whether he wanted to join her and the children for lunch. "Perfect timing, I've just about finished going through the client files and I could do with a break before I make a start on the laptop."

After lunch the children declined a yogurt for dessert and disappeared to watch their favourite cartoon while Andy and Sonya had coffee.

"So have you found anything to help you make your mind up about buying the business?"

"The client files contain recent instructions that Mike had received to rent or sell properties. While they give an indication of recent activity what I really need to see are the accounts for the last three years. Mike had given me some broad brush numbers but we were going to go through the numbers in detail this week. I assume they're on the computer."

"More than likely, Mike was quite meticulous about keeping his financial records up to date."

"Of course, even if I manage to access the hard drive, any secure files, programmes or online accounts will probably have their own usernames and passwords."

They were silent for a moment, both gazing out through the window at the mountains behind the bay. In the distance, clouds were gathering in and around the peaks.

"Finally, it looks like we might get some rain," said Sonya "the reservoirs are down to less than a quarter of their capacity and some properties using underground wells are getting salty water."

"Let's hope it's nice steady overnight rain – although it looks more like a storm brewing. Well I'm going to have a crack at Mike's laptop, but I don't hold out much hope," Andy said, standing up and making his way across the dining room towards the outhouse.

Given what was at stake, Vicente Maldonado was nervous and was sorely tempted to call Peter Roberts to find out if the draft agreements were an acceptable basis for more detailed negotiations. However, it had only been a few hours since he had emailed them to Elena and Joanne so instead, he checked the documents which would be made available to the investors in respect of the first milestone payment for the fourth time.

The deposit agreement was relatively straightforward; it was the share purchase agreement which might require more time to negotiate. Whatever happened, this needed to be in place before the

Urban Planning Committee meeting on the nineteenth of December, even though completion would be conditional upon the land being reclassified.

He made himself another cup of coffee and tried to read the newspaper. Eventually, at half past five, his mobile rang and it was a call from a UK number. He felt his pulse quicken but waited for it to ring three times before answering.

"Sr. Maldonado, its Elena Nuñez here and I'm calling to confirm that, in principle, we and our clients are happy with the draft agreements, although there are some minor drafting issues we need to address."

"Excellent," he replied, trying to keep his voice neutral. "Can we meet next week to agree a final version of the deposit agreement at least?" he continued.

"We've set aside all of Tuesday and, if necessary, Wednesday morning, for meetings in Madrid. I think that should be long enough to finalise the Reservation Deposit Agreement and even make a start on the Share Purchase Agreement."

"Good. Where shall we meet on Tuesday?"

"At Pelayo y Parra's offices."

"Fine. I'll see you there at ten o'clock."

Vicente immediately rang Don Javier to tell him the news and they agreed to meet on Sunday to go over the key points of the agreements. He then rang Fernando Echevaria.

"Good afternoon, Fernando. Good news, the investors want to go ahead so I'm meeting with their lawyers again on Tuesday to finalise the deposit agreement," he said, omitting to mention the fact that twenty-five million euros was being withheld from the purchase price.

"That's excellent news. Let's see if we can bring this transaction to a successful conclusion and get our just rewards for the risks we're taking."

"And are you prepared to continue with the arrangement we discussed in the event the transaction proceeds?"

"Absolutely, I don't see why that hillbilly Enrique Gonzalez should share any of the proceeds. After all, he has no influence over my committee or the Urban Planning Committee."

"Precisely my thoughts and as long as we don't threaten the final outcome or reduce Don Javier's return then I think we can proceed, but carefully. Once we set the ball rolling there's no turning back. So if you're having any second thoughts or doubts, now is the time to tell me, before it's too late."

"None whatsoever, Vicente. Eighteen million euros each is better than twelve and a half million, and Enrique deserves nothing. But are you sure that Johan will deliver his side of the bargain?"

"I don't see any problem there. He's greedy and unscrupulous and one and a half million euros is a lot of money to him. The Cayman Island company is already set up and all I have to do is allocate the shareholdings in the agreed percentages. If Johan delivers his side of the bargain then Enrique's five percent shareholding will be reallocated between me, you and Johan at the appropriate time."

"Is there any way that Javier or Enrique will be able to establish the real shareholding percentages allocated to each of us?"

"Virtually impossible. Enrique won't be around, while Javier doesn't speak or read English and has never been directly involved in dealing with his offshore companies. He trusts me implicitly and I have the relevant Powers of Attorney. Remember, at the end of the day, if the sale goes ahead as planned, Don Javier is not going to lose out financially, we are just redistributing Enrique's five percent."

"Indeed; let's hope we can reach an agreement with the investors."

"Don't worry you can be sure I'll do my best. I'll try and meet with Johan before I go to Madrid to discuss what we are going to do with Enrique."

Mission impossible, Andy thought looking at the log-in screen. With Windows XP, Microsoft had made it virtually impossible to crack log-in codes unless you were the CIA with a Super Cray computer or Bill Gates himself.

The administrator's username, Mike Cameron, was already on screen but it was the password that he needed to gain access to the computer's files and applications. He took a piece of A4 paper and began making a list: first school, mothers maiden name, name of first girlfriend, name of first street, first car make and model, first car registration, parents' names, dates of birth, etc. The list went on and on and he realised that even being able to get half of the information he'd listed would take several days and many phone calls. Still, he had no choice, so he began to write down the information he already knew next to each category on the list.

Two hours later he had tried every potential password he had written down, using both upper and lower case, and all he got each time was the erroneous password pop-up message on the screen.

It was very frustrating but there was not much more he could do until he obtained the information he was missing from Mike's family and friends and went through the same process.

"No joy, I'm afraid Sonya. I have tried every combination I could think of but I need to talk with his family and childhood friends to get some more possible passwords. I'll make a few calls this evening and hopefully I'll be able to have another go tomorrow. Is it Ok to come back tomorrow or can I take the laptop with me and do this from home?"

"Best to take it with you. Saturdays are usually busy with shopping, football and horse riding."

"Ok thanks. I think I'm going to have a restless night; if you have any ideas about potential passwords give me a call."

Once home Andy emailed Cristina Ibañez. "*Nothing in MC's business papers. Unable to access laptop. Will continue attempts tomorrow.*"

He wondered where she was and how soon she or one of her colleagues would read it and hoped she might call him before he went to sleep – if only to hear her sexy voice.

He poured himself a glass of the already open Casa de la Ermita and sat down on the sofa. He had no intention of continuing his battle with the laptop that evening but he thought perhaps a glass or two of wine might give him some inspiration, so he placed a pen and a sheet of paper on the coffee table in front of him.

Half an hour later he had written down a few more categories for passwords. He then turned on his laptop, opened up his Palm Pilot software and began writing down the phone numbers of all those people who might be able to give him the information he had listed and which he did not know.

Naturally, his first port of call was Ann. He told her about the client files and about his failure so far to identify Mike's password. She was able to give him some of the information he required as well as the names and phone numbers of a couple of Mike's old friends who might also be able to help.

"By the way, did you go through his personal papers?" asked Ann, when she had finished giving him the names and numbers.

"Very briefly, but only those files which I thought might have the information I need."

"Did you happen to see if there was a copy of his Spanish Will? I have his English one but I can't access the original Spanish one without his death certificate."

"No Ann, I didn't see anything that looked like a Spanish Will but then I wasn't really looking for that. When you get the papers you can have a look yourself."

"That's true, but Chief Inspector Diaz called me a few minutes ago to say that they have just received the autopsy result and so I'm meeting him tomorrow morning. Hopefully he'll give me the death certificate and then I can locate the original Spanish Will on Monday."

"That's good news re the autopsy. Call me when you know the result," Andy said, without disclosing his own knowledge that Mike had been murdered "and thanks for the information and contact details. I'll let you know if I make any progress over the weekend. If not, I'll have to base my decision on whether to buy the business on what Mike told me and the little information I've been able to gather from the client files I've seen."

He replaced the handset and took a sip of wine. He understood her desire to get Mike's estate sorted out, especially with the amount of money at stake, but couldn't help but feel that there was something odd about the underlying sense of urgency she was transmitting. Oh well, he reasoned, even if they do release the death certificate to her, since Mike's death is officially being treated as murder neither the Spanish or British authorities would release or action the Wills until the case was satisfactorily resolved.

Saturday, 24th November

The rumble of thunder grew louder and longer as the storm approached Los Cipreses on its way out to sea. Andy had been sleeping fitfully and so was quickly awake as the storm reached Los Cipreses. His head was full of numbers, letters, names and dates as he stepped out onto the terrace to experience the power of nature at work.

Massive bolts of lightning briefly and spectacularly illuminated the bay every few seconds, throwing the Punta de Palermo into stark relief against the pitch black sky. Soon wind and rain were lashing the village and its environs. During the regular lightning strikes Andy could see large, white-crested waves rolling inexorably towards the beach. Occasionally he caught glimpses of them crashing into the Punta, their spray climbing high and reaching several of the villas perched high on the headland close to the water's edge. After a few minutes, he returned indoors to towel himself dry and try and get some sleep in preparation for his renewed attempts on Mike's laptop.

A few hours later, he was finishing his cup of coffee and orange juice and bracing himself to start on Mike's laptop again when his phone rang. It was Sonya.

"Hi Andy, I was just tidying up some of the shelves in the living room and I found Mike's palm pilot under some papers. I'm not sure if it's of any use to you but I thought you ought to know."

"Thanks Sonya. It might be useful – it depends on what information he stored in it. Can I come and get it now?"

"Yes, if you're here in the next half an hour."

Andy had introduced Mike to the idea of using a Palm Pilot mainly to keep a back-up of names and addresses of friends, clients, etc., separate from his computer. The advantage was that it could be easily synchronised with the data on the computer. Thus if the computer's hard drive failed or he wanted to travel without it he had easy access to details of his key contacts in the hand-held device.

He drove over to Sonya's to collect the Palm. On his return home, he connected it to Mike's laptop via a USB cable and pushed the on/off button. He tapped on the Contacts logo and instantly an alphabetical list of Mike's contacts appeared. Andy wondered if Mike had marked certain entries as private so that they could only be accessed with a password. He had recommended Mike do this for bank account details such as PINs, online passwords and security codes, etc., and he was just about to find out whether he had taken his advice.

He tapped on the Contacts menu at the top of the screen, then Options and then Security: Current Privacy: "Show Records" the pop-up screen said.

"Bingo!" said Andy out loud. "Now let's see what private information Mike had stored on this little beauty."

Chief Inspector Diaz was not looking forward to his meeting with Ann. While he would be the public face leading the murder enquiry, it was frustrating that he did not know the extent and scope of UDYCO's undercover operation or its possible relevance to Mike Cameron's death.

He had not yet formed an opinion about who might have murdered Mike Cameron but he expected that once his death was officially being treated as murder the pace of the investigation would pick up. The results of the forensic tests on Mike Cameron's keys and the door locks were due next week, and might yield useful clues as to which set of keys had been used to access the office via the garage and storeroom on the night of his death.

His phone rang and he picked up the receiver. "Chief Inspector Diaz, Mrs. Cameron, her daughter and Mr. Macarena are here to see you. They're in the reception."

Chief Inspector Diaz hung up and walked down the corridor to reception to meet them. All three were standing close to the counter and he addressed Ann.

"I'm sorry to disturb your Saturday morning but I thought you would want to know as soon as possible. By the way, I don't wish to be rude but this is a highly personal matter and we usually only discuss autopsy results with immediate family. Maybe Señor Maracena should wait here?" Secretly he hoped Carlos would join them because he wanted to see his reaction to the news that Mike Cameron had been murdered.

"I appreciate that Chief Inspector, but I'm only going to tell him what you tell me so you may as well tell us all together."

He led them to his office and Ann and Emily sat in the two battered plastic chairs for visitors while Carlos stood at Ann's side. Chief Inspector Diaz sat behind his desk and opened the cover of a thick blue file which was resting on top of the desk.

"What I am about to tell you will come as a shock, as it did to me when I received the autopsy report," he said looking at Ann, then Emily and finally Carlos.

"I'm very sorry to have to inform you Mrs. Cameron that your husband's death was not an accident. He was in fact murdered by a person or persons currently unknown."

There was stunned silence for a few moments and then Emily cried out, "No, No" and looked back and forth at Chief Inspector Diaz and her mother, with disbelief and shock on her face. Ann let out an audible gasp and clasped a hand to her mouth, "My God" she said. Carlos too looked visibly shaken, his eyes widening as he looked and listened to Chief Inspector Diaz, but he said nothing.

"Would any of you like some water before I give you the details?"

"No, I'm fine, let's get it over with," replied Ann, while Emily just shook her head and Carlos remained silent.

Chief Inspector Diaz proceeded to tell them the results of the autopsy and that Judge Bustamente would now officially declare the investigation to be a murder enquiry. He explained that this meant they could now get warrants to search premises, seize computers and other material, obtain phone records, etc., and also to begin questioning people who might be able to help them identify Mike's killer or killers.

"Unfortunately, we're still waiting for the results of some forensic and toxicology tests which may help us with our enquiry but, in the meantime, we'll be interviewing a number of people who were close to Mr. Cameron or involved in his business activities over the coming days."

"But who would want to kill Mike? Do you have any suspects?" asked Ann, as Emily sobbed next to her.

"I'm afraid I'm not at liberty to disclose any aspects of the murder investigation other than what I have told you, but if you have information you feel may be relevant to Mr. Cameron's death, however insignificant, I would ask you to tell me now."

"I can't think straight right now but rest assured if anything occurs to me I'll let you know," said Ann. Both Emily and Carlos remained silent. "Do we get a copy of the autopsy report and also the death certificate?" she continued.

"I'm afraid I can't give you either at this stage. The autopsy report is not complete without the toxicology results and a death certificate cannot be issued while the autopsy report is incomplete or until Judge Bustamente authorises its issuance. This will probably be when the case is closed, although it could be sooner if there are some legal justifications for this."

"I see. Is there anything else you can tell us or can we go?"

"I've told you all I can for now and I'm sorry to be the bearer of such unexpected and unwelcome news. I would like to see you all early next week to ask you some questions but I'll call you in advance. In the meantime, if any of you remember anything which may be relevant please call me."

Ann, Emily and Carlos all stood up and followed the Chief Inspector down the corridor back to the reception.

Mike's palm pilot contained a lot of entries and so Andy used the Find function to see which entries contained the words: username and password. There were several, ranging from bank accounts to email accounts and websites such as Amazon, and Andy printed each such entry out.

By the time he'd finished he had over twenty sheets of paper, including one with the password for his laptop. I should have realised he would use a symbolic female but I'd never have guessed it, he thought to himself.

He made another cup of strong coffee and contemplated where to begin. First he decided to email Cristina to let her know that he'd found all of Mike's usernames and passwords. Then he would check Mike's emails, both in Outlook and also in the web-based ones whose details were in the palm pilot.

He typed ElonaGay into the password box and the hour glass indicated that the start-up programmes were being loaded. He opened up Outlook and while the programme downloaded over ten days of emails from Mike's business email account he sent an email to Cristina.

"Success! Have all usernames and passwords. Checking emails and then hard drive. Will advise progress in due course."

He wondered whether she or one of her colleagues would see it first but knew one way or the other that she would be aware of it very soon.

Once Outlook had finished downloading Mike's work emails, Andy went to those emails dated the night of Mike's death. From what Johan Gaards had said Mike had gone to the office that night to check for an email he was expecting from a client. Andy wanted to see if such an email existed and, if so, who it was from. He scrolled down all the emails for the day in question plus the next day to cover any delays in transmission or time zone differences. There were only a few emails and nothing from a client indicating an imminent arrival.

Maybe Johan was mistaken about the email but he doubted it. Mike had definitely had a reason to go to the office that night. Maybe it was not an email from a client, but from Mr. Brown or the investors he was expecting?

Andy turned to the sheets of paper lying on the desk at the side of Mike's laptop. He had identified three different Gmail accounts and it was to these that he turned his attention. One of the accounts was in Mike's own name and Andy knew he used it mainly for personal correspondence, so he left this until last. The second and the third were each set up with a non-descriptive, anonymous address which would not enable the user to be identified. Andy logged in to the first of these and quickly saw that it was an email address Mike had set up for correspondence with Cristina Ibañez and UDYCO, just as he had recently done. A quick scroll through the sent and inboxes revealed little other than intermittent progress reports.

The second of the anonymous email addresses looked as if it had been used to communicate with Mr. Brown or his associates. All the emails in this account either came from, or were addressed to, an anonymous Hotmail address or were to/from Peter Roberts at Moore, Moore & Blackthorn and all referred to the property transaction.

In fact, he knew Peter Roberts from his investment banking days but it had been two or three years since he had any direct dealings with him. He was a very good lawyer despite his bluff manner and Andy was convinced he would not get involved in anything illegal.

The last email from Mike had been to send the reference Peter Roberts had provided regarding the investors to Mr. Brown. This was dated a week before Mike's death but there had been no response. Unfortunately, none of the emails contained names of any of the parties involved, other than Peter Roberts, or specific details of the land in question. Clearly great care had been taken not to disclose any of this information in writing.

Again, no email had been received on the night of Mike's murder. So what email had Mike been referring to?

As Andy pondered this his mobile phone vibrated, indicating he had received an SMS. It was from an unknown number: *"Some important developments re penthouse apartments in phase 2. Can you come to my office to discuss?"*

So curiosity got the better of Ms. Ibañez he thought, as a smile flickered across his face. He looked at his watch. It was just gone eleven and he wondered if Paco or Jose Luis would be in the office. If so, would she agree to come to his place to review what he had discovered and go through the contents of Mike's hard drive? Of course, it would be an excuse to be alone with her in a more informal environment to see if he could get underneath her veneer of professionalism and efficiency. He found her very attractive, not just physically but also because of her obvious intelligence and self-confident manner, and he wanted to get to know her better.

However, he realised that it was unlikely she would have asked him to go to the office if Paco and Jose Luis were there, so he sent her a text message confirming that he would be there in the next thirty minutes.

Ann drove back to Los Cipreses with Emily. Carlos followed them in his car. Emily was still sobbing intermittently but, after the initial shock, Ann had calmed down. "Emily, sweetheart I know you are upset, I am too, but please try to calm down. Crying like this is not going to bring your father back."

"You cold-hearted bitch! He was a fantastic Dad and he didn't deserve to be taken from us like that. Who would want to kill him? He would never hurt a soul."

"You're right, he was a fantastic father and husband despite our recent differences, but the most important thing right now is for the police to catch whoever is responsible. There is nothing you or I can do to bring him back."

"And do you have any idea who might be responsible?"

"None I'm afraid. I had very few dealings with your father in recent months, aside from discussing the divorce, so I don't really know what he was up to or who he was dealing with. Sonya's in a better position to know and I'm sure the police will be talking to her."

"What about your friend back there," said Emily, casting a glance at Carlos in the car behind them.

"Listen, you may not approve of Carlos but why on earth would he want your father dead? We had agreed to divorce and your father was living happily with Sonya – he was not a threat to Carlos."

"Not a threat perhaps but a financial lifeline maybe?"

"How can you say such a thing!"

"Easy. Where did he get the money to buy the bar from?"

Ann paused for a few seconds. "I lent it to him – but it's a business deal and he's going to pay me back."

"I bet, in kind or in cash?" said Emily sarcastically.

"Emily, how dare you talk to me like that. Stop it at once. I am sure the police will quickly find out who did it and that it will be related to your father's business dealings."

They continued the rest of the journey in silence and on arriving home Emily immediately announced she was going to Sonya's to tell her the news. "And don't expect me back until late, if at all, tonight," she said as she left.

"How are you feeling, cariño," Carlos asked Ann, putting his arms round her as they stood in the kitchen.

"I am physically and emotionally drained and I really don't know what to think Carlos."

"Yes, it's been a very difficult morning; the fact that Mike was murdered must have come as a complete shock to you."

"Of course it did and to you too I assume," she replied, pulling away from him and looking him in the eyes.

"Of course, of course, but, after all, he was your husband and you'd been married a long time. I hardly knew him, so the shock would have been much greater for you."

"Yes, and the fact that for more than a week we all thought it was an accident makes today's news even worse."

"You are right, mi amor. Why don't you sit down and I'll bring you some tea. I'm going to have a beer."

Carlos brought the drinks through to the living room and they sat in silence. After a while Ann said: "I'm tired and hungry; let's have an early lunch and then I'm going to lie down."

Samesa's sales office was a reformed cottage twenty yards off the coast road close to the Cerro Grande tunnel. Like most property sales offices in Southern Spain, they were open at weekends, so it was not unusual for Cristina Ibañez to be in the office on a Saturday morning.

Andy walked down some steps and through an open door into a large well-lit room with a model of Samesa's proposed development taking centre stage on a large table. To the right of the model were two desks, each with flat screen monitors and neat piles of papers and files.

As he turned to his left, Cristina Ibañez appeared through an open door located at the other end of the room. She was wearing a navy blue skirt and cream blouse with the Samesa logo as a subtle pattern. Although to all intents and purposes it was a uniform, she still managed to look stunning. Her ash-blond hair was tied back in a neat, high, pony tail which swung gently from side to side as she approached Andy with her hand outstretched.

"Señor Montalvo, welcome and thank you for coming at such short notice," she said in her husky voice.

"My pleasure Ms. Ibañez; I wasn't expecting to see you again quite so soon. Are your two colleagues here?"

"Please call me Cristina, and no, Jose Luis and Paco are not here. Only one of us mans the weekend shifts at this time of year and today I drew the short straw, as I think they say in your country. I've always got work to do and being alone enables me to focus on immediate priorities," she said with a knowing look.

"Of course, and perhaps today I can help you."

"I hope so. Let's go into my office." She turned round and Andy followed her into her office. He plugged Mike's laptop into the mains and Cristina gave him the security code to connect to the Internet via the router in her office.

They went through the correspondence in the three email accounts Andy had already looked at.

"None of this correspondence discloses any new information about the property transaction except the fact that the investors' lawyer is Peter Roberts of Moore, Moore & Blackthorn, who I happen to know quite well from my banking days."

"Yes, we're aware that Mr. Roberts is acting for the investors."

"So why haven't you approached him directly for information about the transaction? I'd be very surprised if he was involved in anything illegal."

"At the moment we have no evidence that the proposed transaction breaks Spanish law or that Mr. Cameron's death is connected to it, so we cannot approach him officially."

"Yes, you'll need some specific evidence for him to break client confidentiality. In the meantime, unfortunately, I haven't found an email from any of Mike's clients on the day of his death in his business email account," said Andy, turning away from the screen and looking at Cristina.

"Ok, that leaves us his personal Gmail account which he used for non-work-related correspondence, so let's have a look at that."

They logged on to Mike's personal Gmail account and saw there were a few unread emails dating from the day of his murder, but they were all newsletters or marketing messages from airlines and other services Mike used, such as Amazon. There was no email from a client on that day, or on either side of it, advising Mike of their imminent arrival.

"Well, that just about confirms it. Mike didn't receive an email from a client that night, but then why did he tell Johan Gaards that he was expecting one?"

"We'll need to check Mr. Gaards' story again. Maybe Mike received a phone call or an SMS while they were drinking in the Cutty Sark? We can get a warrant to access Mike's mobile phone records now so we'll be able to check for ourselves."

"So what's next?"

"Let's go back through two or three weeks of Mike's personal emails prior to his murder to see if there are any clues there. Then we can have a quick look at the hard drive to see if there are any files of interest."

"Sounds like a plan but, notwithstanding the mystery of the missing email, it looks like we might be hitting a dead end."

"Possibly, but let's spend a few more minutes going through the emails. Searching the hard drive could be quite a big job so once we have given it a quick scan I'll get one of our technology experts to do a full analysis."

It didn't take them long to find a series of emails between Mike Cameron and Jonathan Westwood finalising the terms of Mikes' new Spanish and UK Wills and discussing the terms of his divorce settlement. From these, it was obvious that Mike had made new Wills only a few days before his murder which left nothing to Ann.

"Wow, that'll put the cat amongst the pigeons!" exclaimed Andy.

"Why?"

Andy explained how Ann was expecting to inherit all of Mike's estate, aside from the provision for Emily, which was one of the reasons she had offered to sell him Mike's business.

"I also suspect that she's used some of Mike's money to help Carlos buy the bar; I was going to have a look at Mike's bank accounts later. What we need to do is find out where the originals of these new Wills are and ensure that Ann does not get her hands on them."

"Actually the Spanish one will be lodged with a Notary and she won't be able to access it without a death certificate. In any event, if she's not a beneficiary then she won't be able to access it, even with a death certificate. Doesn't your English system work the same way?"

"No. You can leave your original English Will wherever you want but you do need a death certificate to get a Grant of Probate, which in turn enables the executors to act on the provisions of the Will. Listen, I've an idea, let's look in Mike's palm pilot to see if he has made a note of where his Wills are."

Using "Will" in the Find function generated a number of entries which contained the letters "will." Scrolling down the list they quickly came to an entry called UK Will.

Andy clicked on the entry and in the Notes section it said "located in Pensions folder" He thought for a moment. "I remember seeing such a folder yesterday in his desk at Sonya's house. We have to get this before Ann collects Mike's papers from Sonya's and discovers the existence of the new Wills. Shall I call Sonya?"

"Wait a minute. We have to be careful," she replied. "Sonya may not know that Mike was murdered yet. Chief Inspector Diaz was only going to tell Ann a couple of hours ago. She may decide to try and collect Mike's papers from Sonya before we claim them as part of the investigation."

"You're right of course. I'm not meant to know that Mike was murdered so I'll call her and tell her that I have discovered the usernames and passwords and would like to review his files again."

Sonya answered the phone almost immediately. She was crying and Andy asked what was wrong. "Emily's here. She has just got back from seeing Chief Inspector Diaz. Apparently, Mike was murdered."

Andy feigned shock. He comforted Sonya and then spoke with Emily who told him what he already knew; she was clearly also very upset.

"Andy, it's terrible. Who could have done such a thing and why. I wouldn't be surprised if Carlos had something to do with it."

"Now, now, Emily it's not good to speculate and I am sure the police will do everything in their power to find your father's killer.

Would you like me to come round?"

"Yes, you were one of Dad's best friends and Sonya and I would appreciate your presence; it's been a bit of a shock for both of us."

"I'll tell Sonya that Mike's papers will probably be required by the police and that she shouldn't give them to Ann until given permission to do so," he said to Cristina after ending the call.

"That way we should prevent Ann finding the new English Will at least, albeit accidentally, as she thinks she's got the latest version."

Before Andy left for Sonya's they accessed Mike Cameron's bank accounts online to see if there were any untoward transactions in recent weeks. It did not take them long to find the one hundred and twenty-five thousand euros transfer to Ann's Gibraltar account earlier that week.

"That explains where Carlos got the money to buy the bar from," he said. "Of course the transfer is illegal, not only because Mike was dead when it was made but also because, under the terms of his latest Will, Ann is not entitled to the funds in that account."

"Indeed, but if she believed she was entitled to those funds under the terms of his Will it would certainly provide a motive for murder."

Andy considered this for a moment. "I've known Ann for years and I just can't see her being involved in Mike's murder. That doesn't mean Carlos couldn't have had a hand in it; after all it looks as if he is getting money from Ann. Maybe he got greedy?"

"Based on the evidence, we have to consider them both as the prime suspects; I need to get the information about the Wills and the bank transfer to Chief Inspector Diaz ASAP. If they are guilty then it would appear Mr. Brown had nothing to do with Mr. Cameron's death, but we want him to know that we have two suspects as soon as possible."

"Why?"

"If Mr. Brown thinks a murder investigation would reveal his links with Mike Cameron and hence details of the land deal, regardless of whether he was involved in Mike's death or not, then in all probability he'll stop all negotiations. If we already have someone else in the frame for the murder, then hopefully he'll feel comfortable about continuing the negotiations."

"I see, but how do we get this information to him?"

"The best bet is via Johan Gaards, who we know has close links with Mr. Brown. Chief Inspector Diaz can pay him a visit later today to let him know that Mr. Cameron's death is being treated as murder and to confirm some details of his story. He can then let slip that Carlos and Ann are the main suspects."

"From famine to feast in a few minutes, but at least we have two suspects."

"Police work is often like that. Cases are often solved with one crucial bit of information and we may have found it. Now you'd better go to Sonya's."

Andy realised that if Mike's murder was unconnected to the property transaction, once he had obtained Mike's papers and passed them on to Chief Inspector Diaz, then he had no further role to play in the investigation. However, he desperately wanted to get to know Cristina better.

He shut his laptop. "Are you free for dinner tonight?" he asked, as casually as he could.

"That's very kind of you Andy and I'd like to have dinner with you but, unfortunately, under the circumstances, I don't think it would be appropriate for us to be seen eating together in public. Maybe we can have dinner once the investigation is over."

"I'll hold you to that," he said, putting his laptop in its case and standing up.

The doorbell rang. When Carlos opened the door he found himself face to face with Chief Inspector Diaz and two of his colleagues.

"Good afternoon, Señor Maracena."

"Chief Inspector, I wasn't expecting to see you again quite so soon," said Carlos, looking surprised.

"Neither was I Señor Maracena, but there have been some unexpected developments in the case in the last couple of hours and we would like you and Mrs. Cameron to come down to the police station for a chat."

"Unexpected developments, what do you mean," asked a startled Carlos.

"It's better if we discuss that down at the station. Is Mrs. Cameron here?"

"She's asleep. I'll go and tell her you're here."

A few minutes later, while Carlos waited with Chief Inspector Diaz and his two colleagues in the living room, Ann emerged from the bedroom wearing jeans and a sweatshirt.

"Chief Inspector Diaz what's going on? Carlos tells me that there have been some unexpected developments and that you would like us to go down to the station with you. Is that absolutely necessary? Can't we discuss them here?"

"I'm afraid not Mrs. Cameron. The nature of the developments means it's more appropriate that we discuss them at the station."

Ann looked across at Carlos and then back to Chief Inspector Diaz. "It looks as if we have little choice in the matter. Let's go."

Carlos and Ann were driven to the station in El Castillo in separate cars and on arrival were placed in separate interview rooms. Chief Inspector Diaz decided to talk with Ann first and left her alone in the room for a few minutes before entering with a colleague.

"Mrs. Cameron, as you've gathered, we have uncovered some information which may be relevant to your husband's death. On the other hand, it may not be, so I wanted to discuss this with you."

"Chief Inspector, am I under arrest? Should I have a lawyer present?"

"No, you are not under arrest but if you wish to have a lawyer present you can call one."

Ann considered this offer for a moment. "Thank you but that won't be necessary. So what is this new information?"

"In fact there are two things that have come to our attention. Firstly, may I ask you if you have either of your husband's Wills?"

"Yes, I have his latest English Will but, as you probably know, his Spanish Will is lodged with a Notary and I can't get access to it without his death certificate."

"And what is the date of this Will?" asked Chief Inspector Diaz.

"I'm not sure of the exact date but we both updated our Wills about a year ago."

"May I ask what the main provisions of Mr. Cameron's English Will are, the one that you have in your possession?"

"Obviously it's a personal matter but, given the circumstances, I can tell you that I'm the principal beneficiary, although there is a generous provision for our daughter."

"And to your knowledge does your husband's Spanish Will contain similar provisions?"

"Yes."

"Well Mrs. Cameron, it may surprise you to know that an hour ago we found an original English Will dated a few days before his murder, along with a copy of a Spanish Will dated the same day, amongst your husband's personal papers."

Ann looked at Chief Inspector Diaz with a puzzled expression on her face. "Are you saying Mike recently made new Wills?"

"Yes Mrs. Cameron, that's exactly what I am saying."

"I see. And what are the provisions of these Wills?" asked Ann, with more than a hint of concern in her voice.

"I'm not at liberty to say other than you are not a beneficiary of either Will." Ann looked at him open-mouthed, a look of bewilderment on her face.

"And this leads me to the second bit of information," he continued before Ann could recover her composure. "We've discovered that a transfer of one hundred and twenty-five thousand euros was made from an offshore account in your husband's name to a bank account in Gibraltar earlier this week, that is to say, after your husband's murder. Am I correct in assuming that you made this transfer?"

Ann was stunned as the reality of the situation she was in began to sink in. Mike had actually left her nothing. Taking a deep breath she confirmed to Chief Inspector Diaz that she had made the transfer in the belief that she was the main beneficiary of Mike's estate and without the knowledge that he had been murdered.

"Did you ever discuss the provisions of your husband's prior Wills with Señor Maracena?"

"Once, I believe; a few weeks ago he asked me about Mike's Wills when we were discussing the terms of the divorce settlement."

"Did you tell him that you were the main beneficiary of both Wills?"

"I did."

"And did you mention how much money Mr. Cameron had available in his various bank accounts?"

"I think we discussed it in round numbers."

"Which were?

"I believe I mentioned that Mike had just over one million euros in an offshore account, although I discovered after his death that it is actually nearer two million."

"You didn't know it was nearer two million before he was killed?"

"No."

"May I ask what the proposed terms of the divorce settlement were?"

"Mike was offering to pay me a lump sum of six hundred thousand euros and to finance Emily through university."

"So you would have been substantially better off under his earlier Wills?"

"Yes, I suppose I would have been but I never thought of it like that. I can imagine what you must be thinking Chief Inspector but I can assure you I had nothing to do with my husband's death."

Chief Inspector Diaz said nothing for a few seconds. "And can you confirm where you were the night of your husband's murder?"

"As I've told you before, I was alone watching television. I've no witnesses although I did speak with Emily during the course of the evening."

"Thank you Mrs. Cameron and one last question. For what purpose did you transfer the funds from your husband's bank account?"

"It was a loan to Carlos to help him buy a bar."

Chief Inspector Diaz asked her to remain in the room while he went to speak with Carlos who had, by now, been alone in the other interview room for more than twenty minutes; when Chief Inspector Diaz and his colleague walked in they found him pacing around the small room.

"Please take a seat Sr. Maracena. This should only take a few minutes but it'll be more comfortable for all of us."

"What's going on?" asked Carlos, sitting down opposite Chief Inspector Diaz.

"We wanted to ask you a few questions in light of new information that has come to our attention. Firstly, were you aware of the contents of Mr. Cameron's Wills before his death?"

Carlos looked across the table at Chief Inspector Diaz, his eyes narrowing almost imperceptibly. After a few moments he spoke, "No, there is no reason that I would know that."

"I see. And I understand that Mrs. Cameron has loaned you a reasonable sum of money to purchase a bar. Is that correct?"

"Yes."

"Do you know where this money came from?"

Carlos hesitated. "After Mr. Cameron's death she told me that she was the main beneficiary of his Wills and that as a result she now had access to money."

"But you were not aware of the existence of this money before Mr. Cameron's murder?"

"I know that he was offering her a lump sum of six hundred thousand as a divorce settlement so I assumed he had money."

Chief Inspector Diaz put his hands on the table and looked at Carlos intently.

"Sr. Maracena, I'm afraid that what you have just told me is not entirely consistent with what Mrs. Cameron has told us so I'm going to ask you again. Are you sure that you did not know the details of Mr. Cameron's Wills prior to his death?"

Carlos looked increasingly flustered, as he tapped his fingers on the desk and shifted his gaze between Chief Inspector Diaz and his colleague. After a long pause he replied, "Actually, now that I think about it, I do recall discussing Mr. Cameron's Wills briefly with Ann one evening a few weeks ago but it was only a passing reference."

"So you did know that Mrs. Cameron was the principal beneficiary of Mr. Cameron's Wills prior to his death?"

"Yes, I suppose I did, although I'd forgotten about it."

"How very convenient? And were Mr. Cameron's assets discussed during this newly remembered conversation?"

"Ann mentioned something about the lump sum coming from an offshore account but that was all."

"Did she mention how much was in this offshore account?"

"I think she said it was around one million euros."

"Well Sr. Maracena, you may as well know that Mr. Cameron changed his Wills a few days before he was murdered and his wife is no longer a beneficiary. So the money Mrs. Cameron has lent you does not actually belong to her and she will receive nothing from his estate, even if she's not involved in his death."

Carlos looked at Chief Inspector Diaz open-mouthed.

"Now, I think you'll agree that it would not be unreasonable for me to assume that, given the provisions of Mr. Cameron's previous Wills and the proposed terms of the divorce settlement, perhaps you and Mrs. Cameron decided that it would be better if Mr. Cameron were dead?"

"But that's ridiculous," replied Carlos indignantly. "Ann was going to get a decent lump sum; why would she risk her freedom by murdering Mike?"

"Maybe she didn't. Maybe you decided to take matters into your own hands."

"That's even more ridiculous. I wouldn't benefit from Mr. Cameron's Wills so why would I murder him?"

"Not directly, no, but you appear to have enough influence over Mrs. Cameron to persuade her to lend you a significant sum of money."

"Listen, I had nothing to do with Mr. Cameron's death. The night he was murdered I was working in El Boqueron and there are many witnesses."

"Don't worry we'll be checking your movements that evening. In the meantime we'd like to take your fingerprints and a sample of saliva for DNA analysis. Is that alright?"

"Be my guest. Can I go once that is done?"

"We'll see about that," said Chief Inspector Diaz, getting up from his chair.

From his office, Chief Inspector Diaz called the technician to take Carlos' and Ann's fingerprints and saliva samples. He then called his contact at UDYCO and explained what he had discovered.

"I'm convinced that either one or both of them had something to do with Mr. Cameron's death. I'm going to ring Judge Bustamente and ask for permission to hold them for forty-eight hours for further questioning."

After a long phone call, Judge Bustamente agreed and Chief Inspector Diaz went to inform Ann and Carlos that they were officially under arrest on suspicion of being involved in Mike's murder.

Ann became hysterical and it took several minutes to calm her down before taking her to one of the cells. Carlos became angry but had no choice to accept that he would be spending some time in the station.

It was late afternoon by the time the Chief Inspector had completed the formalities for holding Ann and Carlos and as he drove to Johan Gaards' apartment he wondered how easy it would be to find hard evidence to convict them.

He had no particular reason to re-interview Johan Gaards but UDYCO had insisted that he go today to advise him that Mike Cameron's death was now a murder enquiry and to reconfirm his version of events on the night in question. They had also stressed that he must make Mr. Gaards aware that Carlos and Ann were being held on suspicion of Mike Cameron's murder.

Given that it now looked like a straight forward murder-for-money enquiry he wasn't sure why they'd been so insistent about him visiting Johan Gaards today, but assumed it had something to do with UDYCO's undercover operation.

"Good afternoon Chief Inspector, can I get you a drink?" Johan asked, showing Chief Inspector Diaz into the living room.

"No thank you Mr. Gaards. There have been some developments in Mike Cameron's case and I just need to confirm a couple of points in your statement about events on the night of his death. But before I do that I must tell you, if you haven't already heard, that we are now treating Mr. Cameron's death as murder."

"I'm sorry, did you say murder?" asked Johan Gaards, a puzzled expression on his face.

"Yes, I'm afraid so."

"I thought it was fairly obvious that it was an accident. How could anyone have got in and out of the office when the front door was locked from the inside?"

"I can't go into details but the autopsy confirms Mr. Cameron was murdered."

"Can you tell me any more? I love those CSI programmes – its fantastic what modern technology can do."

"No, I'm afraid not, but we do have two suspects under arrest."

"Really and who might they be?"

"I shouldn't really say but no doubt it'll be all over Los Cipreses by tomorrow so you may as well know that it's Mr. Cameron's wife and her boyfriend, Carlos Maracena."

"I suppose I'm not surprised. They say over eighty percent of murders are committed by family members. Have they been charged?"

"No, not yet. Officially they are helping us with our enquiries but hopefully we'll be in a position to charge them in the next few days. Anyway, I just needed to reconfirm two aspects of your statement. You said that when you left the Cutty Sark Mike Cameron said he had to stop at his office to check for an email."

"That's correct."

"And during the course of the evening did he receive a phone call telling him to expect the email?"

"Not that I am aware of. I only left him to go to the gents, and he went once or twice himself, but he didn't mention anything about a phone call."

"I see. And can you confirm what time you left him at the office and what time you arrived at Casa Luque?"

"We left the Cutty Sark at midnight, Pepe was locking up, so we would have got to his office, which is on the way to Casa Luque, about five minutes later. I went straight to Luques, which is about a three-minute walk from Mike's office."

"Do you recall talking to anyone when you first arrived?"

"It was busy and they were showing highlights of Real Madrid's league game against Barcelona. Real Madrid had just equalised when I walked in but I did say hello to Luque and to Antonio, the owner of Restaurante Vista Buena, amid their celebrations."

"Good. Thank you Mr. Gaards and I am sorry to have troubled you so late on a Saturday afternoon," said Chief Inspector Diaz, getting up from the black leather sofa.

"No problem; I hope you can bring the case to a speedy conclusion."

After Chief Inspector Diaz left, Johan sat at his desk and thought about what he had just been told. The fact it was now a murder enquiry was not good news. He rang Don Javier.

"Johan, as you say, the key question is what evidence do the police have to link Carlos and Mrs. Cameron to Mike Cameron's death. I need to discuss this development with Vicente and with my police contact before we decide how to proceed. I'll get back to you as soon as I can."

Javier Urquiza immediately rang Vicente Maldonado.

"Vicente, we are entering dangerous territory. Provided Carlos Maracena and Mrs. Cameron remain the only suspects there should be no reason for the police to delve into Mike Cameron's business activities. But if the evidence is weak and they broaden their investigation then we'll probably need to call off Project Pulpo and take appropriate action."

"Agreed, and there's also the possibility that the investors will pull out when they hear it's a murder enquiry; you need to talk with your contact as soon as possible."

Next Javier Urquiza called Ramon, the son of an old family friend who Javier Urquiza had helped out financially more than once. He had risen through the ranks of the police and was now Chief Inspector Diaz's number two. Javier Urquiza was hoping that Ramon would eventually be assigned to UDYCO so that he could let him know if he ever became the subject of one of their undercover investigations, but to date that had not happened. His usefulness was therefore limited but it was still good to have eyes and ears inside the Policia Nacional.

Don Javier was the only person who knew his identity and who hence had direct contact with him. When Ramon did not answer his mobile Javier Urquiza decided to break his own rules and leave a message.

"Ramon, it's an old family friend who needs to get in touch. Please call me as soon as you receive this message."

It was now late and he was meant to be having dinner with family and friends at one of the better restaurants in El Castillo. He considered cancelling but in the end decided to go. He would take his pre-paid mobile with him and hope that Ramon called him back, and sooner rather than later.

Restaurant Velasco was a long established restaurant which specialised in serving dishes from the Alpujarras – the region on the southern slopes of the Sierra Nevada mountains. It was famous for its choice of cured Serrano ham, hundreds of legs of which hung from the ceiling in the main dining room, and its range of cheeses. Javier Urquiza and his wife were the last to arrive and their companions were already seated at a large table running along the back wall of the restaurant, picking from a selection of cured hams and cheeses.

He gave a general greeting and then sat down at one end of the table, asking the attentive waiter to bring him a beer. As he opened the menu, he felt his mobile phone vibrate against his thigh. He took it out of his pocket, and flipped it open: "Don Javier, its Ramon, I've just heard your message." Javier Urquiza stood up and walked out onto the empty rear terrace.

"Thank you for calling; as you probably realised from my message, I need to speak to you urgently. Ramon, you told me last week that the Mike Cameron case was being treated as an accident but now I understand it has been upgraded to a murder enquiry, is that correct?"

"Yes. It was officially upgraded to a murder enquiry earlier today following the autopsy results."

"And are you involved in the investigations?"

"Yes, until now Chief Inspector Diaz was handling the case alone but now I've been brought in to support him. Today I reviewed the file and sat in on two interviews with the potential suspects."

"Excellent. I'd like to know what evidence makes you suspect murder and also what links these two suspects to the evidence."

"Based on the autopsy report, Mr. Cameron was strangled before the fire started so there is no doubt that he was murdered. However, the fire destroyed most of what physical evidence there might have been.

"And what makes you suspect Mr. Cameron's wife and her boyfriend?"

"This morning Chief Inspector Diaz found Mr. Cameron's latest English Will and a copy of his latest Spanish Will amongst his personal papers. It seems that they were changed very recently to disinherit his wife whereas under the previous versions, which Mrs. Cameron believed were still valid, she was the main beneficiary.

Chief Inspector Diaz believes that she and/or Carlos Maracena killed Mr. Cameron so she could inherit his estate before they were officially divorced."

"Is there any other evidence to support this theory?"

"Mrs. Cameron did transfer some funds from an offshore account in Mr. Cameron's name after his death. She gave this money to Carlos Maracena so he could buy a bar. We're assuming that she felt comfortable enough about inheriting to "claim" the money before the Wills were executed."

"But this is all circumstantial evidence."

"Yes, but we also know that the perpetrator must have accessed the office via the garage at the rear of the building so we are trying to establish who has keys for this garage and also the rear office door."

"I see," said Javier Urquiza thoughtfully. "So how convinced is Chief Inspector Diaz that one or both of these suspects were involved in the murder of Mr. Cameron?"

"Totally, from what I can see. Unfortunately, unless one of them confesses, it's likely to be some time before we find any hard evidence, if we ever do. I think they'll be released on Monday but remain under suspicion."

Javier Urquiza looked pensive. In the scheme of things, this was probably the best news he could expect.

"From what you said earlier you are now directly involved in this investigation?"

"Yes. Chief Inspector Diaz will remain in charge of the case but I will be supporting him and coordinating key aspects."

"Good. I'd like you to keep me informed of any developments, and I mean any developments, as and when they happen."

"May I ask why?"

"You know the rules Ramon – what you don't know you can't tell," replied Javier Urquiza. "Suffice to say, Mr. Cameron was a respected member of the community and I would like to see his murderer brought to justice. Now, changing the subject, have you heard about any investigations by UDYCO into my activities?"

"No. It's all quiet on that front as far as I can tell but, as you know, they operate totally autonomously and are extremely careful about anybody else in the force knowing about their investigations. Like everyone else, we usually read about it in the newspapers or see it on the television once they have completed an operation. Of course, if I hear anything you'll be the first to know."

"Make sure that is so and thank you for the information on Mike Cameron's case. Don't forget to keep me up to date on that."

"I will. Good night, enjoy your evening."

"Thank you, and give my regards to your father."

Before returning to the table, Javier Urquiza called Vicente Maldonado and told him about his conversation with Ramon. They agreed that, while the murder investigation was a blow, it did not appear to pose a major threat at this stage and that they could continue their negotiations with the investors without taking further action. After finishing the call, Javier Urquiza rang Johan Gaards.

"The police are convinced Carlos and/or Mrs. Cameron are behind Mike Cameron's death and that they did it for the money. Provided it stays that way then we're going to continue with Project Pulpo."

On that note Javier Urquiza hung up and returned to the restaurant.

Sunday, 25th November

Chief Inspector Diaz knew the evidence he had was circumstantial and that he needed physical evidence in order to formally charge Ann and Carlos with murder. Otherwise he would have to free them by tomorrow afternoon.

Unfortunately, other than an outright confession, he was relying on the results of the forensic tests to link one, or both of them, to the murder. These would take a few days longer and his priority today was to try and confirm their alibis and to establish what access either of them had to the keys to the garage and rear office door.

He decided to start with Ann and asked that she be brought to the interview room after finishing her breakfast. She did not look well. It was apparent from the bags under her eyes and the pallor of her skin that she had slept very little.

"Good morning Mrs. Cameron. I hope they are looking after you and that you have everything you need," he said to her, as she sat down opposite him and Ramon.

"Apart from my freedom, I suppose so," she replied, with a spark in her voice that did not match her demeanour.

"If I can make your stay with us any more comfortable please let me know, but in the meantime I have a few more questions for you. You've told us that on the night of your husband's murder you were at home alone watching television. Is that correct?"

"Yes."

"You also told us that you spoke with your daughter that evening on the phone. Do you recall what time that was?"

"No, not exactly but she rang me during Desperate Housewives so it must have been between eleven and twelve o'clock. Emily will be able to confirm that."

"And where was Señor Maracena that evening?"

"Working at El Boqueron."

"What time did he return home?"

"Again, I don't remember the exact time but it must have been after half past twelve as I was in bed asleep."

"Did he seem agitated or excited?"

"Not that I recall."

"Can you tell me Mrs. Cameron, do you have either of the keys for the storeroom in your husband's office, or the garage which the storeroom opens into?"

"No, I don't. When Mike left he took all his belongings with him, including all sets of keys. In fact, I never saw or used either of those keys, so I'm not even sure if Mike had them himself."

"Do you know anyone else who might have these keys?"

"I don't, but presumably the landlord would have a set."

"And do you know who that is?"

Ann paused for a moment, "Yes, it's the family that own El Boqueron."

"I see. Thank you Mrs. Cameron, that will be all for now," said Chief Inspector Diaz, signalling to the female officer standing behind Ann to take her back to her cell.

Once Ann had left, Chief Inspector Diaz turned to Ramon. "What do you think?"

"I think she's telling the truth, but I'll check with her daughter about the phone call once we have finished with Señor Maracena and we'll search the house thoroughly for any keys later today." Chief Inspector Diaz nodded and then asked Ramon to bring Carlos to the interview room.

Carlos didn't look as if he had slept much either, but he walked in to the room confidently.

"Good morning Señor Maracena," began the Chief Inspector "I trust you are enjoying our hospitality."

"Not really, but then I don't appear to have a choice, do I?"

"No, not at the moment, but hopefully we can sort this out to everyone's satisfaction this morning."

"The sooner, the better," responded Carlos.

Chief Inspector Diaz held Carlos' gaze for a few seconds. "So tell me Señor Maracena, is it true that on the night of Mr. Cameron's murder you were working at El Boqueron?"

"Yes, I've already told you that."

"What time did you start?"

"The usual time, seven thirty in the evening."

"And what time did you finish?"

"I think the last customer left at about quarter past twelve so I would have left fifteen or twenty minutes after that."

"Was it particularly busy that night?"

"Not especially. There were a few locals at the bar, some regular diners and one or two couples who I didn't recognise."

"Aside from the cook, were you working alone?"

"In the restaurant yes, but Paco and Alvaro, the owner's son, were looking after the bar."

"So these two and the regular customers can confirm you were there all night between seven thirty and about twelve thirty?"

"Yes, although of course not all of the customers were there all night."

Chief Inspector Diaz paused, looked sideways at Ramon and then turned back to face Carlos. "We'll be confirming, of course. In the meantime, do you have the keys to the garage at the rear of Mr. Cameron's office, or to the door inside the garage which opens in the storeroom in his office?"

"Absolutely not, why would I?"

Chief Inspector Diaz ignored the question. "Do you have access to those keys?"

"No."

"And do you know anyone who might have access to them?"

"Not that I'm aware of."

"Would it surprise you to know that the garage and Mr. Cameron's office are owned by the Rojo family, that is, your employers at El Boqueron?"

Carlos barely blinked. "Of course, now that you mention it, that's the garage they use as a storeroom. I didn't realise it was the same one as there are a row of them at the back of that building."

"Your memory certainly seems to require jogging, Señor

Maracena. That's twice now where you've remembered something important after prompting."

"I'm sorry, but this has all been a bit of a shock and I'm tired so I can't expect to remember everything."

"So it seems, but we are dealing with murder and these are significant matters. So, now that we have established that the garage is used by the Rojo family, do you know where the keys are kept?"

"Yes. I think each family member has a set and a set is also kept behind the bar in El Boqueron."

"Good. Now we're getting somewhere. Who uses the set of keys at El Boqueron?"

"Only the family members are allowed to go to the storeroom for supplies."

"But the keys are easily accessible from behind the bar?"

"Yes they are," Carlos replied quietly.

"And have you ever used this set of keys to access the garage?"

"I went a few weeks ago with Alvaro to help him collect some spirits but I can't remember whether he or I used the keys to open the garage."

"That unreliable memory again," remarked Chief Inspector Diaz.

"I honestly can't remember, but it was me that picked them up from behind the bar and I often pass them to whoever is going to the storeroom, so if you find my fingerprints on them that's why."

"How convenient? Do you happen to know if this particular set of keys includes a key for the rear door Mr. Cameron's office?"

"I've no idea."

"Señor Maracena, now that we have established that you had access to the keys are you sure there is nothing else you would like to tell us that might impact on our investigation?"

"Nothing. I was working all night and you should be able to confirm that. Anyway, I had no reason to kill Mr. Cameron."

"Aside from gaining access to large sums of money via his wife," retorted Chief Inspector Diaz. "I think that's all for now but we'll have another chat a little later once we've made a few more enquiries."

Carlos left the room looking rather more deflated than when he entered. Chief Inspector Diaz turned to Ramon.

"He has motive and also the means. The main problem is placing him at the scene of the crime at the time Mike Cameron was murdered. He would only have needed ten, maximum fifteen, minutes so the first thing we need to establish is whether he was at El Boqueron for the entire evening or at least until quarter past midnight."

"So what do you want me to do?"

"Allegedly, the last customers left at quarter past twelve, so try to track them down to see if they remember Señor Maracena being there at that time. Next get the set of keys from El Boqueron and have forensics run tests on them to see if they've been recently copied and if they can isolate any fingerprints. The same applies to Mike Cameron's keys which were in the front door of the office."

"I'll get on to it right away," said Ramon, making his way towards the door. On his way to Los Cipreses he called Don Javier and told him about the morning's events and promised to update him later that day.

Javier Urquiza and Vicente Maldonado were seated on the plush chintzy sofa in Don Javier's study discussing Vicente's forthcoming trip to Madrid to negotiate the deposit and share purchase agreements when Ramon called.

"That was my contact in the Policia Nacional. They've just re-interviewed Carlos and Mrs. Cameron. They've also discovered that Carlos had access to the keys, but it's going to take them some time to check their alibis and complete further forensic tests on the keys."

Vicente looked pensive. "The fact they are focusing on Carlos and Mrs. Cameron is what's important; it should give us enough time to complete Project Pulpo."

"Lets hope so; as long as my contact keeps me informed about developments in a timely manner then we should be able to stay several steps ahead of the police. Now, back to business – what does the timeframe for receiving the first instalment look like?"

"I should be able to finalise the deposit agreement with Peter Roberts and his team on Tuesday. Then it's just a matter of arranging a visit to the secure data room at First City Trust in Zurich for the investors' representative to review the documents. That's a twenty-four hour turn around and then the first million will be released. So I'd say by next Friday or the following Monday at the latest."

"Good, that will give us plenty of time to pay our friends on the Environmental Planning Committee, provided there are no unforeseen delays. What about the second two million?"

"That will be released against evidence that the Environmental Planning Committee has recommended the site be reclassified."

"And how soon can we get that evidence?"

"Fernando says within a day or two of the meeting."

"Which is on the tenth so, again, we should have plenty of time to pay our friends on the Urban Planning Committee before their meeting on the nineteenth."

"Exactly."

"What about the final tranche of two million euros?"

"That will be released when the share purchase agreement becomes effective, which in turn will be conditional upon approval of the PGOU on the nineteenth."

"Do you see any problems with the share purchase agreement?"

"It's going to take longer to negotiate due to the indemnity and the regulatory and legal issues involved, but I'm confident that we can finalise it before the nineteenth."

"Let's hope so, we're very much in your hands. When are you off to Madrid?"

"I'm driving up tomorrow afternoon."

On that note Vicente made his excuses and left Javier Urquiza to enjoy Sunday lunch with his family.

After the progress they had made over the last two days, Andy was trying to have a quiet day to take stock of recent developments. From what he and Cristina had discovered, it seemed obvious to him that Carlos and Ann had a motive to murder Mike. Whether they had had the opportunity was another matter.

Let's see what happens over the next couple of days, he thought, as he selected Samba Pa'Ti on the MP4 player and picked up the Sunday Times. When he'd finished the newspaper he checked his UDYCO Gmail account. To his surprise there was a new email in the inbox:

Witnesses recall JG arriving at Luque's during goals so his alibi looks OK. Main suspects re-interviewed this morning and alibis being checked. CM had easy access to keys so forensics are looking into this. Can you meet me tomorrow morning at 11.00 at Samesa's office as we have a proposal for you?

He was intrigued; what sort of proposal did they have in mind? Whatever it was, he welcomed the opportunity to see Cristina again. He emailed back confirming he would be there and then went to The Lighthouse pub for a late lunch and to watch the big premiership Sunday afternoon game.

Vicente left Javier Urquiza's house and drove to Salar, a town further along the coast. Being closer to Malaga and with direct motorway access it was a popular holiday resort which was busy all year round. He had agreed to meet Johan at Iagos beach restaurant to update him on the latest developments and, more importantly, to discuss their plans for Enrique.

Iagos was famous amongst holidaymakers and foreign residents for its giant paella dish on Sundays and it was packed now that the sun was shining again after Friday night's storm. Its location and clientele made it highly unlikely that anyone would recognise them and the constant noise would ensure that their conversation remained private.

When Vicente arrived he found Johan Gaards already seated at a table on the periphery of the outdoor terrace.

"I'm sorry I'm late, but parking was a nightmare. It never ceases to amaze me how busy this place gets, even in late November," he said, sitting down opposite Johan with his back to the beach and the other diners.

"It's an institution in the area, especially for the foreigners, and what else have they got to do on a Sunday afternoon other than enjoy paella and sangria by the beach," said Johan dismissively. "Frankly, El Tintero is much better and more authentic, but that's another forty minutes in the wrong direction."

"Let's order some paella and a mixed salad then we can move on to business."

"Actually, I took the liberty of ordering just that a few minutes ago. You have to take advantage when you've got the attention of one of the waiters."

Vicente poured himself a glass of still mineral water from the bottle on the table. It was noisy; nevertheless, he kept his voice low.

"Despite the murder enquiry, we're going ahead with Project Pulpo and I expect to finalise the deposit agreement with the investors later this week. If the investors decide to proceed, then the job Fernando and I have discussed with you becomes available. Are you still interested?"

Leaning forwards, he fixed his eyes on Johan's while he waited for his response.

"Absolutely. As it stands, I'm getting nothing if Project Pulpo goes ahead so your proposal makes it much more interesting for me. The last time we discussed this, a fee of one and a half million euros was mentioned. Is this still the case?"

"Yes."

"And how and when is it to be paid?"

"Out of the proceeds from the sale of shares in the Cayman Island company that I'll allocate to you. Naturally, the shares will only be allocated to you when you deliver your side of the bargain but the timing will be crucial."

"Why?"

"Because if something happens to Enrique before the transaction closes in all likelihood Don Javier will ask for Enrique's shares to be reallocated to himself. He may also wonder what's going on if Enrique's death or disappearance is suspicious."

"So what's the solution?"

"Enrique needs to be taken care of after the order to transfer the funds to the Cayman Island bank account has been made but before the funds are paid out again to the shareholders. This will give me time to change the share allocations."

"That's going to be a very small window. What does the timing look like?"

"The Urban Planning Committee is meeting on the nineteenth and the investors will need to see the official minutes so I think the earliest the order to transfer the funds can be made will be on the twenty first, which is a Friday."

"How long will it take for the funds to clear?"

"Normally one working day, so they should arrive in Cayman on Christmas Eve."

"And the transfer out?"

"Don Javier will want it done the same day but I may be able to delay it until after Christmas if absolutely necessary."

"If we stick to the twenty fourth as the drop-dead date, then we'll have a three-day window over a weekend to deal with Enrique. But what guarantee do I have that you'll allocate the shares to me?"

"You and Fernando will come to my office and I'll issue the instructions to the lawyers to change the share allocations before the funds are transferred out of Cayman to the shareholders."

Johan thought about this. It was possible that Vicente would not keep his word. But then what did he have to gain aside from the seven hundred and fifty thousand euros which was his share of Johan's fee and which was a drop in the ocean compared to the eighteen million he was going to receive. Also, if he didn't keep his side of the bargain Johan could tell Javier Urquiza about the double cross.

"So where do we go from here?"

"For the time being, you need to be thinking about arranging Enrique's disappearance."

"Ok, but I'll need to know his movements from the nineteenth through the Christmas period."

"That information should be easy enough for me to get from him directly. After all, he'll want to stay informed as to how the deal is progressing and when he can expect his share of the money."

At that moment, the waiter turned up with two plates of paella, containing a mixture of chicken, prawns and pork, along with a mixed salad. He placed the plates on the table, along with the cutlery wrapped in paper serviettes, and left them alone again.

Forty minutes later, after they had finished their meal and the rest of their discussion, each went his separate ways, Johan Gaards back to Los Cipreses and Vicente Maldonado to Granada.

Monday, 26th November

Ramon tapped on the small rectangular window. Chief Inspector Diaz put the phone down, looked up and beckoned him to enter. He needed a breakthrough and hoped Ramon was about to provide it.

"So, what's the latest news about our two suspects and their alibis?"

"Mrs. Cameron's alibi seems genuine as far as I can tell. Her daughter confirmed that she called her that night at about half past ten UK time and is going to check her itemised phone bill for the exact time. Of course, we don't know what she did after the phone call but I think it's safe to assume that she stayed at home and went to bed after watching Desperate Housewives – after all what else do Desperate Housewives do in Los Cipreses?" he smirked.

"Very funny. What about Señor Maracena's alibi?"

"I've tracked down and spoken with all the diners that evening except for the last two to leave. Their credit card slip was timed at 11.57 pm so we need them to confirm at what time they actually left after paying the bill and if Carlos was still there. They live in the UK and I am hoping to speak with them this morning."

"And Paco and Alvaro?"

"Unfortunately our timing is terrible. El Boqueron closed on Friday for two weeks and Paco and Alvaro, along with Miguel, went on a "boys" holiday to the Dominican Republic on Saturday."

"I assume we can get hold of them via the tour operator."

"Yes, but with the time difference the earliest we can contact them will be this afternoon."

"Have you managed to get hold of the keys in El Boqueron?"

"Yes. I got them from Señor Rojo senior yesterday afternoon. They include a key to the rear office door and I've sent them to forensics."

"Good work. Let's see what the last diners say. In the meantime, check with Pepe at the Cutty Sark to see if he remembers Mr. Cameron receiving a phone call or mentioning the email he was expecting that night. Maybe the fact it's now a murder enquiry will jog his memory."

"Will do boss, I'll get over to Los Cipreses right away.

"Oh, and how long before forensics can tell us whether they were the keys used to open the garage and rear office door that evening and what fingerprints are on the keys?"

"It's unlikely they can tell whether they were used to open the doors that night – it's now nearly two weeks ago and other keys may have been used since, at least to access the garage. They might be able to lift partial prints but then so many people have access to the keys that I'm not sure what they'll be worth even if they can."

"Well, the rear office door should not have been accessed since we finished processing the crime scene and any fingerprints should at least show who's used the keys recently. When will they have something for us?"

"Later today or, more likely, tomorrow."

"Ok, but tell them it's urgent. I'd prefer not to release either of those two this afternoon."

"By the way, have we got warrants for Mr. and Mrs. Cameron's and Señor Maracena's phone records?"

"I was just trying to get hold of Judge Bustamente now and hopefully he will issue them later this morning. Anyway, I'll deal with this while you go to Los Cipreses and chase up the last diners."

"Can I help you with that?"

"Not at the moment, I need something to do on this case," quipped Chief Inspector Diaz with his own attempt at humour. "You work on the alibis, Pepe and the forensics and let's touch base at lunch time to see where we stand. We're going to need concrete evidence linking these two to Mr. Cameron's death if I'm going to persuade Judge Bustamente to formally charge them or at least extend their stay with us for another forty-eight hours."

At eleven sharp, Andy entered the Samesa office eager to find out about UDYCO's proposal and looking forward to seeing Cristina again. Paco and Jose Luis were seated at their desks and Cristina emerged from her office and approached him.

"Good morning Mr. Montalvo and thank you for coming. Shall we go and see the site?" she asked, shaking his hand and leading him back outside to her company-branded BMW X3.

Samesa's site was just off the coastal road on the western side of the Cerro Grande tunnel. As such, it had no view of Los Cipreses bay; however, it looked straight down a pine-filled valley to a secluded beach about five hundred yards away. Aside from the stunning view, the valley was a designated natural park and hence, in theory, no building would be permitted in front of the development.

Despite its stunning location and view, Andy would rather they didn't build the development; nevertheless, it might make a good investment, either for him or for his clients, should he take over Mike's business, so he could claim a legitimate reason for being there with Cristina Ibañez.

"So Johan Gaards' alibi is water tight and it looks as if Carlos and Ann were responsible for Mike's death," he said to her, as they drove up the dirt track to the site.

"It would appear so, but we still need to find out more about the property transaction and Mr. Brown's involvement. It has tax evasion or corruption, or both, written all over it."

Andy remained silent as Cristina pulled over into a large clearing at the end of the track. They got out of the car. The view down the valley to the sea was spectacular and Andy could see why the apartments were flying off the shelf before construction had even started. Here he was alone in a beautiful location with a beautiful woman and they were discussing murder and tax evasion investigations. Not terribly romantic, he thought.

"Not a bad view," he said to break the silence. "Would you buy an apartment here?"

"Fantastic isn't it, but a little too secluded for me."

"Oh, so you like to be close to all the action?" he said, with an amused expression.

"Not necessarily. I like easy access to amenities but I also value peace and quiet. Nevertheless, I'd prefer somewhere a little more anonymous."

"What do you mean?"

"Los Cipreses is a small town and everybody knows everybody else's business. As you know, my job is not one where that is a good thing – quite the opposite in fact. I suppose it would be great as a holiday hideaway but there are so many places in the world to see that I'm not ready yet to invest time and money in a holiday home here."

"I hope you don't tell potential buyers that," he laughed.

"No, we tell them that it's the best investment they'll ever make, whether they want it as their own home or to rent it out and, to some extent, that's true. It just doesn't work for me," she replied, smiling.

A little of the real Cristina Ibañez peeping through, he thought. "So tell me, what's this mysterious proposal?"

Cristina turned to face him, serious once more. "Given that Mike Cameron's murder does not appear to be linked to the property transaction, we'd like you to approach Peter Roberts on our behalf, but in an unofficial capacity."

Andy looked puzzled. "On what basis?"

"That we're investigating Mr. Brown and believe the transaction involves tax evasion, and possibly corruption, and that you are acting for us in a consultancy capacity given your knowledge and experience of offshore transactions and jurisdictions."

"And have you made any official enquiries to cooperating offshore jurisdictions about Mr. Brown?"

"Not yet."

"Why not?"

"Because we don't have enough evidence under the terms of the International Money Laundering Disclosure Agreement."

Andy leant against the front wing of her car and looked down the valley to the sea far below. "What evidence do you have?"

"Nothing that will stand up in court."

Andy looked thoughtful. He knew that without acceptable evidence any approach, official or unofficial, to Peter Roberts was likely to be rejected.

"Peter Roberts must believe that the transaction is legal; why should he tell me anything about it? Lawyers have very strong ethical codes about client confidentiality."

"We can cross that bridge if we come to it, but it's essential that we find out more details about the transaction."

"Ok, I'll give it a try, but don't hold your breath and you definitely owe me a dinner."

"It will be my pleasure."

Fifteen minutes later they were back in the Samesa sales office car park. "I'll call Peter Roberts this afternoon and, by the way, I'm really looking forward to that dinner," Andy said, shaking Cristina's hand.

By lunch time the warrants to access Ann's, Carlos' and Mike Cameron's phone records had been served.

"Of course, if any of them had a prepaid mobile which was bought with cash the phone companies can't help us unless we can prove who the number belongs to," Chief Inspector Diaz remarked to his contact at UDYCO in Seville.

"Do any of them have a prepaid mobile?"

"Mrs. Cameron has one, in fact it is the only mobile she says she has and it was bought in her name so no problem there. Señor Maracena claims he only has a contracted mobile but we're trying to establish if he has a pay-as-you go one too. Mr. Cameron only seems to have had a contract phone."

"When will you get the records?"

"It will take a few days to get the last six months but they're focusing on the last month and we should get those in a day or two."

"What about accessing the data in the phones themselves – the phone companies will not have the text of any SMSs sent, only when they were sent and received."

"That's true, we can access Maracena's and Mrs. Cameron's phones but not Mike Cameron's as it was badly damaged in the fire and we can't even turn it on. Anyway, there's nothing we can do if they've deleted any SMSs."

"Actually, our IT specialists in Madrid have a software package developed by the Metropolitan Police for the Brink's Mat robbery case, which can access the data on the phone's chip, including deleted SMSs, even if it is damaged."

"Really? Is this software available to other units?"

"No. Currently only UDYCO and UCO unit of the Guardia Civil are authorised to use it, but it shouldn't be long before it's available to all forensic units. So if you send the phones to UDYCO's lab in Madrid let's see what they can recover."

"I assume we'll have access to any data recovered?"

"Provided it doesn't prejudice our own investigation but, remember, no one must know about our interest in this case, so please don't mention sending the phones to our lab to anyone. We'll duplicate the chips and get the phones back to you ASAP."

As Chief Inspector Diaz hung up there was a knock on the door; he looked up to see Ramon's face appearing round the door.

"Is it Ok to come in?"

"Yes, please do. So what have you got for me?"

"Nothing on Carlos' alibi yet, but there are a couple of other interesting developments."

"Really, tell me more."

"Well, I tracked down Pepe of the Cutty Sark – another one who is just about to go on holiday, and he told me that he recalls seeing Carlos Maracena in the Cutty Sark the night of Mr. Cameron's murder. Apparently, he went in to get some cigarettes."

"Very interesting, so he probably saw Mike Cameron and Johan Gaards?"

"Yes, if they were drinking and talking at the bar there's a very good chance he saw them, although they may not have seen him."

"Do we know what time this was?"

"Pepe couldn't remember exactly, but he thought it was between eleven and half past."

"So, if Carlos saw them he knew where Mike Cameron was that evening – and he's forgotten to tell us that he popped into the Cutty Sark. Why would he do that?"

"I don't know boss, but I haven't spoken to those last two diners yet and I can't try the Dominican Republic for another hour or two, so right now we can't confirm Carlos' movements towards the end of the evening."

"At least it means I should be able to persuade Judge Bustamente to extend Carlo's stay with us a little longer. What about the keys?"

"Forensics just called. They are still working on the fingerprints but doubt if they'll be able to lift clear prints – the surface area is small and quite a few people have handled the keys. However, they say that the garage and rear office door keys were copied recently."

"Why would anyone want to take copies of those particular keys!" exclaimed the Chief Inspector. "Ok, we need to find out who made the copies, if the copies were used to access the garage and office door that night, and where they are now."

"I'll get forensics to check the two locks and talk with the Rojo family to see if they know anything about copies being made."

"Also organise another search of Mrs. Cameron's house to look for the copies and get Mike Cameron's set of keys to forensics to see if these have also been copied recently, or if they can lift any prints from them.

I'll see if Judge Bustamente will authorise me to keep them for another forty-eight hours; I'll tell him we have been unable to verify Carlos' alibi."

Ramon left and Chief Inspector Diaz rang his UDYCO contact to tell him about Carlos' visit to the Cutty Sark and the fact that the garage and rear door keys had been copied. He was not surprised to hear that they already knew about the copied keys. They obviously had an in with forensics, he thought. An hour later, Judge Bustamente authorised the Chief Inspector to keep Carlos for an additional forty-eight hours, but told him to release Ann.

"Are you sure you don't have copies of the keys to the garage and rear office door?"

"Yes, Chief Inspector, I wouldn't even know where to find the originals."

"Very well Mrs. Cameron, we are releasing you without charge for the time being but we are holding Señor Maracena until we are able to confirm his alibi. I would stress that you remain under suspicion of involvement in your husband's murder and that you are not authorised to leave Spain. You must hand your passport and all mobile phones in your possession to the officer who will accompany you home. If you do have anything you wish to tell me, then now would be a good time."

"Chief Inspector, as I've told you several times, I know nothing about my husband's murder. I've told you everything I can remember which may be relevant, but if I remember anything else I'll be sure to let you know."

"That would be much appreciated Mrs. Cameron; no doubt we'll be talking again soon. Good afternoon."

Andy waited until after lunch before calling Peter Roberts' direct line. He doubted Peter would tell him anything about the property transaction but it was worth a shot, if only to earn his dinner with Cristina.

"I'm sorry I can't take your call and I will be out of the office until Thursday. If your call is urgent please call my secretary Joanne Kirby. If not please leave a message and I'll get back to you as soon as I can," the recorded message said in Peter Roberts' normal bluff and cheery manner.

Andy decided to call Joanne. He had not spoken to her for at least three years and hoped she would remember him.

"Of course I do Mr. Montalvo. How can I help you?"

"Is it possible to talk with Peter – it's quite urgent."

"Unfortunately, he's travelling and won't be back until Thursday but I'll let him know you called and hopefully he'll be able to call you back before then."

"Thank you, that's very kind. I'm in Los Cipreses at the moment so best if he calls me on my Spanish mobile," he said, giving her the number.

He emailed Cristina: *"Peter Roberts out of the office for a few days. Looks like dinner will have to wait a bit longer."*

Ann arrived home in an unmarked police car and found the house being searched by a number of policemen. She entered the house, collected her passport and mobile phone and gave them to the police officer who had accompanied her. She then rang Emily from the landline.

"Emily, its mum. I'm home, where are you?"

"I'm over at Sonya's. What's going on?"

"They've released me but they've kept Carlos for the time being. Why don't you come home so we can talk? There's a police search team here at the moment; I'll call you when they've gone."

When Emily arrived home she gave her mother a quick hug, no more, and then they sat opposite each other on the sofas, separated by the Jali coffee table.

"Mum, did you have anything to do with Dad's murder?" Emily asked Ann without preamble.

"Emily, I swear I had nothing to do with your father's death. I realise now that I made a mistake in lending Carlos the money but I genuinely thought I was entitled to that money. I had no idea your father had changed his Wills."

"But that's the point!" exclaimed Emily "If he hadn't changed his Wills then you would've benefited financially more from his death than from the divorce."

"I know, I know, but I could never have harmed your father. At the end of the day, the divorce settlement was going to be reasonable, so why would I risk losing everything, including you, by killing him?" sobbed Ann.

"Ok, but what about Carlos? He's the one who needed money."

"I've been thinking about that and I suppose I can see why he might be a suspect; but I don't think he is capable of doing such a thing."

"I'm sorry, but I think he's taken you hook, line and sinker, mum. You need to wake up and see him for what he is – an ambitious, self-obsessed slime ball with no morals."

"Let's not go down that route. I'm sure his alibi will be confirmed and then the police can turn their attention to finding your father's real murderer."

"If they release him without charge are you going to let him stay here?"

"I don't know Emily. I think he's innocent; but it might be better if we stayed apart until the police make further progress, and he's officially excluded from their investigation."

"Frankly that would be a good idea and, just to be clear, I'm not staying here if he's released and comes back here."

"Ok, Ok, I understand; let's see what happens over the next day or two. Will you stay with me tonight at least?"

"Yes, if that's what you want."

"Judge Bustamente has authorised us to keep Señor Maracena in custody for a further forty-eight hours but I had to release Mrs. Cameron. How was your afternoon?"

"I've managed to see all of the members of the Rojo family, except Alvaro of course, and none of them recall having had the keys to the garage or the rear office door copied. The search of Mrs. Cameron's house has yielded nothing so far, but I've left a couple of the boys there to continue – it's a big house."

"To be honest I'd be surprised if Carlos, or Mrs. Cameron for that matter, is stupid enough to leave the keys in the house, but you never know. Ok, let's see if we can talk with Paco and Alvaro."

Ramon picked up the handset of Chief Inspector Diaz's phone and dialled a number from his notebook.

"Is that Hotel Playa Sol?" he asked after about thirty seconds. "Good. I'm calling from Spain and would like to speak with some guests who recently arrived on holiday with SpanTours. Their names are Francisco Mayor and Alvaro Rojo." He stopped to listen to the reply.

"Ok, thank you. Can I leave a message for them? Can you ask them to call Ramon Lopez in Spain as a matter of urgency." He repeated his name and the number and then hung up.

"They've gone off on a tour for the day."

"If they don't return your call by tomorrow morning, try and make contact via more formal channels."

"Now, let's get Señor Maracena up from the cells to see what he knows about the copied keys and why his memory failed him yet again."

Five minutes later Carlos was sitting in the interview room facing them.

"Señor Maracena, we've made some progress in confirming your alibi for the night of Mr. Cameron's murder, but unfortunately we have not been able to speak with the last two diners to leave El Boqueron that night, or your friends Paco and Alvaro. As such, we have been authorised to hold you for a further forty-eight hours or until we can verify both these aspects of your alibi."

Carlos glared back at them. "Why haven't you been able to talk with all of these people? Surely it's only a matter of a phone call?"

"You're right Carlos, but your friends are on holiday in another time zone and the English couple are proving difficult to locate. Rest assured we are doing our best to contact them."

"I hope so. I don't wish to spend a minute longer than necessary in this station."

Chief Inspector Diaz got up and walked round the desk and stood behind Carlos. "Putting these people to one side for the moment, Detective Lopez here has made some further discoveries regarding your movements that evening and the keys held at El Boqueron."

Carlos' head and neck jerked round to try and face Chief Inspector Diaz, who had already begun to walk back towards his chair. He looked warily at the Chief Inspector and then glanced across to Ramon, who was standing with his back to the wall behind Chief Inspector Diaz.

"What do you mean, "further discoveries"?" he asked, returning his gaze to Chief Inspector Diaz.

"Well, it appears that your memory is still not functioning properly as far as that evening is concerned; we have it on very good authority that you popped into the Cutty Sark. Mr. Cameron and Mr. Gaards were there, and it's difficult to believe that you didn't see them."

Carlos sighed. "It's true but I didn't think it was relevant. I went in to buy some cigarettes and was in and out in a minute. For the rest of the evening, as I've told you many times, I was at the restaurant until about twelve-thirty, when I went home."

"It may not seem of relevance to you, but it does mean that you were aware of Mr. Cameron's whereabouts shortly before his murder. If we can't verify your whereabouts between five and quarter past midnight then it's not looking good for you."

"Don't worry, I am sure these people will confirm I was at El Boqueron at that time and so I couldn't have murdered Mike Cameron – then you'll have to release me."

"That may be, but for now that is not the case. We also have the matter of the keys to the garage and rear office door. Did you make copies of these keys from the set kept at El Boqueron?"

"No. Why would I do that?"

"I would have thought that would be obvious," said Ramon.

"Well I didn't; you can search the house, or anywhere else you think these copies may be."

"I didn't actually say copies had been made," replied Chief Inspector Diaz, raising his eyebrows "but we are searching Mrs. Cameron's house to see if you or she is in possession of any copies."

He stood up, "I think that's it for now. Hopefully we'll have some news from the Dominican Republic and the United Kingdom in the next few hours. In the meantime, I hope you're comfortable in your cell."

Vicente Maldonado's drive to Madrid was uneventful. The Monday afternoon traffic on the A4 motorway had been relatively light until he reached the outskirts of Spain's rapidly expanding capital city. He continued in ever denser traffic until reaching the Palace Hotel in the centre of the city. He pulled up outside the entrance, gave the keys of the Cayenne to the concierge and then went to reception to check in.

His suite was immaculate, with a king-size bed, a separate area with a sofa, coffee table and desk, and an enormous en-suite bathroom. After showering and changing into something more formal he called some friends to confirm their dinner appointment at El Paseo, one of Madrid's "in" restaurants. They had a table booked for half past nine, which was very early for Madrid, but Vicente didn't want to have a late night, given the importance of his meeting the next day with Peter Roberts and Elena Nuñez.

Tuesday, 27th November

Vicente had breakfast in his room and then caught a taxi to Pelayo y Parra's offices just off Calle Serrano, in Madrid's most sought-after district.

On arrival, he was shown into a large conference room where Peter Roberts and Elena Nuñez greeted him. Peter Roberts turned to a third person in the room, "Let me introduce Juan Miguel Ordoñez, a partner of Pelayo y Parra. He's the one you have to convince that this transaction meets the Spanish authorities' requirements from a tax and money laundering point of view."

Vicente shook Juan Miguel Ordoñez's hand and all four of them sat down at one end of the large rectangular table which occupied the middle of the room. "Before we start on the documents, could you just outline the proposed structure of the transaction for me please, Mr. Maldonado?" Juan Miguel Ordoñez's asked.

Vicente explained that the options over the land were owned by a Cayman Island company and that his clients were proposing to sell the shares in the Cayman Island company to the investors, thus avoiding any transfer of assets in Spain.

When he finished Juan Miguel Ordoñez agreed that, as structured, the transaction appeared to be legal: "but let's get down to the drafting – the devil is in the detail as they say."

They worked on the documents throughout the day, and by late afternoon had agreed all the clauses of the Reservation Deposit Agreement, including the milestones which would trigger the release of the funds, and how the escrow account would operate.

"Excellent, a good day's works," Vicente said when they had agreed the wording of the final clause. He turned to Peter Roberts,

"Can you sign the agreement on behalf of your clients?"

"Unfortunately not. Their internal counsel will want to review and approve the final version."

"How long is that likely to take?"

"Probably a couple of days. They're in London this week so I should be able to get it all tied up by the end of the week."

"Fair enough. The first set of milestone documents will be available at twenty-four hours' notice, subject, of course, to execution of the deposit agreement and receipt of the five million euros in the escrow account."

They agreed to meet at nine the next morning to sign off the agreement with First City Trust, and to continue work on some of the clauses of the Share Purchase Agreement.

After Vicente left Pelayo y Parra's offices, Peter Roberts turned to Juan Miguel Ordoñez: "Are you comfortable that this is a legitimate transaction?"

"Aside from the fact he will not disclose who the principals are, everything appears to be in order, but until we see some of the underlying documentation it is difficult to be one hundred percent certain."

"And is it necessary for us to know the identity of his clients?"

"Necessary, no. Preferable, yes. It would provide us with total protection from a professional indemnity perspective but, if they provide a Certificate of Non-Investigation from the Cayman authorities, then we are not legally required to know who the principals are."

"Ok, but at the faintest hint of a problem then we have to go to the Spanish authorities with details of the transaction so that they can look into it further. After all, if it's legitimate then that should not present a problem to Mr. Maldonado or his clients."

Vicente returned to the Palace Hotel. He was tired but delighted to have achieved his objective. The only fly in the ointment was the delay in the investors being able to sign the agreement and hence pay the reservation deposit.

"This delay could be serious, the very latest we can pay the Environmental Planning Committee members is Friday the seventh and since the sixth is a holiday we must have the first million released to us no later than next Tuesday or Wednesday," said Javier Urquiza.

"I know, but Peter Roberts did say that he should be able to get his client's approval by the end of the week. It will be tight, but there's nothing more I can do."

"I suppose not, but we may need Fernando to reschedule the Environmental Planning Committee meeting – he's being paid enough so I'm sure he'll find a way, if necessary. Still, good work Vicente, it looks like we're on our way."

Vicente Maldonado celebrated by passing the evening with Claudia, a high-class escort he had contacted via the Internet, first dining at the smart, but discreet, restaurant she had recommended and then back to his suite for a nightcap. She was in her late twenties, tall, slim with model-like looks. She was also a qualified civil engineer, but had found the lure of the money she made as a high-class escort to pay for her qualification too hard to resist once she had graduated.

Ramon was sitting in his office, which was much smaller and even more sparsely furnished than the Chief Inspector's; nevertheless, he knew that he was lucky to have an office to himself. He picked up the phone and rang forensics.

"Our analysis indicates that newly cut keys have been used recently to open both locks."

"How do you know that?"

"Firstly, there are traces of metal filings from newly cut keys in the locks. Secondly, like a bullet, each key leaves a unique score on the barrels of the locks and there are recent scores which have not been made by any of the keys you have given us."

"I see. Have you been able to isolate any usable fingerprints on the keys or key ring?"

"We have a couple of partial prints but not good enough to get a match on the database."

"Have Mr. Cameron's keys arrived yet?"

"Yes, they arrived a few minutes ago."

"Good. I need to know if any of them have been copied recently and if there are any prints on them which match those on the set of keys you already have." He put the phone down and walked down the corridor to tell Chief Inspector Diaz the news.

"Do they know how recently the keys were used to open the locks?"

"They can't say for sure but they think they were probably one of the last sets of keys used in those locks."

"Then it's highly likely they were used on the night of Mr. Cameron's murder," mused the Chief Inspector.

"So what's next?"

"Our priorities are to confirm Señor Maracena's whereabouts between midnight and quarter past midnight that evening, to find the copied keys and to see if we can link him to them. So make those calls to the United Kingdom and Dominican Republic and keep looking for the keys. Also, ask forensics to check Carlos' and Mrs. Cameron's clothes for any metal filings which may belong to the copied keys."

"Will do," said Ramon, leaving Chief Inspector Diaz's office. But instead of going to his office he walked through the reception area and out into the street. He took out a Ducados from the packet in his shirt pocket and lit it. Then, while walking down the street, he phoned Javier Urquiza.

"So does this change anything?"

"If we can link the copied keys to Carlos or Mrs. Cameron then we probably have enough to charge them. So we are focusing our efforts on that and confirming Carlos' whereabouts at the time of Mr. Cameron's murder."

"This is good work Ramon and much appreciated. Let me know as soon as you have any more news."

Ann and Emily were eating breakfast in silence, neither of them wishing to initiate a conversation which might result in an argument. Eventually, the silence was broken by the phone ringing. Ann got up from the kitchen table and picked up the handset.

"Good morning Mrs. Cameron, my name is Mr. Burns and I'm calling you from the National Bank of Scotland, Jersey." Ann said nothing and waited for him to continue.

"I'm calling you about a delicate matter but one of some importance. It concerns the transfer of one hundred and twenty-five thousand euros from your husband's account with us to an account in your name at our Gibraltar branch early last week."

Ann remained silent. "Are you there Mrs. Cameron?"

"Yes, I'm here. How can I help you in this matter?"

"Well, it's come to our attention that this transfer was made via our online service after Mr. Cameron passed away. Given the destination of the funds, is it safe for us to assume that you made this transfer?"

"I did, yes," Ann replied in a quiet voice.

"You will appreciate Mrs. Cameron that this account was in your husband's sole name and that upon his death it should have been frozen until his estate is sorted out. Unfortunately, we were not aware of his death at the time the transfer was made, although we understand you were. Technically, therefore, this means you have obtained funds to which you are not entitled. Now I am sure this is due to a misunderstanding on your part, but legally these funds must be returned as soon as possible."

"I see. How long can you give me Mr. Burns?"

"To be honest Mrs. Cameron, the funds should be returned immediately."

"But I don't have access to that sort of sum at such short notice."

"When do you think you will be in a position to return the funds?"

"I don't really know, I need to talk with a few people, but at least a couple of weeks."

"I'm sorry Mrs. Cameron but that's longer than we can give you. My instructions are that the funds must be returned by the end of next week at the latest or we will have to instigate legal proceedings to recover the money."

"Mr. Burns, rest assured that I'll do my utmost to return the funds as soon as possible, but you'll appreciate this has come out of the blue so I'm not sure exactly when that will be."

"Unfortunately that is our position Mrs. Cameron. Let me give you my direct line and also my mobile number. Please call me as soon as you've had a chance to consider how we can resolve this matter."

Ann put the hand set down and looked over at Emily, who was watching her intently.

"Oh God, what am I going to do," she cried. "That was the bank, they want me to return the money I transferred from your father's account by the end of the next week or they'll take legal action."

"Calm down mum. What you need to do is to get the money back from lover boy."

"Yes, but he's already paid for the bar."

"Maybe he's got friends who'll lend him the money?"

"I doubt it, but it's all I can think of right now. Anyway, we're going to have to wait until he's released before talking to him about this."

Later that afternoon, Ramon reported to Chief Inspector Diaz that he had still not heard from Alvaro or Paco.

"So I've asked the local police to pay an unofficial visit to the hotel to stress the importance of them getting in touch with me. The two UK diners are also proving difficult to track down, but Mr. Hornby's secretary has suggested I call first thing tomorrow morning as he will be in the office then."

"Any luck finding the copied keys?"

"No, but forensics will do another search of the house and cars."

Wednesday, 28th November

Claudia left the hotel at two in the morning with a generous bonus, and Vicente fell asleep almost immediately. At eight-thirty, the phone by the side of the king-size bed rang. After four rings Vicente picked up the receiver and an electronic voice confirmed it was his wake-up call. An hour and a half later he was entering Parra y Pelayo's offices.

He was shown to the same conference room as the previous day where Peter Roberts and Elena Nuñez were already seated going through documents.

"Good morning, Mr. Maldonado. I trust you had a good evening?"

"I did thank you. Dinner with a friend, catching up on old times, and a rather later night than I would have liked."

"Good, good. All work and no play makes Jack a dull boy as they say," replied Peter Roberts, with his usual bonhomie. "As far as our little project is concerned, First City Trust has received the deposit agreement and Mr. Marteens will be calling us between eleven and twelve to confirm whether the escrow account arrangements are acceptable."

Juan Miguel Ordoñez joined them and they began to discuss the key provisions of the Share Purchase Agreement. About an hour later, Mr. Marteens rang and Juan Miguel Ordoñez put him on the speaker phone. Mr. Marteens queried a couple of procedural points and then confirmed he was happy with the arrangements.

"Excellent. We're hoping that the principals will be able to sign the Reservation Deposit Agreement by the end of the week and that the funds will be paid into the escrow account on Monday or Tuesday," Peter Roberts told him.

"Assuming this is the case, how quickly can you make the secure data room available?" Vicente Maldonado asked Mr. Marteens.

"Normally we need one working day's notice and there's no reason why that shouldn't be the case here. The biggest delaying factor is usually the interested parties having to make travel arrangements."

"Access will be restricted to a small number of people, so the travel arrangements should not be a problem," replied Vicente Maldonado, turning to Peter Roberts with an enquiring look on his face. Peter Roberts nodded.

"Thank you for your time Mr. Marteens. Please send us the escrow account opening forms by email and we will get them signed and returned to you."

"You can expect them in the next hour and thank you for your business."

Juan Miguel Ordoñez pressed the disconnect button on the base unit.

"Good, as expected, no major problems there. I can sign the account opening forms when they arrive and then you can take them to London for your clients to sign, along with the Reservation Deposit Agreement," Vicente Maldonado said, "then we can give you access to the secure data room at the beginning of next week," he continued.

"That should work. Now, my flight's in three hours so let's summarise the outstanding issues in the Share Purchase Agreement that we need to negotiate next week."

"Given that there are only three weeks until the deadline for the PGOU to be approved, I'd rather continued to negotiate the terms of the Share Purchase Agreement this week," Vicente replied.

"There's some merit in that, but I'd rather wait until my clients have approved and signed the deposit agreement before spending any more time on the Share Purchase Agreement. After all, a few days is not going to make much of a difference."

An hour later, Peter Roberts and Elena Nuñez left for the airport with originals of the deposit agreement and escrow account opening forms, signed by Vicente Maldonado.

That morning Ramon finally managed to speak with Mr. Hornby. He explained who he was and why he was calling.

"That's terrible. We heard about the accident but we didn't know it was murder. Unfortunately, I can't really remember what time we left the restaurant. We'd had a fair bit to drink but I think we may have stayed a few minutes longer after signing the credit card receipt to finish off our aperitifs. I'll have to ask Jayne, she has a better memory for these things than me."

"If you could do that as soon as possible and call me back it would be much appreciated Mr. Hornby."

"She's out of the country at the moment but I'll text and email her asking her to call me ASAP."

"Perhaps you could ask her to call me directly. We'd like to clarify this as a matter of urgency."

"Of course. Give me your number."

Ramon took Mrs. Hornby's call forty-five minutes later. "I couldn't say for certain but I think we stayed another five or ten minutes after paying the bill," she said.

"And was the waiter with you all that time?"

"He was not with us in the sense that he was at our table but he was in the bar area."

"Did you actually see him in the bar between paying the bill and leaving?"

"As you must know, the bar area is separate from the restaurant area so I can't be one hundred percent certain he was there, but he'd been popping in and out of there all night so I assumed that's where he was."

"Did he not accompany you out of the restaurant?"

"No, we walked straight on to the beach from the terrace dining area. It's quicker than going through the bar area, and there were people in the bar."

"But you can't recall whether one of them was the waiter?"

"No, I'm sorry, the windows in the doors are small and I wasn't really paying much attention, but there were several people in there."

"Thank you for calling Mrs. Hornby; we may need to speak with you and your husband again."

"No problem. I hope I've been helpful."

Chief Inspector Diaz was frustrated – they were no further along in confirming or refuting Carlos Maracena's alibi; the Hornby's statements were not conclusive, the copied keys had not been found and, for what it was worth, they had still not spoken to Alvaro and Paco. At lunchtime he took a call from his coordinator at UDYCO.

"We've analysed the mobiles you sent us."

"Did you find anything?"

"Mrs. Cameron's and Mr. Maracena's phones contain nothing relevant to either of our investigations but Mike Cameron received an anonymous SMS at 11.27 pm on the night of his death."

"What did it say?"

"*Arriving tomorrow. Need pick up from airport if poss. Sending email now with full details. Apologies for short notice.*"

"And you have no idea who it was from?"

"No, as I said, it was sent anonymously."

"So if it was intended to lure him to his office it must have been sent by someone who knew he was in the Cutty Sark that evening and close to his office, presumably Carlos Maracena, Johan Gaards or even Pepe, the owner of the bar."

"Yes, that's what we think."

"So what do you want me to do?"

"We'd like you to continue focusing all your efforts on Carlos Maracena. Please do not discuss the SMS or the other potential suspects with anyone else, or you will reveal our involvement in the case."

Chief Inspector Diaz was dumbstruck. He understood that UDYCO were involved in a highly sensitive investigation, but this dual track investigation could lead to misunderstandings and confusion. He couldn't think of what else to say, so he put the phone down and called his boss.

Chief Inspector Diaz's boss listened to his update on recent events and agreed to discuss with his peer at UDYCO the possibility of them sharing more information on their investigation with Chief Inspector Diaz.

"At the end of the day, my job is to catch Mr. Cameron's killer and if UDYCO have information which can assist me in doing that then I need to know. If his murder is directly linked to their investigation then I also need to know to make sure that we do not waste time and resources going down false avenues."

"I'll see what I can do Jose, but don't hold out too much hope; you know how they like to play their cards close to their chests."

Andy was at a loose end until he managed to speak with Peter Roberts so he spent the morning with Sonya, trying to provide some comfort and support. She seemed to appreciate his presence but he couldn't help feeling he was intruding on her grief; and there were only so many times they could discuss the possibility of Carlos and Ann being involved in Mike's murder.

At quarter to two, just as Sonya was preparing to drive down and collect the children from school, his mobile rang. It was a local number which he didn't recognise.

"Hello, Andy Montalvo."

"Andy, hi; it's Maria."

"I'd recognise that voice anywhere. How are you?"

"Fine thanks, but very busy, which is why I haven't had a chance to call you to go for a drink with Tord."

"Don't worry, I've been busy myself – as you probably heard Mike Cameron's death is being treated as murder."

"Yes, and that's why I am calling. Once I heard the news, I decided to see if I could find any transactions in and around the proposed golf course sites over the last couple of years. I'm not sure if there's anything in it but there are one or two transactions which are unusual and I'd like to discuss them with you before potentially raising a false alarm with the authorities."

"Why are these transactions unusual?"

"I'd rather not go into that now, and this afternoon I have to go to Malaga airport to pick up Tord. Tonight we are having dinner with friends; why don't we meet tomorrow morning for a coffee at Samurai? It'll also give me more time to look for other transactions."

"That's fine by me, so long as you think it can wait."

"I only started looking yesterday and what I've found seems legitimate but unusual, so I'd prefer to look at a few more transactions and then see what you think."

"Fair enough; thanks for calling. I'll see you tomorrow morning at say eleven o'clock?"

"Ok, see you then."

Andy slid the phone shut and stood pensively looking through the double French windows at the garden. He heard Sonya enter the room and turned to face her.

"I'll be back in ten minutes," she said. "Sit tight and we'll all have lunch when I get back."

"Sorry Sonya, something's just come up and I need to go."

"Nothing serious, I hope."

"Not really, just some loose ends at work which need sorting out – it seems they still can't function back in London without me," he joked.

Before beginning his drive back to Granada, Vicente Maldonado logged on to the hotel's WiFi network and called Javier Urquiza on Skype.

"It pretty much went to plan today. First City Trust has agreed to operate the escrow account, so it's just a matter of the investors signing the Reservation Deposit Agreement and paying the five million euros as soon as possible."

"What about the Share Purchase Agreement?"

"We've identified most of the key provisions which need further negotiation. Unfortunately, Peter Roberts only wants to continue to work on these once the deposit agreement has been signed."

"I'd probably do the same. We're only talking about a delay of a couple of days at most, aren't we?"

"Yes, but the timing of assigning the options to the Cayman Island company and getting the certificate of non-investigation is vital, so the sooner we can tie up the Share Purchase Agreement the better. Ok, I need to get going, it's a long drive and I don't want to arrive too late. Let's talk later tonight or tomorrow."

Andy felt guilty about leaving Sonya's so abruptly, but it was clear Maria had uncovered something and he wanted to let Cristina know. Once home, he switched on his laptop and checked his UDYCO Gmail account. There were no new messages in the inbox. He clicked on the "Compose Mail" link and wrote:

"No contact with Peter Roberts yet but may have lead into "unusual" property transactions. Am following up tomorrow morning and will let you know if relevant to case."

That should get Cristina's attention, he thought, and wondered how long it would be before he received a reply.

As he sat on his terrace eating a smoked salmon and avocado sandwich, looking out across the empty bay to the Punta de Palmero, he wondered what was "unusual" about the transactions Maria had found. When he finished his sandwich he went back to his laptop and saw that his inbox contained a new email.

"Sounds interesting. Can we meet this afternoon to discuss. Please confirm by return."

He typed: *"Have little to tell you other than source. Should know more tomorrow but happy to meet this afternoon. Your place or mine?"* and clicked on Send.

A minute later he received another email: *"Thanks. Will be in touch shortly to advise location."*

A few minutes later his mobile rang and he slid the cover up to take the call. "Andy, it's Cristina Ibañez from Samesa. With regard to your enquiry about the availability of a penthouse apartment in our new development, it looks as if one of them may now be free. If you come up to our office I can give you the details."

"That's great news. I'll be there in half an hour."

The line was poor, with both static and echo hindering Ramon's ability to hear clearly. Nevertheless, he could hear the person on the other end of the line confirming that they were Alvaro Rojo.

"At last! Thank you for calling me, Señor Rojo. I don't know if you're aware, but we are now treating Mr. Cameron's death as murder and I was wondering if you and Paco could confirm a couple of points for us."

"Yes, my father told me that Mr. Cameron was murdered; but what has this to do with us?"

"One of your father's employees, Carlos Maracena, is a suspect and we are trying to confirm his whereabouts on the night of Mr. Cameron's death. Do you remember that night?"

"Of course, it is not often that someone dies in such a manner in

Los Cipreses."

"So can you recall where you and Sr. Mayor were?"

"That's easy, we were at El Boqueron."

"And was Carlos Maracena working that night?"

"Yes, he started at about seven-thirty if I remember rightly."

"What time did he leave?"

"Probably around twelve-thirty."

"Did he leave El Boqueron at all during that period?"

"Not that I recall. Hang on a minute and I'll ask Paco."

Ramon heard Alvaro Rojo talking to someone. "No, he doesn't think that he left the restaurant until closing time, as I said, around twelve-thirty."

"Are you certain, for example, did he pop out for cigarettes?"

Ramon heard Alvaro Rojo have another brief discussion.

"Carlos was in and out of the bar area all night serving customers in the restaurant, but we don't remember if he left El Boqueron specifically for cigarettes."

"Did either of you two leave El Boqueron after eleven-thirty that evening?"

"No, we were in the bar all night."

"Thank you Señor Rojo. One final question: Did you or anyone else have copies made of the keys to your storeroom garage from the set held at El Boqueron?"

"No."

"That was quick – you seem very sure."

"My father mentioned this when we spoke yesterday. He said that you thought copies of the keys may have been used to enter Mr. Cameron's office via the garage, so I checked with Paco earlier."

"Ok, thank you Señor Rojo I think that just about covers it. When will you be returning?"

"What day is it today ... in another six days."

"Thank you. Enjoy the rest of your holiday, but please call me back if you get a message to call me."

"Will do."

Ramon made his way to Chief Inspector Diaz's office. He had already told him about his conversations with the Hornbys.

"It's unfortunate that we couldn't interview them in person, but we had no choice given the circumstances," remarked Chief Inspector Diaz.

"So it looks as if it's going to be impossible to prove whether Carlos Maracena was or wasn't at El Boqueron between five past and quarter past midnight that evening."

"It looks that way, unless we can find someone who saw him on his way to or from Mike Cameron's office at around that time, or we find physical evidence putting him at the scene of the crime that night. It's a real nuisance; we need to keep looking for the keys and any evidence linking them to Carlos Maracena and/or Mrs. Cameron."

Cristina Ibañez greeted Andy as he entered the Samesa sales office. There was no sign of Paco or Jose Luis as he followed her to her office. She closed the door behind them. Cristina turned to face him and Andy felt himself being drawn to her like a magnet. It might be his imagination, he thought, but could he sense that she too was struggling with her emotions? The spell was broken as Cristina motioned to the sofa in the corner of her office. Still uncertain of how to respond, Andy perched himself in the middle of the sofa while Cristina sat on the armchair which faced the sofa at a forty-five degree angle.

Andy broke the ice. "So what's this about? I don't have very much to tell you yet but you clearly wanted to see me."

"That's a fair analysis. Firstly, we'd like to know the source of information about the "unusual" transactions you referred to in your email just in case it's an avenue we have already explored. Secondly, there've been some developments which, against the better judgment of my superiors, I think you ought to know about. Why don't we start with your source?"

Andy explained how he had asked an unnamed contact in the Notary's office to look for any recent transactions relating to all the proposed golf course sites and that, following the disclosure that Mike's death had been murder, his contact had identified some "unusual" transactions.

"They want to discuss these transactions with me tomorrow before deciding whether to go to the authorities."

Cristina had been listening attentively. "Can I ask who your contact is?"

"I'd rather not say at this stage. It would be best to see what is unusual about these transactions and if they have any bearing on the case."

"Fair enough, but we've already looked at the local land registry records and there are no untoward transactions."

"Interesting, but I understand that until next year Notaries are not legally required to notify changes in ownership of property to the relevant land registry."

"You've certainly been doing your homework! The Notary has informed us that there are no such transactions relating to any of the proposed golf course sites."

"Who knows – maybe he didn't look hard enough. Why don't we wait and see what my contact comes up with. Now it's my turn – what are these recent developments?"

"In fact there have been a few. For example, we have established that copies of the garage and rear office doors were recently used to open the doors – more than likely on the night of the murder."

"That's pretty important – find the keys and you have the murderer."

"In theory, yes, and Chief Inspector Diaz's team is still searching for the copied keys. We've also learnt that Carlos popped into the Cutty Sark on the night of Mr. Cameron's murder to buy cigarettes."

Andy raised his eyebrows. "Then he knew where Mike was that night."

"It looks like it. Also, Mike Cameron received an anonymous SMS at 11.27 pm on the night of his death."

"Crikey, that's a lot of developments in a couple of days. What did this SMS say?"

She passed over a piece of paper and Andy read: *Arriving tomorrow. Need pick up from airport if poss. Sending email now with full details. Apologies for short notice.*

He took a deep breath. "From his email accounts we know that no such email was sent that evening – so it could be that Mike was lured to his death."

"Correct, and the evidence still points to Carlos Maracena,

especially as we can't categorically place him in El Boqueron between midnight and quarter past. Of course, everything I have just told you is confidential."

"That goes without saying."

"Good. Now, unless you hear from Peter Roberts beforehand, why don't we meet here tomorrow morning after your meeting for another site visit," she said, rising from the armchair and opening the door of her office. Andy was sorely tempted to follow Spanish customs and kiss her on both cheeks, but instead shook her hand and walked through the reception area to his car.

"As I've told you before Chief Inspector, the only mobile phone I have is the one I've given you. I'm sure the phone companies have already confirmed that."

"Yes, but they wouldn't have a record of a prepaid mobile would they?"

"I suppose not, but since I don't have one it's immaterial."

Chief Inspector Diaz turned to Ramon. "Ramon, go and fetch Sr. Maracena's personal effects – excluding his mobile phone."

Ramon left the interview room, leaving Chief Inspector Diaz alone with Carlos.

"So you know nothing about an SMS sent to Mr. Cameron on the evening of his murder?"

"Why would I? I don't even have his mobile number in my contacts list, you can check for yourself."

"Ok Carlos, unfortunately I'm going to have to release you, but our investigation into Mr. Cameron's murder is not over by a long way and we'll be keeping a very close eye on you and Mrs. Cameron."

"Feel free, but you'll find nothing that incriminates me," said Carlos, confidently.

Ramon re-entered the room carrying a plastic bag and a paper chit. He handed the bag to Carlos and placed the chit on the table.

"Once you've checked everything is there, you can make one phone call and then Ramon will drop you anywhere you want in Los Cipreses or El Castillo," Chief Inspector Diaz said, as he left the interview room.

"That's very generous of you," Carlos replied, picking up the phone.

"Hi sweetheart, it's me. They've got no evidence linking me to Mike's murder and so they're releasing me. I'll be home in the next hour."

"Carlos, I don't think that's a good idea."

"What do you mean?"

"I need more time to try and figure out what's going on. Your being here is not going to help."

"Sweetheart, you don't think I had anything to do with Mike's death, do you?"

"Right now I don't know what to think, but I do know it would be best if you didn't stay here, at least until we've had time to discuss the situation properly."

"So where do you expect me to stay?" he demanded angrily.

"I'm sure they'll have a room at the Almazara."

"Ok, Ok. I suppose it will do for one night. Why don't I see you there later and we can talk then?"

"Not tonight Carlos. Let's meet tomorrow morning."

Thursday, 29th November

Samurai was a popular café, not just because it was around the corner from the Notary's office, but also because it served, by general consensus, the best hot chocolate and "churros" in El Castillo. It was big for a café – the bar ran almost sixty feet along the right-hand wall and the seating area was over one hundred and fifty square metres.

Unusually, it was virtually empty, and Andy had no problem finding a quiet table. He ordered a freshly squeezed orange juice and waited for Maria, wondering whether this would be the breakthrough they needed.

Maria walked in a few minutes after eleven o'clock and immediately spotted Andy. He kissed her on both cheeks. "Good morning, gorgeous," he said, as she sat down at the table.

"I don't feel gorgeous today," she replied. "It was a late night and an early start to go through the remaining filing cabinets and box files."

"Well you look great. What can I get you?"

"I'd love a chocolate with churros but a coffee will give me more energy."

Andy beckoned the waiter over and ordered two coffees and a plate of churros. "So tell me about these unusual transactions."

"They involve a number of plots in the Rio Seco area but, as I said, they're unusual not illegal, as far as I can tell."

"Is that the site for one of the proposed golf courses?"

"Yes. Not the favourite but one of the top three. Anyway, when I began looking at the title deeds for plots in that area I found some option agreements. That's not unusual, but what attracted my attention was the fact that, in all cases, the option holder was either a Belize or a Seychelles registered company. Normally, if a company is a buyer or an option holder, it's a Spanish company or one from another EU country – it's very rare to use offshore companies."

"So don't you have to report these transactions to the Spanish authorities?"

"Actually, no. Notaries will only be legally required to report transactions involving companies in tax havens from January."

"Interesting. Are there option agreements for all the plots that make up the site?"

"No, only for the bigger plots as far as I can tell but, remember, it's not a legal requirement to notarise an option agreement."

"So there may be more option agreements?"

"Yes, but we've no way of knowing without asking the current owners."

"But for those option agreements which have been notarised, we know who the sellers are but not the buyer or buyers?"

"That's right – as I said, using companies is a common enough practice, but not ones from these jurisdictions. What do you think, should I go to the authorities?"

"Actually, the authorities have already been in touch with me about the golf course deal Mike was working on. Of course, I couldn't help them, but if I give them this information they can decide if it's relevant."

"Relevant to what?"

"An investigation they're carrying out. I can't say any more than that."

Maria looked surprised. "Which authorities and why didn't they come to us first?"

"I can't say who I'm dealing with but, apparently, they asked the Notary to look for any unusual transactions relating to all of the proposed golf course sites; he told them there weren't any."

"That doesn't surprise me – his wife's family are the owners of one of the bigger plots."

Andy raised his eyebrows. "That explains it then."

"So do you think there is something funny going on?"

"I suspect so. In my experience, people usually only use these particular jurisdictions for tax evasion or money laundering purposes. How many option agreements have you found?"

"Five so far and I've looked at most of the title deeds now."

"Can you take copies of them?

"Yes, but it may take a while. I don't want to raise any suspicions."

"Ok, first let me tell the authorities, and then I'll let you know if they need copies."

They both stood up, their coffees and churros untouched and now cold.

"Maria, it may or may not be relevant but I really appreciate you looking into this. I'll call you as soon as I've talked to my contact," Andy said, leaning over to kiss her on each cheek.

Ann was agitated and trying not to raise her voice. "Carlos, surely you can see why the police think you might have murdered Mike and why I have serious doubts myself?"

"Darling, I didn't murder Mike. I was at the restaurant all evening until half past twelve, apart from popping out for a couple of minutes for cigarettes, and that was well before midnight," Carlos replied forcefully.

"That's what you and your mates say, but the police haven't been able to confirm that yet."

"Listen, I didn't murder your husband and there's no evidence to support that theory, which is all it is."

Ann looked doubtful. "But you did ask me about Mike's Wills and then you borrowed the money to buy the bar from me once he was dead."

"Just unfortunate coincidences, no more. Believe me. Now can I come home?"

"No. I don't think that's a good idea until they find Mike's murderer."

"But it would look bad if we aren't living together."

"No worse than living together while we're both under suspicion."

They sat in awkward silence, Ann avoiding Carlos' eyes while sipping her coffee. She put her cup down.

"Carlos, there is something else we have to deal with as a matter of urgency."

"Like what?"

"The bank called me yesterday and they want the money I transferred from Mike's account back by the end of next week."

"That's impossible. I used all of it and more to buy the bar!"

"I know, but can't you borrow it from one of your friends, using the bar as security?"

Carlos thought for a moment. "The only person I know who might have that sort of money is Johan Gaards – I suppose I could ask him."

"You could also try and get a mortgage on the bar."

"I don't think either of us have enough provable income to qualify for a mortgage of that size. Anyway, even if we did, valuations of commercial premises are usually quite low and the banks will only lend up to fifty percent of the valuation, so it wouldn't be anywhere near enough."

"Well, we need to do something, otherwise they're going to take legal action and that may include embargoing the bar, as the funds were used to buy it."

"Let me talk to Johan."

"Ok, but do it today."

An hour after leaving Samurai, Andy met Cristina Ibañez in the clearing next to Samesa's site. The area surrounding the clearing was covered in pine trees, which grew denser further away from the clearing. The sun was high in the sky and Andy could just catch the scent of the pine trees in the light breeze. It would be much stronger in the full heat of summer and would also be mingled with the smell of dry, baked earth. Nevertheless, it was enough to evoke childhood memories of happy summers in Los Cipreses spent exploring the mountainsides with his friends.

"We must stop meeting like this," he said jokingly "people will begin to talk."

"Don't joke about it – if we need to continue meeting face-to-face then we'll have to formalise a business relationship."

"And how do you propose we do that?" enquired Andy, with a bemused look on his face.

"The easiest way would be for you to put a holding deposit on the penthouse apartment and then we can negotiate the purchase contract, including the fitting out of the apartment to what, I'm sure, are your very exacting standards."

"And UDYCO will reimburse all of my costs?"

"Of course, but let's not jump ahead of ourselves. Tell me what you've found out about these unusual transactions."

Andy proceeded to tell her what Maria had discovered. When he'd finished Cristina paced a few yards up and down in the clearing, obviously thinking through the implications.

"Using options is clever because it fixes the price in advance and gives the option holder two ways of selling the land, either by exercising the option and then selling the land or by selling the option to a third party for a premium and letting them exercise the option," she said to Andy.

"That's right and, since the options are held by offshore companies, we have to assume that the intention is the latter, in order to avoid taxes in Spain."

"So, the question is whether Mr. Brown or any Spanish residents are the beneficial owners of these companies."

"And," Andy interrupted, "using Belize and Seychelles companies makes that impossible to prove!"

"But, as you've said before, Peter Roberts must be comfortable that the transaction is legal – otherwise surely he would have advised us."

"That's right, and you know that the only way to do that is to get a certificate of non-investigation concerning the *bona fida* owners of the companies. The problem is that neither the Belize nor the Seychelles authorities will provide this as they've not signed the International Money Laundering Disclosure Agreement."

"So Vicente Maldonado must have somehow convinced Peter Roberts that the transaction is legitimate."

"That's the only explanation I can think of."

"Then we need to see if the option agreements shed any light on the matter."

"Agreed. I'll call my contact this afternoon and see if they can get us copies."

The Buena Vista hotel had been a boutique hotel long before the concept of boutique hotels had become fashionable. It was a two-storey restored farmhouse on a hill behind Los Cipreses, with a courtyard and multi-level terraces and gardens on its southern side, facing the bay.

The six double rooms were all on the first floor, two each on the northern and southern sides of the courtyard and one each at the northern and southern ends. The lounge and bar areas were on the ground floor and there were two alcoves adjoining the bar area, one of which had double doors leading to a terrace.

Carlos arrived shortly before six-thirty and sat in the more private of the alcoves with a beer. The bar and lounge were deserted, apart from Harry, one of the owners, who was on reception and bar duty.

A few minutes later Johan Gaards walked into the bar and spotted Carlos. He ordered a mineral water from Harry and then joined Carlos.

"So they've released you then."

"Yes. They've got no evidence connecting me to Mike Cameron's murder so they had no choice."

"And obviously you didn't do it," Johan said half jokingly, but in a tone which required a response.

"Of course not."

"Do you have any idea who did?"

"No, and anyway I didn't come here to discuss Mike Cameron's death."

"So what do you want to discuss?"

"It's about the loan. I was wondering if you could make me another and if we could also renegotiate the repayment terms."

Johan Gaards looked at Carlos with a surprised look on his face. "I'm confused. You told me that you would be able to repay the original loan in thirty days and now you want to increase it and change the terms. Why?"

"Unfortunately, the funds I thought I'd have access to are no longer available. At the same time I have to repay Mrs. Cameron one hundred and twenty-five thousand euros as soon as possible."

Johan let a few seconds pass. "Tell me, why do you owe Mrs. Cameron one hundred and twenty-five thousand euros, and why do you have to repay it as soon as possible?"

"Mrs. Cameron lent me the money to buy Bar Salamander and the bank wants the money back."

"I don't understand; why does the bank want the money back?"

Carlos looked uncomfortable. "Actually, the money came from one of her husband's accounts."

"I see. So you need one hundred and twenty-five thousand euros so Mrs. Cameron can return the money to Mr. Cameron's bank account?"

Carlos nodded glumly.

"And assuming that I agree, how do you propose to repay me one hundred and sixty-five thousand euros?"

"By selling a share in the bar to some partners or even selling it, if absolutely necessary."

"How much did you pay for it?"

"Officially, one hundred thousand, unofficially one hundred and fifty thousand."

Johan considered this for a moment. "What partners did you have in mind?"

"Paco, Alvaro and Miguel."

"Have you spoken to any of them about this yet?"

"No. I only found out about the bank today and they're on holiday until next week."

"Ok, let me think about it. I'll call you in the next couple of days with my decision."

"Johan, I need an answer as soon as possible. I know you can afford it and I swear I'll repay you."

"Slow down Carlos. What makes you think I can afford it? "

"I know that you must earn you a pretty penny from your nocturnal activities."

Johan's eyes narrowed and his face darkened. "I thought I'd made it clear that this was a subject we would not be discussing again," he said glaring at Carlos.

"I'm sorry, but I'm desperate," responded Carlos defiantly.

Johan took a deep breath. Project Pulpo was at a delicate stage and he couldn't afford to run the risk of alienating Carlos just yet; who knew what he might tell the police? "Ok, let's forget it for now. As I said, I'll call you in the next couple of days, I'm sure the bank can wait – I hope I don't have to lend you the money to pay for the drinks," Johan said, as he put down his glass, stood up and left.

Vicente Maldonado had spent the entire day nervously waiting for Peter Roberts' call. At five to eight his phone rang. "Good evening Mr. Maldonado, I'm sorry to call you so late but I thought you'd want to hear the news," Peter Roberts said in his usual jovial manner.

"Definitely, so tell me, do we have a deal?" he said, trying to sound as casual and relaxed as possible.

"We do. My clients signed the Reservation Deposit Agreement half an hour ago and will instruct their bank to transfer the five million euros to the escrow account tomorrow. The cleared funds should be there by Monday."

"That's great news, my clients will be delighted. I'll advise First City Trust to look out for the money and instruct them to set up the secure data room."

"Good. Elena will fly to Zurich on Monday evening and go to the bank's offices first thing on Tuesday morning. In the meantime, my secretary will email you and Mr. Marteens scanned copies of the signed agreements first thing tomorrow morning."

Vicente Maldonado immediately called Javier Urquiza.

"Good but the timing's getting tight, remember we need the first million of the reservation deposit released by Friday at the very latest if we are to pay our friends on the Environmental Planning Committee."

"I know, but if all goes according to plan, the funds will be released on Tuesday afternoon or Wednesday morning – which just about gives us enough time. If not, either Project Pulpo is virtually dead in the water or, as you said, Fernando will have to reschedule the meeting."

Friday, 30th November

Emily and Ann were adjusting slowly to the new situation and were beginning to bond again in Carlos' absence. They avoided talking about Carlos or even Mike, preferring instead to discuss Emily's experiences at university, her plans for the future, cooking and watching television or DVDs of old films.

Nevertheless, Ann was tired and stressed and, in the end, she'd asked her doctor for some Valium, which he'd been happy to prescribe "but only one week's supply," he cautioned. "Come back and see me again next week and we'll see how things are."

Emily had taken to answering the phone, not only because her mother could be spaced out thanks to the Valium but also to intercept any calls from Carlos. So when the phone rang at lunchtime Emily answered the call.

"Hello."

"Good afternoon. Could I speak with Mrs. Cameron please?"

"Who's calling?"

"It's a personal matter."

"I'm her daughter; if you'd like to speak with her then I need to know who you are."

"Of course, of course. Please tell her it's Mr. Burns from the National Bank of Scotland."

Emily considered this for a moment and then decided it was best if her mother spoke with Mr. Burns. After all, the issue of returning the money was not going to go away and her mother seemed calm.

"Mum, its Mr. Burns from the National Bank of Scotland," she said to Ann, passing over the handset to her mother.

Ann looked lost for a moment but she took a deep breath and put the phone to her ear. "Hello Mr. Burns, how can I help you?"

"Good afternoon Mrs. Cameron. I was wondering what arrangements you've made to return the funds to your late husband's account?"

Ann hesitated for a moment. "Mr. Burns, it's very short notice and I'm still trying to make suitable arrangements. In fact, I'm expecting to hear something later today or tomorrow."

"Well our lawyers are still insisting the funds are returned by the end of next week."

"Believe me Mr. Burns, I want to get this sorted out as soon as possible but I don't think I'll have any news for you until later this afternoon at the earliest and more likely over the weekend."

"I see. Well I must warn you that our lawyers are preparing to serve papers to embargo all of your assets and also Mr. Maracena's bar."

"Perhaps that's the best solution. After all, I don't have any assets and the bar should at least be worth one hundred and twenty-five thousand euros."

"We would rather try to settle this amicably before taking legal action but I am under pressure given the circumstances surrounding your husband's death."

"I understand, but I'm doing all I can. I'll call you as soon as I have any news."

The reality was that Carlos appeared to be her only hope; all her friends had seemingly abandoned her.

"I know Carlos talked with Johan Gaards yesterday evening about lending him the money, so I'd better call him to see if Johan's got back to him yet."

Chief Inspector Diaz was not happy. All in all it was a bad end to the week. Ramon and his team had failed to find the copied keys and forensics had been unable to find any metal filings from the copied keys on Ann's or Carlos' clothing or even any usable fingerprints on Mike Cameron's keys. As a result, they still couldn't place Carlos Maracena at the scene of the crime.

As a last resort he'd asked forensics to re-examine what was left of Mike Cameron's clothing to see if they could find any foreign

DNA or fibres which were not his or part of his clothing. Unfortunately, even if they found something, until Granada's new fully equipped forensic lab was completed next year, all DNA tests had to be sent either to Seville or Madrid, usually resulting in significant delays.

The final straw had been when his boss told him that UDYCO would not be sharing any information about their investigation with him for the foreseeable future.

He was certain that Carlos Maracena was guilty of Cameron's murder but, as it stood, he was currently at a dead end. However, with luck, next week would bring a much needed breakthrough, he thought to himself.

It was mid-morning and it had been four days since Andy had left a message for Peter Roberts, who was meant to have returned to the office yesterday, so he called him on his direct line. He picked up the phone almost immediately.

"Peter, hi, it's Andy Montalvo."

"Andy, good to hear from you. I'm really sorry for not getting back to you but I've been very busy working on a deal and it completely slipped my mind, pressure of work and all that."

"I understand. I'll be in London next week and there's something important I'd like to discuss with you; I was wondering whether you're free on Tuesday?"

"Hang on a second. Yes, I'm free from one. Why don't we have lunch?"

"I'd rather see you at your offices, if that's Ok."

"Sounds serious, can you tell me what it's about?"

"To be honest it's sensitive and I'd rather not discuss it on the phone but it's to do with a land deal I believe you're working on in Los Cipreses."

"Ah, I see. You know I can't breach client confidentiality."

"Yes, I realise that but let's have a chat about it anyway."

"Fair enough, I'll see you on Tuesday at one then."

Andy immediately went online, and sent Cristina an email confirming the meeting with Peter Roberts. Half an hour later she rang him.

"Andy that's great news. Have you got copies of the option agreements yet?"

"No, but I'm expecting to get them later today."

"Perfect. When you have them can you scan them and email them to me?"

"Will do."

"Good. Why don't we meet tomorrow to discuss the arrangements for the London trip and go through the option agreements?"

"Which place do you have in mind this time?" he asked with a chuckle.

"The Ruta de Veleta restaurant at the Sol y Nieve ski resort? By all accounts the snow is poor and it's forecast to be windy, so there shouldn't be too many people and it's only a ninety-minute drive from the coast."

"That sounds like a good idea – not quite the same as dinner but I'll see you there at around two o'clock."

Later that day, as the sun began to sink towards the horizon, Maria rang Andy and told him that she had copies of the option agreements. "I'm leaving the office now; why don't we meet at Luque's for a sundowner in half an hour. Tord will be there so you can meet him too."

"Great, I'll see you there."

The wind was picking up and the forecast was for an unsettled weekend with the possibility of heavy showers, both on the coast and inland. Consequently, Luque had pulled down the plastic awnings to protect the external terrace.

This protection from the elements, and the fact that it was sunset on a Friday evening, meant most of the terrace tables were occupied, but Andy managed to find one which was free and sat down. Luque came over to greet him and took his order for a non-alcoholic beer. A few minutes later Maria appeared, accompanied by a tall man with floppy blonde hair and pale blue eyes – a stereotypical Scandinavian, thought Andy as Maria introduced Tord.

They sat down and Andy and Tord made polite conversation for a couple of minutes before Maria removed some papers from the briefcase at her side and handed them to Andy.

Tord raised his eyebrows and glanced at both of them. "Business on a Friday evening?"

"Andy's thinking of buying Mike Cameron's business and these are copies of the company's constitution and articles of association."

"Yes, I need to make sure there are no hidden liabilities or agreements with third parties before buying the shares, and Maria very kindly offered to bring me copies of the documents on file."

"Surely the easiest thing would be to buy the assets and not the shares."

"Probably, but there are very few assets, mainly goodwill in fact, and the company may have some tax losses which I can use so it's worth a look."

"Anything to minimise taxes – God knows they are high enough in Norway!"

They continued chatting for a while until Tord suggested they go for a pizza at Pomodoro.

"I'd love to but I need to get back to go through these documents."

"Tonight?"

"I'm afraid so. I've got a deadline of this weekend to decide whether to buy the shares in the company or just the assets, so I really need to review these documents and discuss them with my lawyer tomorrow morning."

"Lawyers working on a Saturday, that's unheard of!" exclaimed Tord.

"He's an old friend and in fact tomorrow morning is the only time he can go through this with me," said Andy standing up. "Anyway, great to meet you and maybe we can do dinner next week. I'll be in touch with Maria and don't worry, I've got the drinks."

When he got home Andy studied the option agreements. Apart from the fact that the option holders were Belize and Seychelles companies, they looked like standard agreements. He noted that in all cases the exercise price per square metre of land was very low, which meant the potential profits were enormous if the land was reclassified.

When he had finished noting down the key details he scanned the documents and emailed them to UDYCO. At the same time he sent an SMS to Cristina Ibañez advising her he'd done so.

Saturday, 1st December

Once past El Castillo, Andy turned north onto the main road to Granada. As he approached the outskirts of the city he took the road sign posted Sierra Nevada. It was a good road, but one which got steeper and steeper as it climbed towards the Sol y Nieve ski resort. Grey dense clouds hung over the resort and, as he got closer, it began to snow. Won't be much of a view today, he thought, but then lunch with Cristina Ibañez would more than compensate for that.

He parked in the main car park, took his brief case containing copies of the option agreements and made his way to the Ruta de Velta restaurant.

Cristina Ibañez was already seated at a table and she rose to greet him. She was casually dressed with a patterned knitted crew neck wool jumper, black jeans and brown suede boots, and wore her almost trademark pony tail.

"You look as lovely as ever Cristina," he said, while kissing her on both cheeks.

"Thank you, that's very kind of you Andy."

They sat down and discussed their respective impressions of the resort while looking at the menu. Once they had ordered, Andy put the copies of the option agreements on the table.

"So what do your legal eagles think?" he asked, patting the agreements.

"If we can demonstrate that the ultimate owners of these companies are Spanish nationals and that these companies have received, or are planning to receive, monies not declared to the Spanish authorities, then that's tax evasion."

"Which I assume brings us back to Peter Roberts?"

"That's right. The fact that he is willing to meet us is a big step in the right direction and I think these agreements should persuade him to give us more detail about the deal."

"Let's hope so. So when is my flight to London?"

"We have separate flights booked on Monday afternoon. Here are your tickets. We're staying at the Hilton Tower Bridge."

Andy looked surprised. "So you're coming too?"

"I wouldn't miss it for the world," Cristina replied, smiling. "No, seriously, an UDYCO representative needs to be there and in this case that's me. Do you have a problem with that?" she asked, tilting her head and raising her eyebrows.

"On the contrary and maybe I could take advantage and show you a few of the sights," Andy replied, with a hint of a smile on his face.

"Nice try but I'm familiar with London. But if you're free on Monday night I'll treat you to that dinner I owe you at the Oxo Tower. It's only a short hop down from the Hilton."

"Hmm, I'll have to check my diary but I think I'm free."

Over lunch they swapped skiing stories and then discussed how they would make their case to Peter Roberts for his unofficial cooperation with UDYCO's investigation. The snow was continuing to fall and the light was beginning to fail, as the clouds clung to the surrounding peaks and enveloped the resort, so they chose to skip dessert and head back down to Granada.

"Is eight-thirty Ok for dinner at Oxo Tower?" Andy asked as they left the restaurant.

"A little early for us Spaniards, but we can have a cocktail or two beforehand."

"Great, I'll call you when I arrive and confirm the arrangements."

"I'm looking forward to it already," replied Cristina smiling.

Once home, Andy called the Oxo Tower restaurant and made a reservation for Monday evening. He knew the *maître de* quite well as he had used the restaurant regularly, so getting a table with a view across the Thames over to the City was not a problem.

As Andy and Cristina were going their separate ways, Carlos and Johan Gaards were ordering coffees in Bar Madrid in Los Cipreses.

"So will you lend me the money?" asked Carlos as the waiter

walked back to the bar.

"That's very direct Carlos, don't you want to make polite conversation until at least the coffees have arrived?"

"Let's face it Johan, neither of us is into niceties. You know the situation and I need an answer."

"Ok, let's get down to brass tacks then. The answer is no, Carlos. If I lend you another one hundred and twenty-five thousand euros that will make a total of one hundred and sixty-five thousand euros you owe me, with no guaranteed means of repayment. The bar is probably worth a maximum of one hundred thousand euros in a fire sale situation, which leaves you sixty-five thousand plus interest short."

Carlos shook his head. "But if Miguel, Paco and Alvaro buy into the bar I can probably raise one hundred and twenty thousand. The balance I can pay back from cash flow."

"Not a chance Carlos. That would still leave you owing me forty-five thousand euros plus interest. The bar is in a good enough location, but trade is so seasonal that you've got no guaranteed cash flow. I'd want to be repaid within a year; that's over five thousand euros a month, including interest. Anyway, who says Miguel, Paco and Alvaro will want to buy into the bar and then what?"

Carlos had already thought about this. "You could take a charge over the bar and I'll repay you over three years. That way you'd also have some security."

"Sorry Carlos, it's too risky and I don't want to own any assets in Spain."

The waiter placed their coffees on the table and moved away. Carlos leant across the table towards Johan. "I was hoping it wasn't going to come to this but I really don't want to lose the bar, so you leave me little choice."

Johan looked at him questioningly as Carlos continued. "Lend me the money and I'll repay it, plus interest, in two years and, in the meantime, the authorities will be none the wiser about your nocturnal activities."

Johan regarded Carlos with a surprised but bemused look on his face. "Are you threatening me?"

"I'd prefer to say that in return for a loan I'll help to protect your business interests."

"Are you ready to play with the big boys Carlos?"

"As ready as I'll ever be Johan."

"So be it. Let me give it some thought."

"Don't think too long, I need to get the money to the bank in a few days."

"I'll call you tomorrow," said Johan, rising abruptly from his chair and leaving the bar.

As he drove home, Johan knew that the most sensible thing for him to do was to leave Spain now, never to return. However, the money he stood to make from his arrangement with Vicente Maldonado and Fernando Echevaria was far too large a sum to pass up, so he had to find a way to stay to see that through.

On reaching his apartment he called Javier Urquiza and told him about his conversation with Carlos.

"It puts your night-time operations at risk as well as leaving me open to more blackmail in the future. What should we do?"

"It seems we have little choice. Agree to lend him the money and then make arrangements to silence Mr. Maracena as soon as possible – preferably before you have to give him any money."

"That's what I was thinking, but it's very risky. His death may cause the police to refocus their investigation into Mike Cameron's death and we don't want that, especially at this stage of Project Pulpo."

Javier Urquiza was silent for a few seconds. "That's true but, on the other hand, it may actually do the opposite."

"What do you mean?"

Javier Urquiza went on to explain his idea.

"That would be a very neat solution," Johan agreed "and, come to think of it, I have an idea of how that could be arranged."

"But you don't have much time if you want to avoid handing him the money."

"I know, but I have to wait until the boys are back from the Dominican Republic."

"And when's that?"

"Tuesday morning, which should give me just enough time to make suitable arrangements. I'll tell Carlos that I need a few days to get that amount of cash together."

The next morning Johan called Carlos with the good news.

"He says he'll have the money in cash by next Friday, so why don't you call the bank and tell them we'll pay the money in cash in Gibraltar tomorrow week," Carlos told Ann.

Monday, 3rd December

Zurich was not one of Vicente Maldonado's favourite European cities. He went two or three times a year to visit various banks and to place or remove documents from a number of safety deposit boxes, but he found it dull compared to Granada, London or Seville. Its advantage was that it was outside the European Union and maintained strict banking secrecy laws, both attributes which Vicente Maldonado and his clients appreciated.

As he entered First City Trust's non-descript offices just off Bahnhofstrasse, he knew the next two days would be crucial. If the investors pulled out now it was highly unlikely that the Environmental Planning Committee would recommend the site. The site would then remain as rustic land and be virtually worthless.

Mr. Marteens handed Vicente an electronic pass key. "You can change the combination to suit yourself and the secure data room is just down the corridor from the safety deposit boxes."

Vicente descended in the lift to the secure floor, changed the combination of the data room lock and then spent several hours blanking out any information which might be used to identify the site and its owners from the notarised copies of the option agreements and title deeds. When he finished he replaced all the documents in the safety deposit box and went back to Mr. Marteens office.

"Have you received the reservation deposit yet?"

"Yes, Mr. Maldonado, it arrived a few minutes ago."

"Excellent. Ms. Nuñez should be here at nine o'clock tomorrow morning and I'll be here an hour earlier to set up the data room. I'll see you then."

Given its location, the Hilton Tower Bridge was an extremely popular hotel with financiers, lawyers and deal makers doing business in the City, but the lobby and reception area were empty when Andy checked in at quarter past seven.

"Has Ms. Ibañez checked in yet?" he asked at the check-in desk.

"Yes sir, a few minutes ago. Would you like me to put you through to her room?"

"Yes please."

"Hi there, welcome to London, you've arrived safe and sound. Are you still Ok for dinner?"

"I'm looking forward to it; it's been a while since I had dinner there."

"Me too. I'll see you in reception at eight then."

Andy watched as she emerged from the lift at five past eight. As usual, she was wearing simple but elegant clothes, this time a plain black dress with a cream-coloured satin T-shirt underneath. The dress showed her athletic figure off to full effect but without being too tight. Unusually, her hair was loose, reaching just below her shoulders; she looked striking.

Andy was nervous. This was the opportunity he'd been waiting for. He found Cristina very attractive and he wanted to find out if she was as attracted to him as he was to her. She had always been professional and polite but occasionally he had caught glimpses of mischievousness or teasing on her part, and they certainly seemed to be on the same wavelength. However, neither did he want to jeopardise their professional relationship – it would be a delicate balancing act.

"What can I say? You look fabulous," he said, holding her at arm's length, before giving her the two obligatory kisses on the cheeks.

"That's more than enough, thank you," she said, her green eyes twinkling.

He helped her on with her coat and they made their way to the taxi, which was already waiting outside. On the short journey to the restaurant she told him that she had eaten there a couple of times when she had been posted to London during another case she had worked on.

"I'm surprised we haven't met before then."

"It was three or four years ago, before you joined the serious fraud squad."

"So your host would have been my predecessor?"

"Not necessarily," she replied with a mischievous smile.

"Tell me more," Andy said, returning her smile.

"Maybe later," she rejoined, as the taxi pulled up outside the Oxo Tower building.

After an aperitif at the noisy bar they were shown to their table. It was one of the best in the restaurant, with stunning night-time views across the river to St. Paul's and the City and down the river to the London Eye and Waterloo Bridge just beyond it.

"Great table Andy. I never managed to get this one."

"Ah, well you obviously came with the wrong person!"

They spent some time studying and discussing the menu and then, having chosen their courses, Andy asked for the wine menu. He realised that this would be the first time they would drink wine together.

"They do have a reasonable selection of Spanish wines but, to be honest, I'm a bit of a New World fan myself. How about you?"

"It may surprise you to know that I'm a convert to New World wines too. The problem is that it is very difficult to get hold of them in Spain so I can't indulge as much as I would like."

"Great, since we both are having fish why don't we have a New Zealand Sauvignon Blanc?"

"Perfect. Let's go for the Cloudy Bay, I see they have this year's vintage."

"I'm not about to complain. You obviously know your wines!"

Conversation between them was easy and relaxed as they discovered common interests and avoided discussing the case which had brought them to London. It was late when they arrived back at the hotel and Andy escorted Cristina to her room on the fourth floor.

He sensed something special was happening between them and when she turned to thank him he was strongly tempted to draw her towards him and kiss her, but he sensed now was not the time or the place for such a move. In all likelihood she would reject it and it would not only taint their professional relationship but also might destroy any possibility of developing a closer personal relationship with her once the investigation into Mr. Brown was over.

"We don't have to be at Moore, Moore & Blackthorn's until one and their offices are close by, in fact we can walk, weather permitting.

I'm going to pop into the serious fraud squad; why don't we meet in the bar here at half past twelve?" he said, moving away from her slightly.

"Sounds good to me. Thank you for a lovely evening, it was fun to forget about work and relax with good company."

"My pleasure, I only hope that it won't be our last."

Cristina laughed as she opened her door. "Don't worry; hopefully it won't be too long before we can have a proper off-duty dinner. Good night, see you tomorrow."

Tuesday, 4th December

Vicente led Elena Nuñez down a well-lit corridor in the basement to a small ante room.

"All the notarised copies of the documents relating to the first milestone payment are in there," he said pointing to a door "but before we go in can I ask you to leave your overnight bag, brief case, blackberry and any other electronic devices on this table? They'll be perfectly safe, as you know; this whole floor is a secure area."

Elena Nuñez nodded and did as he asked. He inserted the electronic pass key into a reader on the wall, punched in a six-digit code and pushed open the door. In the middle of the room was a rectangular metal-framed table which had several piles of papers laid neatly on its top. There was one chair on either side of the longest part of the table.

Vicente pointed at the documents lying on the table. "Each pile comprises an Option Agreement, Land Registry Certificate and Title Deeds for each of the twenty-two plots which make up the site. The two ring-bound documents are the architect's official project and the Environmental Impact Study prepared by the Junta de Andalucia's Environmental Department."

Elena sat down in the chair on the far side of the room facing the door. "I'll start with the architect's project and then the Environmental Impact Study," she said, taking one of the ring-bound documents.

Vicente sat in silence as she went through the two documents. An hour later, she indicated that she had finished reading both files.

"Do you have any questions?"

"No. The project is very thorough. According to the Environmental

Impact Study it meets all the relevant environmental requirements."

"Good. Let's move on to the Option Agreements and Title Deeds. You'll see that I've blanked out the information which would enable you to identify who the current owners or option holders are."

"Is that absolutely necessary? After all we have signed a confidentiality agreement and we already know that the options are being sold by a Cayman Island company."

"That's true but, as I told you in London, my clients prefer to remain anonymous. As agreed, I'll provide the name of the Cayman Island company upon signature of the Share Purchase Agreement."

Elena nodded. "I'll start with the paperwork for the biggest plots and work my way through, but it's going to take a few hours."

"Take as long as you need, I'll stay here. Would you like me to order coffee and sandwiches?"

"No thanks, I'm fine," she replied, taking the first set of documents and placing the Option Agreement, Land Registry Certificate and Title Deeds side by side. She checked that the description of the plot was the same on all three documents and also where the plot was located on the project plan. She then read the option agreement and checked that there were no charges or embargoes on the plot in the Land Registry Certificate.

She worked quickly once she got into a routine. Nevertheless, it was nearly two o'clock by the time she finished crosschecking and reviewing all twenty-two sets of documents.

She placed the last documents in a pile and removed her glasses. "A very thorough job, Mr. Maldonado; everything seems in order. I'll call Mr. Roberts and let him know. He can then authorise the release of the first one million euros from the reservation deposit."

"Excellent. Do you want to call him from here?"

"No thank you. I need some fresh air so I'm going to grab a sandwich. I should be back shortly."

"Very well. I'll wait for you in Mr. Marteens' office."

Elena found a café a block away from the bank and ordered a black coffee along with a sandwich. Then she called Peter Roberts. "All the documents look fine from a legal perspective but all names, dates and amounts have been blanked out."

"Did Mr. Maldonado say why?"

"To protect his client's anonymity. He'll give us the relevant details upon signature of the Share Purchase Agreement."

Peter Roberts was expecting Andy Montalvo at any moment and wondered what relevance the information he wanted to discuss with him might have on the transaction.

"I must say I'd prefer a greater level of disclosure – they should at least be prepared to give us the name of the Cayman Island company. Nevertheless, we either have to assume they're acting in good faith or we walk away now, before it costs our clients one million euros. Ok Elena, I want to think about this for a while so tell Mr. Maldonado I'm in a meeting and that you've been asked to call me back in a couple of hours."

"He won't be very happy."

"A couple of hours won't make a difference one way or the other," Peter Roberts replied, putting the phone down. A few minutes later his secretary told him that Andy Montalvo and a guest had arrived. Peter Roberts had been expecting Andy to come alone but he asked Joanne to show them both into his office.

"Hello Andy, good to see you."

"Good afternoon Peter, and thank you for seeing us. Can I introduce Cristina Ibañez of UDYCO, the anti-corruption and money laundering unit of the Spanish National Police?"

Peter Roberts looked suitably impressed. "Pleased to meet you Ms. Ibañez, I've heard of UDYCO but never had the pleasure, if I can call it that, of being paid a visit by one of their members."

"Well this is an unofficial visit but one which I hope will lead to cooperation between your firm and UDYCO."

"Sounds intriguing, so what's this all about?"

"Perhaps it would be better if Andy explained the situation," Cristina said, looking over to Andy. Andy cleared his throat.

"Peter, UDYCO suspect that the property transaction in Los Cipreses which Mike Cameron introduced to you involves tax evasion, and possibly corruption, so they would like to know more about the structure of the transaction and the principals involved to see whether this is in fact the case."

"That's quite an opening statement Andy. Do you have any

evidence to back this up?"

"We've obtained copies of some of the option agreements covering plots which make up part of the site your clients are negotiating to buy. These are held in the name of Belize and Seychelles registered companies. As you know, these are non-cooperating offshore financial centres and if these companies are controlled by Spanish nationals any undeclared payments to these companies would constitute tax evasion."

Peter Roberts considered this information for a minute. "Can I see copies of these option agreements?"

"Of course," said Andy, handing Peter copies of the five agreements Maria had given him. "They're in Spanish but you can clearly see the names of the companies and their registered addresses."

Peter Roberts flicked through the documents. "Tell me, what do these amounts and dates signify?"

Andy and Cristina looked at the clauses he was pointing out.

"Those are the payment terms for the option. In this particular case there were two payments, one of five hundred thousand euros in June last year and the balance in June of this year."

Peter Roberts looked through all of the agreements, making notes in his Black n' Red notebook. When he had finished he turned to Andy and Cristina, "Do you mind waiting outside for a minute while I make a phone call?"

When he was alone he called Elena Nuñez. She was still in the café waiting for his call. "Elena, are you sure that none of the option agreements had the name of the option holder on them?"

"Yes. They were all blanked out."

"And what about the payment terms for the options?"

"They were also blanked out."

"Ok thanks. Stay where you are and I'll call you back shortly."

He asked his secretary to show Andy and Cristina back into his office. All three sat back down round the coffee table.

"Ms. Ibañez, let me assure you that my firm would not knowingly be involved in anything illegal and, until now, we were satisfied that this transaction was legitimate."

"And why was that, if I may ask?"

"Firstly, because the transaction does not involve the passing of title of any assets physically located in Spain – my clients will be buying shares in a Cayman Island company which in turn owns options over land in Spain.

Secondly, because prior to completion, we will receive a Certificate of Non-Investigation from the Cayman Island authorities with regard to the *bona fide* shareholders of the company owning the options. As you know, legally that's sufficient for us to proceed with any transaction via Cayman without having to notify the Spanish authorities.

Finally, we're receiving an indemnity in an amount of twenty-five million euros in the event any tax authorities decide to make a claim."

Andy and Cristina looked at each other. "Clever," said Andy "and it works – if the options are owned by a Cayman Island company. So the main questions are, how and when will the options be acquired by the Cayman Island company, and are the owners of any of the companies involved Spanish nationals?"

Peter Roberts looked at both of them. "Please bear in mind that we did take legal advice on the Cayman Island structure from Pelayo y Parra. They signed off on it, subject, of course, to receiving the Certificate of Non-Investigation."

"Don't worry Mr. Roberts, we didn't think you'd be involved in anything illegal but, given what we've told you, can you give us more information about this transaction?"

"Yes, I think based on these documents we need to be asking a lot more questions."

"Good. So can you tell us who you are dealing with?"

"A lawyer from Granada called Vicente Maldonado. Do you know him?"

"Yes, he is known to us but we have nothing concrete on him yet. He is one of several people that we are planning to ask all cooperating offshore financial centres to investigate."

"Has Mr. Maldonado given any indication of who his clients are?"

"No. He's quite adamant that they wish to maintain their anonymity and that he'll be able to provide a Certificate of Non-Investigation which will enable them to do so."

"And at what stage are the negotiations at?" asked Andy.

"Actually, a crucial one," and he went on to explain about the reservation deposit and the milestone payments and the fact that Elena Nuñez was currently in Zurich waiting for his approval to release the first million euros from the reservation deposit.

"So the milestone payments are linked to approvals in the planning process and completion is conditional upon the approval of the new PGOU, including reclassification of the land in question?"

"Correct."

"Didn't this link between payments and planning approvals strike you as suspicious?" asked Cristina.

"Not really. Virtually every greenfield site property deal is conditional on various planning approvals being granted. We were also told that the funds from the reservation deposit would be used to make outstanding payments under some of the option agreements."

"But, as you can see from these option agreements, which cover the largest plots and therefore presumably involve the largest payments, all the payments should have been made several months ago, so this doesn't ring true," said Andy.

"We also believe that the planning process is being influenced. If that's true we could bring corruption and money laundering charges, as well as tax evasion, against the relevant individuals," Cristina continued.

"Why money laundering?" asked Peter Roberts.

"Under Spanish law any proceeds obtained from a criminal act automatically fall into the category of money laundering. If the planning process has been influenced and the people concerned have profited from the increased value of the land then those proceeds will have been obtained fraudulently."

Cristina paused to allow Peter Roberts to absorb everything she and Andy had told him. He looked thoughtful as he scanned the notes he had made, underlining certain words and phrases. When he reached the end he wrote a few bullet points and then addressed them.

"Ok, it certainly looks as if there is something strange going on here so I am going to advise my clients to pull out of the deal."

Andy and Cristina were prepared for this reaction. "Mr. Roberts, let's not be too hasty, we need your clients to continue with this transaction," Cristina said. Peter Roberts looked at her enquiringly.

She continued. "We need to establish whether the principals behind the proposed transaction are Spanish nationals. In order to do that, we need the name of the Cayman Island company and, from what you say, you won't be given this until the Share Purchase Agreement is signed."

"That's correct – but by the time we get that far my clients could be five million euros out of pocket and could be considered to be aiding and abetting one or more criminal offences!" Peter Roberts exclaimed.

"If this transaction is illegal and we are able to prove it with your help then the Spanish authorities will indemnify your clients for any loss as well as reasonable costs incurred. We will also give them immunity from prosecution."

Peter Roberts considered this, "That sounds fair, but you understand that I'm going to have to consult with some of my partners."

After several phone calls to Madrid and Seville they reached an agreement on how to proceed. UDYCO's lawyers also agreed that Cristina and Andy should request the cooperation of the Cayman authorities.

"I think the evidence we have, even without the Share Purchase Agreement, is strong enough to provide reasonable cause," Andy had told UDYCO's head lawyer. "Anyway, I have very good connections in Cayman and I've worked with them before on the same basis, so I'm confident they'll agree."

Peter Roberts called Elena Nuñez in Zurich and confirmed that he had authorised Mr. Marteens to release the first million. He did not mention his meeting and agreement with UDYCO.

"When you speak with Vicente Maldonado, agree a date for meeting in London or Madrid later this week or early next to finalise the Share Purchase Agreement," he asked Elena before hanging up.

Vicente Maldonado was getting increasingly nervous as he waited for Peter Roberts to confirm that his clients were going to proceed to the next stage. He didn't know whether to kick his heels in Mr. Marteens' office or to go for a walk. Eventually, at four o'clock he decided to go for a walk. Although Mr. Marteens would remain in his office until six that evening, it would no longer be possible to transfer the money from the escrow account today.

He made sure that Elena Nuñez had his mobile number and then wandered down Bahnhofstrasse in the direction of Lake Zurich and Belvoir Park. Just as he was returning to the bank an hour later, his mobile rang. It was Elena Nuñez confirming that their clients would proceed to the next stage and that Peter Roberts had authorised Mr. Marteens to release the first milestone payment.

Vicente breathed a huge sigh of relief.

"Now we'd like to finalise the Share Purchase Agreement. Would it be convenient to meet later this week?" she asked.

"Of course. Where and when would you like to meet?"

"Preferably Madrid or London on Thursday or Friday."

"Thursday is a national holiday in Spain and I'll be meeting with my clients to update them and get further instructions regarding the Share Purchase Agreement; why don't we say Friday in Madrid?"

"Good. Let's meet at Pelayo y Parra's offices at ten."

"Perfect."

"Thank you; I look forward to seeing you on Friday."

He had missed the last flight to Malaga so he made his way to his hotel and checked in for an extra night. He then called Javier Urquiza and told him the good news.

"Excellent. When are you back?"

"I'm withdrawing the cash first thing in the morning and catching the midday flight, so I should arrive at about three."

"Come back via Los Cipreses and we'll make the arrangements to pay the Environmental Planning Committee members. I'll be at the house all day but call me on the mobile once you've landed."

The taxi dropped Miguel off last and he found Johan Gaards waiting for him.

"Hi Miguel, welcome back. Had a good holiday?"

"Fantastic; wine, women and song – what more could you want? But it looks like there have been some developments in the Mike Cameron case while I've been away. What's going on?"

"Unfortunately it's being treated as murder instead of an accident. I thought you said you'd been very careful."

"I was, but maybe I used a little too much force. Anyway, how could we know that forensics would be so hot on the keys?"

"Well, it's very unfortunate and we need Carlos to be the only suspect – even if they can't convict him."

"I couldn't agree more."

"Good and I think there's a way we can do this. It means a little bit more risk for you, but you'll be well rewarded and, if done properly, that should be the end of the matter."

Johan outlined his idea. "But it's essential that this time it's definitely seen to be an accident. The problem is the timing – the sooner the better."

"That would be a neat solution. So what's in it for me?"

"Double what you got for Mike."

Miguel considered this, his beady eyes darting around in his pock-marked face. "Ok, I think that's acceptable. Now here's how I think we can do it," and he told Johan his plan.

Later that evening, after a few rum and cokes, Carlos readily agreed to Miguel's suggestion of a celebratory party with some of the girls from Queens Club – he was ready for some fun and female company after the events of the last week. Melanie's place was perfect, a walled-in villa tucked away in a cul-de-sac on the Punta, with stunning views, a large garden and the added bonus of a heated indoor pool.

Wednesday, 5th December

Vicente Maldonado walked through the arrivals lounge at Malaga airport with one million euros in cash in his laptop carry case. He preferred not to transport such large sums of cash, but there were no security checks on arrivals so all he had to do was to get through customs. As usual, the Civiles were chatting amongst themselves – they only ever really spot-checked intercontinental flights, especially those from the Americas, so in ten minutes Vicente was in his car and heading towards Los Cipreses.

How does the Share Purchase Agreement look?" Javier Urquiza asked him once Vicente had shown him the cash and the signed agreements.

"In good shape. The only two major outstanding issues are the mechanics behind verifying that the Cayman Island company owns the option agreements and obtaining confirmation that the PGOU has been approved."

"Will we have a problem with either of those?"

"No. I'll assign the option agreements to the Cayman company using my power of attorney as soon as the Environmental Planning Committee recommend the site to the Urban Planning Committee."

"What about proving that the PGOU has been approved?"

"Fernando says that he will be able to get a copy of the signed minutes of the Urban Planning Committee meeting by the following day at the latest."

"Excellent. Miguel has a plan for dealing with Carlos, so with luck that problem will be solved tonight."

"Good; we can't afford for him to make any mistakes this time."

"Quite. Now, what about delivering the payments to our friends?"

"The problem is that tomorrow's a holiday and I've got to be in Madrid first thing on Friday morning, so I'm not going to have time to make the deposits. Shall I ask Johan to do it on Friday morning?"

"Can we trust him with that much cash?"

"If he feels he is being looked after then we won't have a problem," replied Vicente.

"I've promised him a bonus, but events are moving more quickly than we expected and he may decide to cut and run."

Vicente Maldonado smiled to himself. He knew that Johan was too interested in the million and a half euros he and Fernando had promised him for dealing with Enrique to run off with cash.

"Provided Miguel does his job properly tonight there's no reason for him to abandon ship," he said to Javier Urquiza.

"You'd better be right. A million euros is a lot of money and if it doesn't reach our friends on time Project Pulpo will be dead in the water."

"The alternative is for you to drop the cash or for me to delay my trip to Madrid."

"No, none of those is viable so have Johan do it.

"Will do."

At police headquarters in Seville, Cristina was briefing her boss while Andy waited outside the office. He was not overly familiar with Seville, but the two weekend breaks he had enjoyed there in the past had whetted his appetite, and he was looking forward to a couple of days there with Cristina, even if it was for work rather than play.

"So, what's the plan?" he asked her, when she eventually came out of her boss' office.

"It's going to be a busy few days."

"You mean no time for flamenco, tapas and a guided tour of the city?" Andy asked in an exaggerated tone of disappointment.

"I'm afraid not. Later this afternoon we're meeting with UDYCO's lawyers to formalise your position as a consultant to us and then to prepare the paperwork for the Cayman Island authorities. What has been agreed is that you and I will go to Cayman in person to request their cooperation."

"First London, now Seville, next Cayman; where will it end!"

Andy exclaimed, with a huge grin on his face. "Now, closer to home, what about dinner this evening?"

"You're out of luck – strictly business. We're dining with UDYCO's head lawyer and the head of the forensic accounting unit. They want to get to know you and also pick your brains."

"Sounds like fun! And tomorrow? After all it is a national holiday."

"Tomorrow my team and I will start our investigation into the assets of the members of the Environmental and Urban Planning Committees."

"Is there anything I can do to help?"

"Thanks for the offer, but I don't think so. We have our own systems and processes for such investigations. It may take several months to get all the results but we need to set the ball rolling ASAP, starting with applications for the relevant warrants."

"I guess I'd better go back to Los Cipreses for the long weekend then, but at least I've got Cayman to look forward to."

"That's true, I've never been and maybe this time there'll be time for you to show me the sights," she replied, with a twinkle in her eyes.

Tonight is going to be fun with a capital F, Carlos thought, as he drove back from El Castillo after buying the drink and sourcing some cocaine.

Miguel, Carlos and Paco met at El Burro at eight-thirty before heading off to the villa – Alvaro had cried off due to a family engagement. The villa was spread over a single storey and the living room comprised two large rooms on slightly different levels, separated by an archway and three steps. Carlos had bought several bottles of Grey Goose vodka, Havana Club 7-year-old rum, various mixers as well as the cocaine. Paco and Miguel had also brought several grams of cocaine, so there would be no shortage of stimulants, even if the girls didn't turn up.

"Don't worry, they'll be here. They're being well paid and these girls like to party, if you know what I mean," Miguel said, winking, as Carlos put on his favourite El Camaron flamenco CD.

"Great, now pour me a vodka and red bull while I do a line,"

Carlos replied, while cutting some cocaine on the glass-topped coffee table.

By the time the three girls from Queens Club arrived Carlos and Paco were already well on their way, but Miguel was carefully moderating his consumption. Two hours later, fuelled by frequent intakes of cocaine and several bottles of vodka and rum, all six were dancing in the centre of the lower living room.

"Let's go for a dip," shouted Miguel above the music at the gyrating bodies and pointing towards the French windows in the corner of the room leading to the indoor pool.

Before long only thongs and briefs were in evidence as they dived and jumped into the pool. After a few minutes of horseplay they dried off and returned to the lower living room. Carlos prepared six lines of cocaine, each with a vodka shot, and they raced to see who could finish first. Paco then manoeuvred the tall blond to one of the sofas in the upper level room, leaving Carlos and Miguel dancing with the remaining two girls.

"Hombre, let's finish the Charlie and then maybe you should have a romantic dip before some more vigorous exercise – if you know what I mean," Miguel whispered in Carlos' ear.

Carlos grinned. "Good idea – line up the Charlie!"

Miguel waited for peace to descend on the house and then rose slowly from the sofa, careful not to disturb the girl at his side, who was in a deep slumber. He climbed the three steps to the upper living room and peered in. He could hear laboured breathing and just made out the shape of two bodies on the sofa. He turned round and made his way to the pool room. The water was still and the pool lights reflected off the tiles to create a turquoise glow which gradually faded into darkness at the edges of the room.

He could easily see Carlos sprawled naked across two sun lounger mattresses close to the edge of the pool. For a moment he couldn't see the girl but, as his eyes adjusted to the light, he saw her curled up on the seat of the A-frame swing a few feet behind Carlos. He padded over to the A-frame swing. He knew he would have to be careful not to wake the girl but, like the others, she looked totally out of it. After all the cocaine and booze they had consumed he was not surprised, but then that had been the intention.

Then he moved a few paces back to Carlos. He was only a couple of feet away from the edge of the pool but Miguel knew that lifting a dead weight of over eighty-five kilos and putting it in the pool would be difficult and might wake the girl. He crouched down next to Carlos.

"Carlos, Carlos are you alright?" he whispered in his ear, shaking him gently. Carlos did not respond so he tried again without raising his voice.

Carlos' eyes flickered open. They were glazed and unfocused. "Carlos, come on you don't look good hombre. Let's get in the pool to freshen you up."

Carlos grunted and shifted his body slightly. Miguel slid his arms under his armpits and pushed his legs over the edge of the pool.

"What's going on?" Carlos mumbled.

"Just trying to get you straight hombre," Miguel replied, slipping into the pool with Carlos.

Carlos struggled briefly as Miguel pushed and held his head under the water but he didn't have the strength to withstand Miguel and soon his body went limp. Miguel released his head, but held Carlos by one arm as he looked over to where the girl was lying. She had not moved. He turned Carlos' body over so it was face down and quietly left the pool via the aluminium ladder on the side nearest the door. After drying himself with one of the towels scattered nearby he went back to the lower living room, found his jeans on the floor by the sofa and removed a bunch of keys from the belt hook.

He unhooked a wire clasp containing two keys and then quietly walked to the entrance hall where Carlos had left the house keys when they had entered the property earlier that evening. He joined the wire clasp with the two keys to the main key ring containing the house keys and then used the towel he had brought with him to thoroughly wipe the two new keys he had just added to the set.

He sent an SMS to Johan and then, having completed this final task, returned to the sofa, snuggled up to the sleeping body and closed his eyes.

Thursday, 6th December

Chief Inspector Diaz arrived at the house shortly after Ramon and his team. It was barely daylight and Ramon had gathered the occupants of the house in the upper living room. He took Chief Inspector Diaz down to the pool room where Carlos' body was being examined by the assistant pathologist.

"Looks like they had a bit of a wild party last night to celebrate Miguel's and Paco's return, and Carlos' release from custody. Lots of cocaine and alcohol. The girls are from Queens. They paired off and then crashed out between three and four in the morning. The one with Carlos woke up about half an hour ago and found him floating face down in the pool."

"Where were the others?"

"Paco and his bit of skirt were in the top living room and Miguel and the blonde were there," replied Ramon, pointing through the door at the sofa in the lower living room.

"No Alvaro?"

"Apparently he was at a family function."

Chief Inspector Diaz turned to the pathologist. "Cause of death?"

"Looks like a clear cut case of drowning while under the influence of drink and drugs."

"Of course, the question is how or why did he get into the pool? He may have got up and slipped and fallen in or he may have decided to take a dip."

"I can't find any evidence of a bang to the head or any other force being applied."

"So it could have been an accident?"

"Yes, but I'll have to reserve judgement until we do a full autopsy and get the toxicology results."

"And when will the autopsy be done?"

"Not until Monday or possibly Tuesday. Juan Luis is away for the long weekend and I'm not authorised to undertake one by myself yet."

"These god damn holidays are always interfering with our work," exclaimed Chief Inspector Diaz. "Just make sure it's top of Juan Luis' list when he returns.

Ramon, go and finish taking their statements. When you talk with Paco, reconfirm Carlos' whereabouts on the night of Mike Cameron's death between twelve and twelve thirty. Then go and see Alvaro and do the same. I'm going to pay a visit to Mrs. Cameron."

Ann heard a car pull up outside the house. She opened the front door just as Chief Inspector Diaz was poised to ring the bell.

"Good morning Mrs. Cameron, I hope I am not disturbing you at this early hour," he said, noting that she looked tired and was not wearing any make up.

"No, I've been up a while. To what do I owe the pleasure?" she said with a hint of sarcasm.

"I'm afraid I have some bad news. Can I come in?"

"Why not." and she led him wearily to the living room.

"I'll try and be brief," he said, going on to describe how Carlos had been found dead earlier that morning. "While it appears that Mr. Maracena's death was an accident, are you aware of anyone who would want him dead?"

Ann had remained calm as the Chief Inspector imparted the news but now began to sob quietly. "Carlos was not the easiest of people sometimes, but I don't know of anybody who would want to kill him."

"Was he in trouble financially? For example, we know that he bought Bar Salamander with money from your husband's estate, which you now need to repay to the bank. How was he planning on repaying you?"

"He had arranged a loan from a friend. In fact he was expecting the money today."

"Do you know who this friend is?"

"Yes, it's Johan Gaards."

Chief Inspector Diaz was taken aback. "I didn't realise they were close friends."

"They're not – it was a business arrangement, but now I won't be able to repay the bank and God knows what they'll do."

"I'm sure they'll be reasonable given the circumstances."

Ann carried on crying. "I wouldn't be so sure, especially since I'm still a suspect in Mike's death."

Chief Inspector Diaz picked his words carefully.

"That's true, Mrs. Cameron; and if Carlos killed your husband then you may be an accomplice but I no longer believe that is the case."

"What – that Carlos killed Mike or that I was an accomplice?"

"It still looks likely that Carlos killed your husband, but at the moment we're unable to prove that beyond reasonable doubt. In fact, we may never be able to do so now that he's dead but, unless we discover new evidence, I'll be recommending that we drop our investigation into your possible involvement."

This was not something he had formally discussed with his boss, but his gut instinct told him Ann was an innocent victim of Carlos' machinations.

"Well I must say that's a relief. On top of losing my husband, my inheritance and being duped by my lover, all I needed was to be implicated in a murder I knew nothing about."

Chief Inspector Diaz could think of nothing else to say so he rose from the sofa. "Thank you for your time Mrs. Cameron. I'll be in touch when I have some more news."

Andy left Seville straight after breakfast. As he approached the junction with the A7 which would take him back to Los Cipreses his mobile buzzed, signalling he had an SMS. He waited until he was on the motorway before picking up the phone to view the message.

It was from Cristina: *"Carlos found dead this am. Call me when convenient."*

He pulled in at the next service station to call her. She answered immediately and told him the circumstances of Carlos' death.

"Any sign of foul play?"

"Apparently not, but we need to wait for the autopsy results, which won't be until Monday or Tuesday."

"Well it doesn't affect our investigation, but hopefully it will bring the investigation into Mike's murder to a close."

"I hope so; let's wait and see what conclusions Chief Inspector Diaz reaches. The big day for us is tomorrow."

"You can say that again. If they agree the terms of the Share Purchase Agreement then a trip to the Caymans beckons."

"Yes, but for all the wrong reasons," she replied.

When Ramon finished talking to Alvaro Rojo he rang Don Javier.

"Ramon, I'm certain Mr. Maracena's death was an accident and that you'll reach the same conclusion. You should also take a look at the keys to the house, you may find something interesting."

"Thank you for your advice Don Javier, but this is getting a little messy and I need to be careful not to compromise my position."

"Don't worry Ramon. I think you'll also find that your investigation into Mr. Cameron's death can now be cleared up to everyone's satisfaction, but don't forget to keep me informed." Javier Urquiza hung up and Ramon walked down the corridor to Chief Inspector Diaz's office.

"Hi boss, I've taken statements from everyone."

"And?"

"As we thought, they'd been on a cocaine and drinks binge and all the evidence points to Carlos drowning while under the influence of drink and drugs."

"What evidence did you find?"

"The remnants of cocaine, drink and various items of clothing. Forensics should have gathered all the physical evidence by now and I'll go through it with them tomorrow." He decided to say nothing about the keys until he had had a chance to study them himself.

"What did Paco and Alvaro say about Carlos' whereabouts the night of Mr. Cameron's murder?"

"They're ninety-nine percent certain he was at El Boqueron all night, although they admit it's possible he left the premises for a few minutes for cigarettes. In any event, Carlos was in and out of the bar and restaurant areas serving customers, clearing tables, etc., so he wouldn't have been visible to them all of the time."

"So we can't confirm his whereabouts at that time, one way or the other."

"I'm afraid not. What did Mrs. Cameron have to say?"

"She doesn't know of anyone who would have wanted Carlos dead, although she did say that Johan Gaards had agreed to lend him money so he could repay her."

"Is that significant?"

"I'm not sure, but I'm interested as to why Johan would lend Carlos a substantial sum and also where he gets that sort of money from, so I've left a voicemail for him."

Taking advantage of the departure of many Granadinos to the coast for the long weekend, Vicente Maldonado had arranged to meet Johan for lunch at a taverna located in the Albaicín, Granada's famous Moorish quarter. He had with him a non-descript sports holdall containing two thousand of the notorious "bin Ladens," as five-hundred euro notes were known in Spain. This nomenclature had arisen due to their invisibility – despite the fact that over thirty percent of all the European Union's five-hundred euro notes were estimated to be in Spain.

"I hear Sr. Maracena is no longer with us," Vicente remarked to Johan.

"Yes, that problem has been solved and Miguel assures me that this time the police will treat it as an accident."

"Let's hope he did a better job this time, because if they latch on to him we could be in serious trouble; Los Cipreses is in danger of becoming Spain's murder capital. Ok, let's put that to one side for now. Our priority is to pay our friends on the Environmental Planning Committee before Monday. The money's in here," he said, sliding the holdall under the table to Johan.

"There are three bundles and I want you to place one in each of the following safety deposit boxes by close of business tomorrow," and he proceeded to give Johan details of the banks, two in Malaga and one in Antequera, along with the codes to open the safety deposit boxes.

"Consider it done," Johan said, his hands firmly fixed round the handles of the holdall.

"Good. Now, assuming there are no unforeseen problems, we should be finalising the legal agreements with the investors over the next few days. That means we have to start planning Enrique's disappearance."

"Have you asked him about his plans for the Christmas period?"

"Yes. He's officially taking holidays from Christmas Eve to second of January. He says he is going to stay in Los Cipreses until he receives his share of the proceeds."

"And the earliest the money will be received in Cayman is still Christmas Eve?"

"Yes."

"Good, that means our three-day window from the twenty-first remains in place. Do you know his movements over those three days?"

"He says that, at the moment, the only social function he is going to that weekend is a lunchtime barbeque on the twenty-third being held by Mrs. Nicklass."

"You mean the rich bitch with the house at the top of Cerro Grande?"

"That's the one."

"That may be a good opportunity," remarked Johan. "Who's going?"

"The leading lights of the expat community, along with the mayor and Enrique – so surely it's too public a place for anything to happen to him."

"That depends on what happens and also when and where. It's a very steep and windy road to that house and a few years ago the son of Jose Luis Roca died when he lost control of his car coming down that road from a party."

"Yes, I remember. It was quite a sensation at the time, rich kid dying at wheel of a Ferrari. Do you think something similar could be arranged?"

"It's just a thought; we're going to have to look at a number of options, but that's a good one to start with. Anyway, I'll give it some thought over the next few days and get back to you."

Vicente drove back to Granada, showered, changed and then left immediately for Madrid. He made the journey in record time as the roads were virtually empty and he was able to drive the Cayenne at an average of 160 km per hour all the way. It had been a long day and he was tired so, unfortunately, a night with Claudia was out of the question. He needed his energy for the negotiations the next day but, if they were concluded successfully, then he would have something to celebrate with her tomorrow night. So after a quick snack at the bar he went straight to bed.

Friday, 7th December

On arriving at Pelayo y Parra's offices the next morning he was shown into a conference room, where Peter Roberts, Elena Fernandez and Juan Miguel Ordoñez greeted him.

"Here we are again," Peter Roberts said, shaking his hand. "Let's see if we can knock this agreement into shape today."

"There's no reason why we shouldn't be able to," replied Vicente. "I think the only outstanding issues are mainly procedural."

"True enough but they're important, especially verifying that the Cayman company is the owner of the options and that the land has been reclassified. Not forgetting the Certificate of Non-Investigation."

After some discussion, they agreed that Peter Roberts, together with a Cayman Island lawyer of his choice, would review the relevant documents to ensure that the Cayman Island company had legal title to all the option agreements.

"We'll provide the Certificate of Non-Investigation by the nineteenth, which means that the sale of the shares can take place as soon as you receive the signed copies of the minutes of the Urban Planning Committee," Vicente said.

"When do you expect that to be?"

"The meeting is on the nineteenth, so we should get them the next day or the twenty-first at the very latest."

"It's going to be very tight if there are any delays, remember Christmas Eve is a half day in London and Cayman, and the twenty-sixth is also a holiday."

"I don't foresee a problem. On Tuesday I'll send you a copy of the Environmental Planning Committee's recommendation so that the second instalment of the deposit can be released. When do you think your clients will be in a position to sign the Share Purchase Agreement?"

"I'm happy with it and, given time is of the essence, I'll ask their internal counsel to review it over the weekend. If he's happy with it then we can sign it on Tuesday, after we receive the Environmental Planning Committee recommendation."

"Perfect. Let's print four originals and I'll sign and initial all of them to save time. If we need to make changes we can do it via fax."

Once Vicente had signed and initialled the agreements he left, declining an invitation to dinner later that evening. He was looking forward to celebrating with Claudia.

Peter Roberts turned to Elena and Juan Manuel, "Many thanks and well done – a good job. Elena, can you bring Richard Drew of Bodden & Walker up to speed so he can make the necessary arrange-ments. Tell him we'll probably be there next Thursday. We should be able to do the due diligence on Friday. Then it's just a matter of waiting for the Certificate of Non-Investigation and confirmation that the PGOU has been approved."

He excused himself and went to a private office which Juan Miguel had reserved for him. He placed a memory stick with the new draft Share Purchase Agreement into the USB port of the computer on the desk, logged on to his email account and typed an email to Cristina and Andy.

"All terms and conditions of Share Purchase Agreement agreed. I attach copy signed by Vicente Maldonado for your perusal. Name of Cayman Island company to be provided when Mr. Maldonado receives copy signed by me on behalf of clients. I'll do this as soon as we receive a copy of Environmental Planning Committee recom - mendation."

He clicked on Send, removed the memory stick and returned to the conference room.

Ramon arrived at the station mid-morning. It had been a late night in the bars of El Castillo and he felt tired and hung over. The first thing he did was to visit forensics to review the evidence they had gathered from the house where Carlos had died the previous morning.

Only Antonio, a junior member of the forensics team, was there. The rest of them, like virtually everyone else, were taking advantage of the long weekend. Antonio laid out several plastic bags containing items such as trousers, shirts, shoes, empty bottles, glasses, etc., on the worktop at the far end of the room.

"We'll be processing these for prints and any trace elements on Monday then they'll be sent to Seville for DNA testing," he said to Ramon.

"Do you have the keys to the house?"

"Yes, here they are."

Ramon put on a pair of latex gloves and took the small plastic bag from Antonio. "Can you bring me the keys from the Mike Cameron case."

Once Antonio had retrieved Mike Cameron's keys, Ramon compared the keys on both key rings. "Bingo! The keys to the garage and the rear office door are on the same key ring as the house keys Carlos had," he said to Chief Inspector Diaz a few minutes later.

"Good work. That's a big step in the right direction. Get forensics to check if they're the copies that were used to open the two doors and if there are any prints on them. If they're the same keys then I think we've found Mr. Cameron's killer!"

"Will do, but I don't need to tell you that it won't be until Monday at the earliest."

Vicente returned to the Palace Hotel. Once in his room he called Javier Urquiza and told him what had been agreed.

"Excellent. As soon as we receive the second instalment of the deposit we can pay our friends on the Urban Planning Committee. Talking of which, has Johan made the drops today?"

"I assume so. I'll call and check with him in a minute. What's the latest news concerning Carlos?"

"My source confirms everything points to an accident. The copied keys have also been found and the Chief Inspector is now aware of this fact. That should enable him to close the Cameron case as well."

"Let's hope so; we can't afford to have the police sniffing around any more, even if they weren't on the right track."

"By the way, when you talk to Johan tell him Chief Inspector Diaz wants to talk to him regarding his loan to Carlos and, while it's impossible for them to link Carlos' death to that transaction, he needs to be careful what he says," Don Javier said.

"Will do."

"Good. Now, can you update the others regarding the Share Purchase Agreement?"

"Of course. I'll email them once I've spoken with Johan."

In Los Cipreses the weather had settled back into its previous pattern of clear blue skies and daytime temperatures in the low twenties. The truth was that they needed rain, and plenty of it, to replenish the reservoirs and avoid water restrictions the following summer, but there was none in sight.

Rather than hang around all morning waiting to hear from Peter Roberts, Andy went for a long bike ride up in the mountains. Four hours later he was back at his house and was ready for a long soak in the bath before checking his email.

When he logged into his UDYCO Gmail account he found Peter's email with the revised Share Purchase Agreement along with an email from Cristina:

"Looks like all systems go, subject to EPC recommendation. Have a great weekend."

He clicked on the Reply link:

"Fingers crossed for Monday. Assuming EPC approve we need to make arrangements for Cayman trip. Are you free to discuss over dinner this weekend?"

He knew she'd said that she would be working over the weekend but it was worth another try he thought to himself. A few minutes later he received a reply:

"Staying in Seville for EPC on Monday and will confirm travel arrangements then but, as per London trip, we will travel separately."

Short and to the point he thought, but then he understood that her colleagues also had access to the email account and, after all, this was business.

Monday, 10th December

Cristina Ibañez was tired. It had been a long three days; but at least they had made some progress in identifying and reviewing the personal bank accounts and Spanish assets of the members of the Environmental and Urban Planning Committees.

The vast majority of them seemed to be living within their means. One or two had assets which were inconsistent with their salaries but Cristina knew from experience that this might be explained via an inheritance, family or spousal wealth or legitimate business interests. She also knew there were many ways to hide ill-gotten gains, whether in Spain or abroad; far more detailed investigations would be required.

However, today was going to be crucial. If the Environmental Planning Committee recommended the Los Cipreses site then they could progress their investigations into Project Pulpo. If not, then they would be at a dead end, as without evidence that the committee may have been subject to undue influence, they were unlikely to be granted the necessary search and disclosure warrants.

The committee had convened at eleven that morning. It met in private and was not obliged to make public the results of its deliberations, but UDYCO's source on the committee had undertaken to inform them of their decision, so now it was just a matter of waiting.

"Check with forensics about the keys and if they have re-examined Mike Cameron's clothing yet. Then call Juan Luis and see when he's doing the autopsy on Carlos."

Ramon walked over to forensics, which was in an annex to the main building.

"These are definitely the same keys that were recently used to open the two doors, so that's a step in the right direction. Unfortunately, we've not been able to find any fingerprints on them."

"What about Mike Cameron's clothing? It's been over a week since we asked you to re-examine that for any foreign fibres or DNA."

"Yes, but it was a short week and we've been busy and under-staffed so we haven't had a chance to do that yet. It'll be done as soon as we finish processing the evidence in Mr. Maracena's case – unless you want it done first. Of course, if we find any samples containing DNA they will have to be sent to Seville or Madrid for analysis, depending on who's busier."

"Ok. Finish what you're doing and then do it." Ramon returned to his office and dialled the pathology lab. Juan Luis answered.

"Perfect timing, I've just completed the autopsy on Carlos Maracena."

"And what are your conclusions?"

"He drowned. I won't get the full toxicology results for a few days but from what I've seen he ingested a lot of cocaine and alcohol so I'm not surprised. He must have been virtually comatose when he entered the water and there's no evidence that force was applied."

"Thanks. I'll let Diaz know."

At half past one Cristina received confirmation that the Environmental Planning Committee had agreed to recommend the Los Cipreses site for reclassification and redevelopment. She asked for the names of the members who had voted for the project and then emailed Andy and Peter Roberts:

"Los Ciprese site approved by EPC. Arriving in Georgetown on Thursday evening on flight from Miami. Staying at Cayman Reef Resort condominium on 7 Mile Beach. Andy, best if you travel via New York and book each leg of the journey separately. Also recommend you rent a condo and not stay in a hotel."

Andy immediately set about checking flight availability and decided to fly to New York via Barcelona. As he had nothing to do in Los Cipreses he chose to fly the next day, stay overnight in New York, and then fly to Grand Cayman on Thursday, arriving a few hours before Cristina and Peter Roberts.

He knew Cayman Reef Resort well from previous visits. It was a well-protected, high-quality complex in a prime location on the famous 7 Mile Beach. He wanted to be close, but not too close to Cristina, so, after some online research, he rented a two-bedroom condo at the northern end of the beach.

He wanted to hear Cristina's voice before he left, so he called her on her Samesa mobile. She answered almost immediately. A good sign he thought.

"I've rented at Silver Sands. It's a couple of miles north of Cayman Reef Resort. Peter's staying at the Marriott, which is between the two complexes so we'll all be within easy reach of each other."

"It's crucial that Javier Urquiza, or any of his associates, do not know that either of us is on the island, so we can't meet with Peter. Also, I think we should meet Doug James of the Cayman Island Monetary Authority at your condo."

"I agree. Doug's an old friend so I'm sure that'll be fine. Have you made any progress with your investigations into the committee members?"

"We're slowly but surely pulling a lot of loose ends together but there's still a lot to do so I'll update you on Thursday evening, unless something important happens in the meantime."

"Ok. So are you looking forward to it?"

"Yes, and I'm glad we'll be spending a few days there instead of an overnighter."

"Me too. It's become a bit too touristy in recent years but it still has a fabulous beach, warm water and great scuba diving and we should have some time to enjoy the facilities."

"That would be nice but business first, pleasure second," she replied.

"Naturally; but we're there for the weekend, and it would be a shame to waste the opportunity."

Vicente Maldonado received the news direct from Fernando half an hour after Cristina Ibañez.

"Excellent. When can you scan and email me the official

minutes?"

"My secretary will circulate the minutes this afternoon and I'll get them signed off by mid-morning tomorrow."

"The sooner you can get them to me, the sooner we can make the necessary payments to our friends on the Urban Planning Committee meeting."

"Don't worry, you'll have them as soon as I get them. So what's next?"

"The investors sign the Share Purchase Agreement, I allocate the shares in the Cayman Island company and then we request the Certificate of Non-Investigation."

"What about our friend Enrique?"

"That's in hand, but nothing's going to happen to him until the investors instruct the transfer of funds."

"Which will be when?"

"If all goes smoothly, the twentieth or twenty-first."

"Then what?"

"If Johan delivers his side of the bargain, then both of you will come to my office so we can reallocate Enrique's shares before the cleared funds leave the account. I assume you'll be available."

"Of course."

"Good. In the meantime, why don't you tell Don Javier the good news while I call Peter Roberts?"

When Vicente finished speaking with Peter Roberts he called a number in Georgetown. "Jim, it's Vicente Maldonado here."

"Hi Vicente," a voice with an American accent replied. "I've been waiting for your call. Are you ready to push the button on Carrington Investments?"

"Yes – I'm about to fax you the signed authority to assign the option agreements to Carrington. Then I'll email you what the initial share allocations will be. Once that is done you can request the Certificate of Non-Investigation."

"What's the timing on this, Vicente?"

"Close of business your time on Wednesday. Is that a problem?"

"No, it shouldn't be."

"Good. I'll also email you details of the lawyers who'll be under-taking due diligence on Carrington Investments but, as discussed, you are not under any circumstances to disclose the names of the shareholders, is that clear?"

"Yes. Anyway, that's normal practice if a Certificate of Non-Investigation is involved."

"Ok. Email me as soon as the formalities are complete. Any doubts or questions then either call me on Skype if I am online or on the mobile number I gave you if I'm not."

"Thank you for coming in," Chief Inspector Diaz said, showing Johan Gaards into his office.

"Anything I can do to help," he replied, sitting down in one of the battered plastic chairs in front of the Chief Inspector's desk.

The Chief Inspector focused his piercing blue eyes on Johan. "Good. As you know, Carlos Maracena was found dead last Thursday and I understand you were friends?"

"I wouldn't say friends. More like acquaintances. Why do you ask?"

"I believe that you had agreed to lend him a large sum of money."

"Yes, he needed to repay the money he had borrowed from Mrs. Cameron to acquire Bar Salamander and so he approached me for a loan."

"Did he say why he needed to repay Mrs. Cameron?"

"Apparently there are some complications regarding her inheritance following her husband's death."

"Why did you agree to lend him the money?"

"It was a business proposition. I think Bar Salamander has great potential if managed properly."

"I'm not so sure, but then I'm not a businessman. Still, one hundred and forty thousand euros is a lot of money. Do you mind telling me where you obtained this sum?"

"I don't see the relevance of the question but, as you know, I've been here for many years, had a few businesses and owned several properties so I have capital."

"And did you give him the money?"

"No, I was going to give it to him on Friday."

"Were you aware that he and his friends were having a party on Wednesday evening?"

"No. I don't mix socially with any of them."

"One last thing. When did you last speak to Carlos?"

"Let me think," replied Johan, pausing for a while. "Yes, it would've been a week ago on Sunday when we finalised the terms of the loan."

"And you didn't see him after that?"

"No. We'd agreed to meet on Friday morning so I could give him the money.

Ok, thank you Mr. Gaards; I think that covers everything."

"Good, but feel free to call me if you have any more questions," Johan replied, rising from the chair and making his way to the door.

Chief Inspector Diaz looked thoughtful. There was something about Johan Gaards that bothered him. He couldn't put his finger on it but his general air of arrogance and nonchalance didn't help. Unfortunately, since the Policia Nacional were not responsible for Los Cipreses he had never had any dealings with him or had a reason to look into his activities. Nevertheless, he felt certain that he was part of UDYCO's undercover operation and it was very frustrating that they wouldn't tell him more about their investigation and Johan Gaards' role in it.

Tuesday, 11th December

London was dull and drizzly as winter took its grip and Peter Roberts was looking forward to spending a few days in the Caymans. Aside from a welcome break in the sun, it was quite exciting to be on the inside of a major criminal investigation, whatever the outcome.

The familiar ping of an incoming email interrupted his thoughts. It was from Vicente Maldonado, and the scanned copies of the minutes of yesterday's EPC meeting were attached.

He forwarded it to UDYCO and Andy and then to Elena Nuñez, asking her to review the EPC minutes. A few minutes later she rang him to confirm that the minutes seemed to be genuine and that the committee had recommended the Los Cipreses site for the proposed golf course development.

"In which case can you confirm to Mr. Marteens at First City Trust that the second tranche of the reservation deposit can be released and I'll sign and fax the Share Purchase Agreement to Mr. Maldonado."

A couple of hours later Peter Roberts sent UDYCO and Andy another email.

"*SPA signed and scanned version attached. Tranche two of reser - vation deposit authorised for release. Name of CI company confirmed by VM as Carrington Investments. Only UPC approval and CNI required to make SPA effective. See you both in Cayman. Have a safe journey.*"

While he was waiting for Ramon to bring him the forensics report on Carlos Maracena, Chief Inspector Diaz reflected on Mike Cameron's death and his discussion the previous afternoon with Johan Gaards.

UDYCO had not provided any further information about the

mysterious SMS on Mike's phone. So, although the copied keys had no fingerprints, he was prepared to accept that their presence in Carlos' possession, along with the fact that they had been unable to confirm Carlos' whereabouts between twelve and quarter past that night, made it highly likely that he had killed Mike Cameron.

As far as Johan Gaards was concerned, he wondered if it was a coincidence that he had been involved with both Mike Cameron and Carlos Maracena not long before their deaths. There didn't seem to be a connection, but was he missing something, or were UDYCO covering something up?

There was a knock at the door and he beckoned Ramon to enter. "Forensics say there's no physical evidence to suggest Carlos' death wasn't an accident."

"No real surprise there after the autopsy. I suppose it's probably safe to assume that Carlos murdered Mike Cameron but it would be helpful if forensics could find some concrete evidence placing Carlos at the scene – have they re-examined Mike Cameron's clothes yet?"

"They say it's a delicate job given the condition they're in but he expects to complete it by the end of the day. Maybe they'll find something."

Chief Inspector Diaz shook his head resignedly. "It's a long shot and we've probably just about got enough to put Carlos in the frame, but I'm still not entirely convinced. Anyway, I've got to go to Granada this afternoon so call me as soon as forensics give you their findings."

In Seville, Cristina Ibañez and her team were putting the finishing touches to the applications for warrants to the Spanish authorities and Interpol requesting disclosure of financial information on, and assets held by, members of the Environmental and Urban Planning Committees.

The evidence looked compelling and she felt it should be more than enough to convince the relevant authorities to issue the warrants. However, she knew that for a speedy resolution it was vital to convince the Cayman Island Monetary Authority to provide the names of the shareholders in Carrington Investments, preferably before the Urban Planning Committee meeting on the nineteenth.

She therefore emailed the application to Andy:

"Please use attached to help make our case to CIMA. Let me know if you need any further information. Happy translating!"

Definitely from her he thought, looking at the last two words and exclamation mark. He had picked up the two emails from Peter Roberts earlier in the day and already made a start of summarising the evidence for Doug James. Nevertheless, UDYCO's application for warrants would allow him to dot the I's and cross the T's.

As he reviewed the document Cristina had sent him, Andy noted that it named Vicente Maldonado and all the EPC and UPC committee members, but that two names had been left blank. No doubt one was Mr. Brown's, but he was not sure who the other might be, so he sent her an email asking for the two missing names.

"Not appropriate to disclose now. Let's discuss on Thursday in Cayman."

At seven o'clock that evening Jose, the head of forensics, called Ramon, who was in a bar round the corner from the station having a beer and a cigarette. "I've found something interesting. Why don't you come by and I'll explain?"

A few minutes later he was telling Ramon about the two strands of hair he had found on the back of Mike Cameron's fleece which did not, on first examination, belong to Mike Cameron.

"The fact that they were on the back of the fleece could be significant, since the killer strangled Mike Cameron from behind. Given the condition of the samples I'll have to send them to Madrid for the DNA profile as they are the only ones with the necessary equipment."

"How long will it take?"

"With this poor quality sample usually at least two weeks, but I know how important this is to Chief Inspector Diaz and I'm conscious we should have picked up on this first time round, so I'll see if I pull some strings in Madrid and get it done sooner."

"The hairs could belong to the murderer, or to anybody else who was in close proximity to Mike Cameron before his death," Chief Inspector Diaz said to Ramon, who had called him with the news. "So if forensics can get a decent sample and it's not Carlos' and they can't match it to samples on the national DNA database, then ask them to check it against samples from Ann Cameron, Sonya, Pepe of the Cutty Sark and Johan Gaards."

"Yes boss, but I think we only have a DNA sample from Mrs. Cameron as she's the only one of them who has been arrested as a suspect."

"So tomorrow ask the others to volunteer samples. If they've nothing to hide then they shouldn't have a problem. If any of them refuse then we'll have to look into their alibis in more detail. This investigation may not be over yet Ramon."

Ramon called Javier Urquiza and gave him this latest news.

Wednesday, 12th December

The deliberately irritating jingle from his mobile phone woke Andy at six o'clock. He struggled out of bed, made his way to the bathroom and showered. It was still dark when he left the house but, as he drove to Malaga airport, the twinkling stars faded away as the night sky was gradually replaced by the soft orange glow of the sun's rays emerging from beyond the horizon.

It was four o'clock New York time when the classic yellow cab dropped him off at the W hotel on 42nd street. It was a typical mid-December afternoon, cold and grey, with dusk rapidly approaching. The festive season was very much in evidence, with hanging light displays, well-lit trees and other decorations occupying what seemed like every store front and many lamp posts. People were bustling up and down and across the major streets, in and out of shops, many carrying multi-coloured, multi-sized shopping bags.

Although he had many friends and business contacts in New York, he had made no arrangements to meet or have dinner with anyone. Instead, he intended to take advantage of the weak dollar to do some Christmas shopping and then have an early night before flying to Cayman the following day.

Before heading to Fifth Avenue he checked his emails. It had been twelve hours since he'd been able to do so, and he was pleased to see an email from Doug James confirming he would be at Andy's rented condo at eleven o'clock on Friday morning. Andy forwarded the email to UDYCO, along with the presentation to CIMA, which he had finished on the plane, and then hit the shops.

As Andy was checking into his hotel, Vicente Maldonado and Johan Gaards were meeting in Granada at the same taverna as the previous week. It was beginning to fill up with a combination of tourists, locals and what looked like university students, but the noise and low lighting suited their purpose.

Earlier, Vicente had received confirmation that the second instalment of two million euros from the reservation deposit had been paid into the designated Swiss bank account. Now he needed to agree a plan of action for Enrique with Johan. Unfortunately, for once, Johan was quite agitated.

"I had no choice but to give them a DNA sample. I very much doubt it's going to match the hairs they've found on Mike Cameron's jumper, but if they match them to Miguel then we potentially have a serious problem."

"Don't worry Johan. Firstly, Miguel's DNA isn't on the police database and secondly, our source tells us they haven't been asked to collect a sample from him, so, even if the hairs are his they can't match the DNA to him."

"Let's hope you're right, because if there's any chance of me being in the frame for Mike Cameron and Carlos Maracena's deaths then I'm out of here, Project Pulpo or no Project Pulpo."

"Listen, it's unlikely the police are going to make any further progress but if they do we'll know in advance from our source and can act accordingly. We're only a week away from the Urban Planning Committee meeting and it would be a real shame if you were to lose out on your one and a half million euros bonus."

Johan thought about this for a few seconds and then nodded. "You're right. If necessary, we should be able to buy enough time to complete Project Pulpo."

"Good. So what are you going to do about Enrique?"

Johan explained his idea in detail. Vicente agreed it was feasible and promised to get Johan what he needed. Then he left the taverna and returned home to call Jim Dexter who confirmed that all the formalities regarding Carrington Investments had been done.

"By the way, Peter Roberts of Moore, Moore & Blackthorn is arriving in Georgetown tomorrow to undertake due diligence, so expect a call from him," Vicente told him before clicking on the red Skype button.

Vicente was pleased with how smoothly things were going. Provided the Certificate of Non-Investigation was issued by the nineteenth, all that remained was for the Urban Planning Committee to deliver their approval. Given that he was going to transfer two million euros to various offshore bank accounts tomorrow he did not expect that to be a problem.

Thursday, 13th December

Before leaving the W hotel for JFK and his flight to Cayman, Andy checked his emails and saw that overnight Cristina had sent him an email signing off on the presentation to CIMA. It ended: *"Suggest we meet for a working breakfast tomorrow before our meeting with Doug James. Is 8.30 at your place OK? Best to email me your response."*

"8.30 at my place is fine. Any special requests for breakfast," he replied before logging off and turning off his laptop.

On its approach to Georgetown, the plane flew down the length of 7 Mile Beach, giving Andy and the passengers on the left-hand side of the aircraft an eagle eye's view of the famous white sand and the turquoise Caribbean Sea. He had been a relatively frequent visitor, both in his banking days as well as during his spell at the serious fraud squad, and so was familiar with Grand Cayman. In truth, in terms of geography the island itself had little to offer, being small, virtually flat and, for the most part, narrow. Its fame was due primarily to 7 Mile Beach, the scuba diving and, of course, its status as one of the world's leading offshore financial centres and, since signing the International Money Laundering Disclosure Agreement, it was slowly shaking off its public image as a centre for money laundering and tax evasion.

Andy emerged from the plane and was immediately hit by a blast of warm air, his sunglasses instantly misting up as condensation formed on the lenses. It must have been at least thirty degrees, and the humidity was palpable as he made the short walk across the tarmac to the air-conditioned terminal.

Given his recent role at the City of London Police, immigration formalities were completed quickly and smoothly and once he had collected his hire car he was at his rented condo within thirty minutes. The unit was on the first floor of a three-storey block and comprised two bedrooms, each with an en-suite bathroom, an open plan kitchen/living area and a terrace overlooking the beach, which was no more than thirty yards away. Andy quickly unpacked his holdall, put on a pair of swimming trunks, grabbed a beach towel and went for a swim. The sea was warm and crystal clear and he luxuriated in it for a while before returning to the condo.

By the time he had showered and changed it was five o'clock. He assumed that Cristina had arrived in Miami and was waiting for her connecting flight to Cayman so he checked his emails, but was disappointed to see that there was not one from her.

He decided to drive to the supermarket to stock up with various items. On the way back he picked up a pizza and rented a DVD of Casino Royale. Might provide some ideas on how to behave in a difficult situation, he thought jokingly to himself. By the time he finished watching the film two hours later he very much hoped his personal little adventure would involve no violence but that he got the girl.

There was still no email from Cristina who, he assumed, had arrived on the island by now, but before retiring to bed he rang Peter Roberts.

"Hi Peter, Andy here. When did you arrive?"

"About an hour ago. How about you?"

"Oh, I've been here long enough to swim, shop, eat and watch a movie."

"Lucky you, hopefully I'll get some R and R over the weekend. What are your plans tomorrow?"

"I'm meeting with Cristina first thing then with Doug James at eleven-thirty to make our case for their cooperation. You've seen the presentation and I'm not expecting any problems."

"Yes, the evidence is compelling; do you need anything else from me?"

"No. In fact, as we discussed, it would be best if we have no face-to-face contact while you're here. Vicente Maldonado and his accomplices may be keeping an eye on you. Carry out the due diligence as agreed and we can swap notes by phone or email."

"Fair enough. I've arranged to meet their lawyer, a Jim Dexter, at eleven tomorrow morning to start the due diligence. My sources say he operates just on the right side of the tracks, if you know what I mean."

"No surprise there. I can almost picture him wearing a white or cream linen suit and a panama hat."

Peter Roberts laughed, "I hope not because that's what I'll be wearing!"

Friday, 14th December

Andy got up at seven-thirty. He didn't have much to do, but he wanted to be ready just in case Cristina wanted breakfast. At eight-thirty sharp he heard a knock on the door.

"Welcome to my humble abode," he said, waving her in. "Did you have a good journey?"

"Yes, no problems; just a four-hour lay over at Miami International, so I eventually got in at ten-thirty last night."

"Have you had breakfast?"

"No, I was hoping you might do the honours."

"Well, since you didn't reply to my email all I've got is some coffee, orange juice and toast. Will that do?"

"It'll have to," she replied, looking a little surprised and even, he thought, disappointed.

"Of course, I could rustle up some scrambled egg with smoked salmon to put on the toast if you prefer and I might even manage a fresh fruit salad. How does that sound?"

A smile lit up her face. "That sounds wonderful."

"Good. You sit out here on the terrace and I'll do the "honours" as you so neatly put it. There's coffee in the cafetiere, but if you want some tea let me know."

After placing a bowl of freshly sliced and diced tropical fruits and a jug of freshly squeezed orange juice on the table Andy disappeared to the kitchen. A few minutes later he returned carrying two plates, each containing a piece of toasted sesame bread covered with a mixture of scrambled eggs and smoked salmon.

"Voila! My only breakfast trick. No champagne I'm afraid as it's a working day," he said, placing a plate in front of Cristina.

"That looks and smells fantastic, Andy. What have I done to deserve this?"

"Just being here is enough. Now tuck in and then afterwards you can tell me who the two missing names are and update me on the latest developments."

"Javier Urquiza and Johan Gaards," Cristina told him after they had cleared the table and began to discuss the case they were going to make Doug James of CIMA for their cooperation.

"I'd guessed Johan might be one of them but I've never heard of Javier Urquiza."

"No reason why you would have done. He's originally from Granada but has been living in Los Cipreses for a number of years. He keeps a low profile but is wealthy, outwardly from property development but, as you know, we also suspect he is involved in the drugs trade."

"Well, if he's behind this little scam he could make an awful lot of money if he manages to get away with it."

"If he is behind it then I think he's going to be spending a lot of time behind bars."

Andy inserted the two names into the document they were going to give CIMA and printed off three copies on the printer the Silver Sands administration office had supplied. He placed one of the copies, along with supporting documents, in a clear plastic folder, ready to give to Doug James.

Cristina then told him that the autopsy on Carlos had concluded his death was an accidental drowning and that they had also found the two copied keys with the set of keys to the house he had died in.

"I suppose that pretty much confirms Carlos murdered Mike then."

"It looks that way, but Chief Inspector Diaz still can't definitely place him at the scene of the crime and we haven't traced the source of the SMS. However, on re-examining Mr. Cameron's clothes earlier this week, forensics found two small hairs on the back of his fleece which don't belong to him. They've been sent for DNA analysis to see if we can identify who they belong to. If they're Carlos' then the case is closed. If not, then there are still some questions that remain unanswered."

"And how long is that going to take?"

"They're poor quality samples and need special treatment but hopefully we should have the results by the middle of next week."

The sound of the door buzzer interrupted their conversation and Andy went to let Doug James in. He was tall and skinny, with receding wavy blonde hair. He looked very formal in a pin-stripe navy suit, a white shirt and dark red tie, but he had a very healthy tan which served to set off his bright blue eyes. After introducing Cristina, the three of them sat down and Andy explained the purpose of their visit, going through the presentation and supporting documentation.

Doug James sat patiently listening to Andy without asking any questions, but occasionally jotting notes on the documents Andy had given him. When Andy finished, Doug remained silent while he flicked through the documents. Andy and Cristina waited expectantly. After a while Doug said:

"It's a very well-structured transaction and if you can prove bribery is also involved then you have them over a barrel. The problem is that no offence has been committed yet, as far as we are aware."

"That's true but it would be amazing if Spanish nationals were not involved and the use of the Belize and Seychelles companies makes the intention to evade tax look strong," Andy replied.

"So essentially you want us to let you know whether the individuals named herein," he said, tapping the documents, "are shareholders of Carrington Investments?"

"Yes, that's it."

"Ok, based on what I've seen, I'll recommend that we cooperate with you, but I'm unlikely to get formal approval until Monday lunchtime at the earliest."

"So long as we have an answer before the nineteenth, which is when the Urban Planning Committee meets, that would be fine Mr. James."

"I think I should be able to manage that. I'll set the ball rolling this afternoon. It was a pleasure to meet you Ms. Ibañez and, contrary to what the popular press would have people believe, the Cayman Islands do not condone, encourage or support money laundering or tax evasion, so I hope we can help UDYCO to bring this case to a speedy and successful conclusion," Doug James replied, rising from his chair.

A little later, after tying up a few loose ends, Cristina also left, as she had work to do.

"So how did Peter Roberts get on?" she asked him a few hours later.

"Quite well it seems. The articles and memorandum of association of Carrington Investments seem to be in order, as does Vicente Maldonado's authority to enter into any agreements on behalf of the company. Apparently the Belize and Seychelles companies have assigned the options over to Carrington Investments so all he's waiting for is the Certificate of Non-Investigation."

"Good. Have you heard from Doug James?"

"No, and I don't really expect to until Monday."

"So now it's just a matter of waiting."

"I'm afraid so, but it's only a couple of days and there are worse places to spend a weekend. I realise we can't be seen together in public but there's no stopping you coming over for a BBQ this evening. What do you think?"

"I'd love to but I have to check in with Seville again and the jet lag is kicking in. Can we do it tomorrow?"

"Understood; I'm feeling a little tired myself. Shall we say eight-thirty sharp." In truth, Andy was disappointed that he couldn't see her that evening. Another missed opportunity, he thought, while reluctantly accepting that work and rest would have to take precedence over his desire to get closer to Cristina.

Saturday, 15th December

Andy spent most of the day lazing around on the beach – reading, snorkelling and listening to music. He was looking forward to spending the evening with Cristina and as he finished preparing a mixed leaf salad with mushrooms and king prawns he wondered how the evening would go. Earlier he had placed a large tenderloin steak in an olive oil, soy sauce and honey marinade and now all he needed to do was to set the table, shower and wait.

Cristina did not disappoint. She was excellent company and the conversation, like the wine, flowed easily between them. Andy had chosen a Ravenswood Zinfandel to accompany the meal, knowing that the wine would compliment the marinated steak. Cristina had approved and before long they were on their second bottle.

"So how come you've never married? Do you like to play the field or just not found the right person?" she asked him in a teasing tone, her green eyes sparkling, "

"The latter. Earlier this year I broke up with my long-term girlfriend. We had some great times but marriage never seemed to be a priority and we slowly drifted apart. How about you?"

"Oh, I'm one of those divorce statistics on a government chart. Married my university sweetheart, both set out on our careers and ended up as virtual strangers. He wanted children, I didn't, so we decided to call it a day last year before it got nasty."

"I'm sorry to hear that."

"Don't be. It was for the best. I love my job and having a family has never been high on my list of priorities. It sounds selfish but I see it as being realistic. I think children need at least one full-time parent, and I can't see myself in that role, while my ex was not about to give up his career."

"A true career woman then."

"It looks like it, doesn't it, but then you never know what's coming up round the next corner."

"I'll drink to that," Andy replied, raising his glass with a smile and a wink.

They were sitting on the terrace. A few scattered clouds were drifting slowly across the night sky and they could just catch the sound of the sea gently lapping against the sand.

Andy cleared away the plates and brought out the chocolate fudge cheesecake he had purchased earlier that day. "Not one of my own creations, I'm not very good with desserts, but it looks pretty good."

"Andy if I continue to eat like this I'm going to have to spend all day tomorrow exercising!"

"A small piece won't hurt you. We can always go for a midnight walk along the beach to work off the calories."

"That sounds like a marvellous idea, but I need to be getting back soon. I'm booked on a trip to Stingray City tomorrow and I need to be up quite early."

"Sounds like a poor excuse to me, but we could always sprint a couple of hundred yards instead to save time!"

Cristina laughed. "You're incorrigible. I'd love to walk along the beach with you, but we both know that now is not the right time."

"If not now, when? We are on a Caribbean island thousands of miles from Spain and off duty."

"Andy, if only it were so simple. You know that being seen together here by any of Javier Urquiza's accomplices would sabotage the investigation. It's a very small island and it's not worth the risk. I'm sure there'll be other opportunities once this is all over."

They finished their dessert in silence, and when Andy returned from the kitchen they stood a couple of feet apart, leaning on the balcony, watching the sea. Andy turned to face her and took a step forward. She turned towards him and he placed his hands on her elbows. He looked straight into her eyes.

"Will there be other opportunities? This investigation will finish one way or the other in the next few days and our paths may never cross again. I can't help but I feel there is something special happening between us and I don't want to lose the opportunity to find out what that is."

Cristina looked up at his face. "I feel it too, but we have to be patient. If it's real we'll find the right moment."

"Carpe diem," Andy said, pulling her gently towards him and placing his lips on hers. For a brief moment she resisted. But soon she was returning his embrace and kisses with equal passion. Their bodies interlocked, shifting and twisting to enable the maximum contact between them.

"Andy, stop" she said, gently pushing him away. "I want this as much as you do but not now, not here."

Andy held her at arm's length. "As usual, you're right. It will have to wait, though not too long I hope. Probably a good idea if you go before we change our minds."

Cristina nodded and broke free from his grasp. "Why don't you call me a taxi while I go and freshen up," she said walking towards the bathroom.

Sunday, 16th December

As Andy set off on a hybrid bike to tour the west side of the island, Cristina was stepping onto a glass-bottom boat which would take her and nineteen other tourists to the sandbank that was Stingray City, one of the Cayman Islands' leading tourist attractions.

Since the early 80s, when a few locals had swum with, and tamed, some wild stingrays, it had grown into a massive tourist operation which involved hundreds of tourists swimming with, feeding, and handling large number of stingrays, some with a wing span of more than two metres. It was compelling and unusual, if somewhat increasingly tacky.

She wished Andy was with her so they could enjoy the experience together, but knew they had to sacrifice their own personal feelings for the sake of the investigation. It had been a long time since she had felt so attracted to a man and she hoped they would be able to carry on where they left off the night before in the not too distant future.

"So how was your day?" Andy asked her later that evening.

"Fantastic. Stingray City may be very commercial but what an experience! I never thought I'd get so close to, let alone handle, a stingray. It's amazing how soft and velvety their skin is and how tame they are."

"Yes, it's quite something standing on a sandbank half a mile from shore surrounded by scores of friendly stingrays, not to mention braying tourists! What about the rest of the day?"

"A siesta, then a walk down the beach followed by some snorkelling."

"Ah, ha, I thought it was you walking briskly past me listening to your iPod, lost in thought."

She laughed. "And I thought you were sleeping off the effects of all that wine!"

Andy told her about his bike ride and how much the island had changed in the few years since Hurricane Ivan. They bantered for a while longer and then agreed to meet at her condo the following day.

"By then I'll have had an update from Spain and should be hearing from Doug James."

"Yes, a big day tomorrow, so sleep tight."

"You too," she said hanging up.

Monday, 17th December

Late the next morning Andy walked the two miles along the beach to the Cayman Reef Resort. It had been built in the eighties but was still one of the top developments on 7 Mile Beach due to its location and high-quality construction. Cristina's apartment was a top-floor penthouse just yards from the beach.

"No expense spared then," he said to her when she'd finished showing him round.

"It's actually the only gated private development on 7 Mile Beach and there were no other units available, so I'm not complaining," she replied with a wry smile.

"I wouldn't if I were you, but it's a shame you're not staying longer to be able to enjoy it to its full potential. So what's the news from HQ?"

"No major developments. Forensics are still working on getting a decent DNA sample from the hairs found on Mike's fleece, while my team are waiting for CIMA to confirm the names of the shareholders in order to request warrants."

"Ok, let's call Doug to see if he has any news for us."

Andy talked for a couple of minutes with Doug James and then hung up, giving the thumbs up sign to Cristina. "They're in and he'll call us in couple of hours to confirm whether any of the suspects are shareholders in Carrington Investments."

"Fantastic. If Javier Urquiza and any of the others are the beneficial shareholders we'll have enough to request arrest warrants. If not then we are back to square one," she said.

"We'll know soon enough. In the meantime let's see if Peter has finally finished the due diligence," replied Andy as he logged in to his UDYCO Gmail account.

"Satisfied documentation is in order. Have been advised CNI should be available tomorrow. So all systems go subject to UPC. What is situation with CIMA?" Peter's email to them read.

Andy typed, *"Confused with all the TLAs? CIMA cooperating and will confirm whether VM and Co are shareholders in Carrington Investments in next couple of hours. Will call you once we have heard."*

He looked at Cristina.

"What are TLAs?"

"It's a bit of joke in the business world that everything is reduced to Three Letter Acronyms," Andy replied smiling. "Ok to send?"

Cristina nodded and he clicked on the Send button. They treated themselves to a beer while they waited for Doug James' call. They chatted easily, the chemistry between them evident, but they were both secretly relieved when the phone rang. Cristina picked up the receiver.

"Ms. Ibañez, Doug James here. I hope you are enjoying your stay on Cayman and that Andy is looking after you."

"Very much so to both Mr. James. I'm just sorry that I can't stay longer."

"Oh well, I am sure your work will bring you back again. Talking of which, we've checked the names you gave us and I can confirm that Javier Urquiza, Vicente Maldonado, Fernando Echevaria and Enrique Gonzalez are all shareholders in Carrington Investments."

"Nobody else, for example, Johan Gaards?"

"No, only those four individuals."

"And what proportion do they hold the shares in?"

"Give me a second. Ah, here it is. Javier Urquiza has eighty-five and the others five percent each."

"Thank you so much Mr. James. If the PGOU is approved and the investors transfer the funds we'll have a prima facia case for charging these four individuals with tax evasion at the very least."

"It would appear so and, as agreed, we'll issue the CNI tomorrow. We'll be in touch then but do give me advanced warning next time you plan to visit; I'd be delighted to take you out for dinner."

"I'll do that and thank you once again."

"So Johan Gaards is not involved then?"

"Not directly it seems. We think he's more involved in the drug-running side of the business. There's no need for him to be involved at this level, and he's probably paid in cash or via an offshore account."

Andy was punching numbers into a calculator as Cristina spoke. "Based on the share holding percentages, Javier Urquiza stands to receive just over one hundred and ninety-one million euros and the other three just over eleven million each. Not bad, even if they've had to pay out a few million in bribes."

Peter Roberts was not surprised at the news. "I'm going to stay to receive the CNI and oversee the transfer of funds. Mr. Maldonado assures me that I'll have the official minutes of the Urban Planning Committee meeting by Friday morning at the latest, which means I should be in a position to order the transfer of funds later that day."

"Perfect. I'm flying back to Spain this evening and Andy is leaving first thing tomorrow, so it would be better if you email us when you've received the CNI."

Tuesday, 18th December

Vicente Maldonado had asked Johan to come up to Granada, and they met in one of the many bars in Calle Elvira, just off the Gran Via. Although the sky was clear, the temperature was close to freezing. There were a few people in the bar having their traditional mid-morning coffee break, but Vicente and Johan found a quiet corner where they could talk without being overheard.

"Well Johan, things are progressing smoothly and tomorrow is the big day. If that goes according to plan then by this weekend the funds should be on their way to the Cayman Islands, which means it will be down to you to fulfil your side of the bargain."

"Don't worry, provided you have what I asked for then it shouldn't be a problem."

"I hope not, there's a lot of money involved," replied Vicente sliding a ubiquitous Zara carrier bag under the table. "Everything you asked for is in this bag. Just don't lose or mislay it."

Johan looked inside the bag and took out two smart boxes, each about 15 cm long by 6 cm wide and 4 cm deep. They were finished in what looked like leather and had hinged lids. He discreetly opened each box, checked the contents and then closed them and put them back in the bag.

"Was it difficult to get?"

"Let's say I had to pull a couple of favours and grease some palms. So is the plan the same as we discussed a couple of weeks ago?"

"Yes. It's a perfect opportunity and I've got myself the perfect cover."

"Excellent. Then I'll leave it in your very capable hands."

"What about the reallocation of the shares to me?"

"Come to my office at lunchtime on the twenty-fourth and I'll instruct the Cayman lawyer to change the allocations before the funds are transferred out again to the shareholders. I assume you want your share transferred to your account in Belize."

"Yes. Is there anything else I need to do or know?"

"No. We're in the hands of the Urban Planning Committee now, but I'm not expecting that to be a problem. I'll be in Seville tomorrow and I'll let you know as soon as I have any news."

Wednesday, 19th December

Andy arrived back in Los Cipreses tired but excited after a twenty-hour journey involving three flights, but today he would survive on adrenaline as he waited for the results of the Urban Planning Committee meeting. He wasn't expecting any surprises but once the PGOU was approved and the funds transferred Cristina could make her move.

He had not called Cristina when he had landed at Barcelona, reasoning that she would not appreciate a wake-up call at five o'clock in the morning, so he called her now on her Samesa mobile number. It went straight to voicemail so he left a message.

After showering, he checked his emails for the first time since leaving Cayman and saw that Peter Roberts had confirmed receipt of the Certificate of Non-Investigation.

Just as he went to the kitchen to make another cup of coffee, his phone rang. It was Cristina.

"Good morning Ms. Ibañez. How was your trip back?"

"Good morning to you too Mr. Montalvo. It was uneventful. And yours?"

"Much the same. Everything went smoothly and I just got home an hour ago. Have there been any developments?"

"Nothing of any importance. Today the final piece of the jigsaw should fall into place."

"What about the arrest warrants?"

"On their way to Judge Bustamente as we speak."

"When do you think you'll be able to arrest them?"

"As you know, we have to wait until the order to transfer the funds to Carrington Investments had been made, so if Peter orders the transfer on Friday we'll have a six-day window until the twenty-seventh, which is how long Doug James has agreed to hold up the funds.

"That should be plenty of time."

"Yes, but, ideally, the arrests must be carried out simultaneously so we need to establish the movements and whereabouts of all five of them over that period and pick a suitable day and time. We're currently working on that but keeping tabs on five people 24/7 involves a lot of manpower and careful coordination."

"I know – I've been involved in a couple of similar operations myself. So what time is the Urban Planning Committee meeting?"

"What a lot of questions – I hope you're not like this every morning!"

"I'm usually docile and receptive to any reasonable suggestions in the mornings but this is business!" Andy replied laughing.

"Fair point. To answer your last question, the Urban Planning Committee meeting should start any minute now and, to pre-empt your next question, it's expected to go on until two o'clock, if not later. The Los Cipreses PGOU is the only thing on the agenda but it is very controversial so there's likely to be a heated discussion."

"Nothing new there then, lots of raised voices, arm waving, interruptions and then, by the end of it, they'll all be best friends!"

"Something like that, but the noise level and time taken will also depend on how much influence Javier Urquiza has bought, so we'll just have to wait and see. Ok, I must go and update my boss. Let's touch base later."

Javier Urquiza was very nervous. Although he had paid over two million euros to various committee members, it only needed one to have a change of heart and Project Pulpo could be dead in the water. He had suggested to his wife, in a manner not to be questioned, that she spend the day Christmas shopping for their daughters' and grandchildren's presents, so he was alone in the house waiting expectantly for a call from Fernando or Vicente.

Eventually, at twenty to three, his prepaid mobile rang. It was Fernando.

"All systems go Don Javier. The PGOU, including the reclassification of the land, has been approved."

Javier Urquiza let out a sigh of relief. "Well done Fernando. It looks as if you are going to be a rich man."

"Not as rich as you Javier, but I'm not complaining."

"When will the official minutes be signed?"

"We're breaking for lunch while the secretary prepares the minutes. We'll review and hopefully sign them later this afternoon. Nobody wants to reconvene tomorrow; anyway the Junta wants to make an official announcement as soon as possible in order to quell any speculation."

"So you'll give a signed copy to Vicente this evening?"

"Yes. We've arranged to have dinner tonight in Jerez."

Cristina told Andy the news shortly afterwards. "Now it's over to Peter Roberts. When he pushes the button so to speak we can plan the arrests."

"Have you any idea when that will be?"

"We have a couple of options but we're still trying to confirm the whereabouts of all the suspects. In any event, you'll appreciate that I can't disclose that information to you."

"Of course, but will you be involved?"

"No. I don't want to blow my cover, and anyway we have special teams that handle these types of high profile arrests."

"So what are your plans for the weekend and Christmas?"

"Apart from coordinating the arrests? Paperwork, meetings; paperwork, meetings, more paperwork and more meetings – there's still a lot to do."

"Any chance of having Christmas lunch with me? I'd be delighted to drive over to Seville."

"Thank you for the offer and I'd love to but I'm on duty. I promise you we'll have plenty of time for dinner once this operation is over."

"Somewhere hot and away from prying eyes I hope," Andy said with a chuckle.

"I'm sure that can be arranged."

"I'll start making plans and there'll be no escape. Good luck and let me know when the funds have been transferred so I can switch on the television."

"I will, but we're going to try and keep the arrests low-profile, so don't expect it to make the national headlines."

When they finished talking, Cristina emailed Peter Roberts and Doug James:

"UPC have approved PGOU. Peter should expect minutes within next 24 hours. Official announcement to be made by close of business on Friday. Peter, as discussed, please delay transfer of funds until Friday pm."

Thursday, 20th December

Chief Inspector Diaz was getting increasingly frustrated; the forensics lab in Madrid had still not come up with the results of the DNA tests. However, at twenty-five past eleven he received the call he was expecting.

"We've finally managed to extract a good enough sample to run a check against the samples you gave us, as well as the national DNA database, but we can't find any matches."

This was a blow; Diaz knew that he still had to try and establish who the hairs belonged to before closing the case. He thought for a moment.

"If we get you some other samples how long will it take you to run another check?"

"Assuming the samples are of good quality, less than twenty-four hours, the hardest part was extracting a decent DNA sample from the hairs."

"Is that realistic?"

"I can promise you that if the samples are here before six o'clock tomorrow evening you'll have the results by close of business on Monday. I can't give you any guarantees for the rest of the week as we have skeleton staffing, but I'll get it done as quickly as possible."

"Thanks, I appreciate it," Chief Inspector Diaz said, putting the receiver down. Now he regretted that he had honoured Ramon's long-standing request to take the day off to do some Christmas shopping, so he called him on his mobile.

"Ramon, Madrid called. There is no match to the DNA from the hairs so as a last shot I want you to get samples from Paco and Alvaro, and for good measure Miguel as well, and make sure they get to Madrid by six o'clock tomorrow evening."

"But boss, I'm on my way to Malaga and won't be back until late this afternoon."

"I know but call one of your team and get it organised." Ramon called Don Javier straight away on his prepaid mobile to tell him the news.

"Don't do anything and turn your official mobile off. I'll call you back on this mobile in the next half hour." Thirty-five minutes later Ramon took another call from Don Javier.

"Listen carefully. I need you to delay collecting these new samples until tomorrow morning, and none of the three must know in advance that you're going to be asking them for samples. The first thing to do is to keep your mobile switched off and tell Chief Inspector Diaz that the battery ran out before you could contact any of your team. After that make up what you like but you must delay this."

"But this could seriously damage my career."

"Don't worry; I'll make it worth your while. Just do it."

Andy was delighted to hear Cristina's voice. Although he had only spoken with her yesterday, he hadn't realised how much he missed her.

"This is an unexpected but welcome surprise; I assume this isn't a social call?"

"I wish it were, but I'm afraid not. We've been unable to match the DNA hair samples found on Mike's fleece to Carlos so, as a last resort, Chief Inspector Diaz has decided to get samples from Paco, Alvaro and Miguel."

"That's very disappointing. So the case is still open?"

"Yes, but remember Paco and Alvaro are singing from the same hymn sheet as to their whereabouts that evening and I don't think Miguel has even been questioned, so it's conceivable that one, or all three of them, was involved in Mike's death."

"True, but why would any of them do Carlos' dirty work?"

"Who knows; money is a big motivator."

"Let's hope Chief Inspector Diaz can make a connection, I really want to see Mike's killer caught. How are your arrest plans going?"

"Slowly but surely. We have the warrants and all the surveillance teams and remaining phone taps should be in place sometime tomorrow. Hopefully by Saturday or Sunday we should be in a position to make an informed decision as to when to act. What are your plans for the weekend?"

"Why? Are you free?"

"Andy, you already know the answer to that!"

"It was worth asking. Actually I'm having dinner with friends on Friday night and a party up on Cerro Grande on Sunday lunchtime. Other than that just lazing around and maybe some cycling, but rest assured I'll be thinking of you."

"That's nice; I wish I could join you."

"Well at least I have something to look forward to after Christmas. That will keep me going."

"Me too. Have fun, be good and we'll make plans when this is all over."

Johan Gaards arrived at Javier Urquiza's house just before two o'clock. Something must be up, he thought. It was unusual to be summoned at such short notice and for the meeting to be held at the house. As instructed, he had ridden over on a scooter borrowed from the pizza delivery service owned by Don Javier, and wore a full-face crash helmet which he did not remove until he was safely inside the house.

Javier Urquiza led him to his office, where they joined Vicente Maldonado on the sofa at the far end of the room. Vicente looked tired. Johan knew that he had been in Seville yesterday and that he had had dinner with Fernando before returning to Granada. He must have driven down from Granada this morning so it was definitely something important.

Javier Urquiza turned to Johan. "Johan, as you know, yesterday the final hurdle in Project Pulpo was passed and we expect to receive the money in the next few days. Unfortunately, it has come to my attention that the police will be asking Paco, Alvaro and Miguel for DNA samples tomorrow, to see if any of them match those of the hairs found on Mike Cameron's jumper."

Javier Urquiza stopped, allowing what he had told Johan to sink in. Johan stared at him with narrowed eyes. "I was afraid of this. If they match the hairs to Miguel's DNA there's a good chance he'll implicate me in both Mike Cameron's and Carlos' deaths."

"Exactly; and none of us want that."

"So what do we do?" asked Johan, looking at the two of them.

"Dead men can't talk, so Miguel needs to be neutralised before they take a DNA sample from him," replied Vicente.

"And I suppose you want me to deal with him?"

"Given that time is of the essence, I can't see any alternative, can you?" Javier Urquiza said.

Vicente and Javier Urquiza looked anxiously at Johan. Eventually he said: "Not really, but then I'm running an even greater risk by getting directly involved, so I think a bonus would be appropriate."

"Yes, Vicente and I have already discussed that and here's the deal – provided that Miguel has been disposed of and you go to Belize straight away, we'll pay you one million euros as soon as we receive the funds from the investors."

Silence filled the room while Johan thought. If he got it right he could make at least two and a half million euros, one million for Miguel and the one and a half million for Enrique, which Don Javier was not aware of.

"Ok, I think I can deal with Miguel, but I want five hundred thousand euros paid into my offshore account now, and the balance once you received the money from the investors and I confirm I'm in Belize."

Don Javier glanced at Vicente, who nodded imperceptibly.

"I think we can go ahead on that basis, but you need to sort Miguel out ASAP and then make yourself scarce."

"As soon as you transfer the money I'll be on my way to deal with Miguel. I was planning on leaving the country next week anyway so I'll just bring it forward."

Javier Urquiza stood up and moved across the room to his desk, on which a laptop stood open. "Give me a couple of minutes to log on and make the transfer and then I'll print out a confirmation."

A few minutes later Johan left the house wearing the full-face crash helmet and made his way down from the Punta to the Old Town.

"Do you think he'll do it?" Javier Urquiza asked Vicente.

"Yes. He's a greedy, cold-hearted son of a bitch and he'll be set up nicely for retirement with all the money you've paid him over the last few years, plus this extra million."

"True, and he won't want Miguel implicating him in either Mike Cameron's or Carlos' deaths. The problem is that he knows too much and if the police latch on to him he could cause us big problems. Maybe we should get rid of him once he has dealt with Miguel; after all we don't need him after that."

"I don't think we can risk yet another body turning up or even disappearing in Los Cipreses at the moment," replied Vicente, knowing full well that he needed Johan alive, at least until Enrique had been taken care of. "If necessary, we can deal with him in Belize," he continued."

Vicente used Javier Urquiza's laptop to check his emails and saw that, as promised, Fernando had emailed a scanned copy of the signed minutes as they had not been ready the previous evening when they had met for dinner.

"Signed minutes attached and official announcement will be made by the Junta tomorrow morning."

He printed two copies out and gave one set to Javier Urquiza. Although, there were some amendments to the PGOU, the Project Pulpo land reclassification had been approved as originally presented.

"These look fine. I'll email a copy to Peter Roberts and ask him to confirm when the funds will be transferred." Vicente said to Javier Urquiza once they had both finished reading the minutes.

By the time Vicente arrived back in Granada he had received an email from Peter Roberts *"Thanks for signed minutes, but have been instructed by my clients to wait until official announcement is made tomorrow before transferring funds."*

Vicente cursed and rang Fernando.

"The press conference is at eleven tomorrow and a press release will be posted on the official website immediately afterwards."

Vicente emailed Peter Roberts with the url of the website and asking him to check it first thing in the morning. He then rang Javier Urquiza.

"There's not much we can do; Cayman is six hours behind so it might not be until lunch time tomorrow before we get confirmation that the funds have been transferred."

Johan knew that Miguel would probably either be at home or in El Boqueron. He hoped he was at home, which was his first port of call.

He was in luck. Miguel opened the door; he was unshaven and wearing a scruffy T-shirt and a pair of briefs. "Hombre, I've just got up. Come in. I'll get dressed then we can go and grab some lunch."

"Actually, I've got a better idea. I'm bored with all this Christmas business; how do you fancy doing some boar hunting tonight?"

It was a long shot, but Johan had been hunting with Miguel on several occasions, so the request was not unusual.

"Well, I'm not working again until Saturday night and the hunting is meant to be particularly good this year." Miguel said pensively. "Ok; what the hell, why not? If we can bag a boar it'll make a great Christmas meal."

"Good. Why don't I pick you up in half an hour. You pack some cans of fabada and I'll bring some bread, cheese and Serrano ham. Let's take your tent and hide and I'll bring my binoculars and my new third-generation night vision scope – I've been dying to try it out."

Half an hour later Johan returned in his 4 X 4 and helped Miguel load his 30-calibre Winchester rifle and rucksack, along with the tent and hide, into the back of the jeep, where his own gun and backpack were already stored.

"I see you've bought the Leupold."

"Yes. It's much better for close distance shots and I've adapted it for my new night vision scope."

The Sierra de Tejeda y Almijara was less than an hour's drive from Los Cipreses and there was little traffic, so they found themselves at the main entrance to the hunting ground just before four o'clock. On the drive up Johan had persuaded Miguel to try a spot off the Camino del Pino.

"It's a bit off the beaten track, but it's close to a trail the boars are known to use."

Both were experienced hunters and knew that at night in a wooded area they would usually hear the boar before they saw them. Johan's night vision scope could then be used, instead of the traditional torch, to turn the target area into virtual daylight without fear of scaring the boar.

As they bumped their way slowly along one of the dirt roads down into the valley below, the road became narrower and the pine trees thicker and thicker. Johan was keeping a careful eye out for parked vehicles in the small clearings which occasionally appeared on either side of the road, but he saw none. After about five kilometres the road widened slightly and Johan turned down an even narrower dirt track leading through the pine trees on the right.

"It's about a kilometre down here. We can just about make it in the jeep," he said to Miguel.

"Sounds good to me. We need to be setting up the hide and tent before it gets too dark."

Johan drove carefully, but could not stop the overhanging branches occasionally scraping and banging against the roof and doors of the 4 X 4. In a few minutes they reached a small clearing and Johan stopped. They got out and Miguel followed Johan to a spot just in front of the vehicle.

"See how the trees thin slightly and the slope is gentle for the first thirty yards, but then falls away sharply? The boar forage for food on this flatter stretch, which also serves as a trail through the valley. If we set the hide up here facing this trail we should catch some coming along here later tonight."

Miguel nodded. "Yes, I can see why this is a good spot. Secluded with good cover – perfect terrain for foraging. I'm surprised there's no one else here."

"Fortunately it's a Thursday, and I think it's only known by a small number of people. No one else is likely to turn up at this hour, so hopefully we'll be undisturbed. Anyway, the light's fading fast so let's get a move on."

First, they set the hide up a few metres to the front and left of the jeep, facing the trail and the valley below. Then, under the glaring headlights of the jeep, they erected the tent, a few metres behind the hide.

As darkness descended, silence engulfed the Sierra de Tejeda y Almijara and a pale, luminous, almost full moon was already high in the night sky. The temperature was dropping quickly, so they lit the portable gas unit which provided both heat and light, while they checked and loaded their guns inside the tent. Once Johan had mounted his new night vision scope on the Leupold, he handed it to Miguel.

"Have a look through that – it's awesome. No need for you to hold a torch while I take aim."

Miguel took the shotgun and took imaginary aim at a spot in the woods. "Wow. I hope you're going to let me use this tonight, otherwise you'll have an unfair advantage."

"Of course, we'll take turns, but let me have the first shot. Let's just hope the boar are active. Come on, turn off the lamp – let's go hunt."

The hide was a green plastic sheet which had a clear plastic window, approximately half a metre high, running along the longest side of the rectangle at head height. Johan and Miguel unzipped the window and folded it upwards, using hooks to keep it from flopping back down, and then sat next to each other.

Although it was a clear night, the pine trees prevented most of the moonlight reaching the forest floor, and they could see little beyond ten metres other than shadowy blackness. Johan and Miguel watched and listened in silence for the sound of boar. The animals usually moved fast along trails unless they stopped to forage for food, and Johan hoped the acorns they had scattered on the trail in front of the hide would attract them. If boar turned up it would make his job easier, otherwise a bit of improvisation would be required. In any event, he had Miguel alone now and nobody knew where they were.

After an hour they had heard and seen nothing but, suddenly, there was a rustle in the undergrowth ahead of them followed by some crunching. Johan raised the Leupold and aimed it in the direction of the noise. He looked through the scope and could immediately see a boar sow surrounded by a number of piglets about twenty metres ahead. He gave Miguel the thumbs up and took aim. The Leupold was very effective at distances of up to fifty metres, but he only wanted to cripple the sow so he aimed for her rear leg. There was a loud retort and almost instantly the sow fell and began to squeal.

"Shit! It's a good size sow but I missed her neck; now she's injured and on the ground half under a bush, and I can't get a clean shot from here. Why don't you go down and finish her off with the Winchester, it'll be cleaner and neater than the Leupold. You've got a torch, haven't you?"

"Yes, but do you think it's safe to go out there. There may be a male about and he could be angry."

"I didn't see one and chances are he's miles away by now. Anyway, I'll cover you using the night scope."

Miguel left the hide holding his torch in his left hand and rifle in his right. He turned round the front of the hide and began to walk tentatively down the slope, shining his torch on the ground in front of him. It had a powerful beam and he soon spotted the sow. As he moved towards her, Johan was lining up his shot. His pulse was racing and adrenaline flooded through his body, but his hand remained steady. He pulled the trigger and Miguel was suddenly propelled forward for a few feet before falling on his face, close to the injured sow. Johan waited. Miguel did not move but the sow continued to squeal.

He left the hide and located Miguel's rifle and torch using the night vision scope. Then he shot the sow with the rifle and turned back to survey Miguel's body. He could leave it where it was and claim it had been an accident, but then he would have to report it to the police as soon as possible. The alternative was to roll the body onto the steeper slope beyond the trail where it was unlikely to be found, by humans at least.

He decided on the latter, as he didn't want the police investigating yet another death. If the body was found there would be nothing to link him directly to Miguel's death once he got rid of the Leupold. In any event, he would be out of the country in a few days and setting up his yacht-chartering business in the Caribbean under a new identity.

Once he had rolled Miguel's body into the valley, he did the same with the sow, as he didn't want other hunters finding her and investigating why such a prize had been left. She weighed more than Miguel and by the time he had finished he was sweating profusely despite the cold. He brushed the area with a pine branch to cover signs of tonight's activity and returned to dismantle the hide and change into the clean clothes he had brought with him.

By midnight he was on his way back to Los Cipreses. He disposed of the gun and his hunting jacket in one of the many agricultural water tanks which littered the countryside on the way down to the coast. Once in Los Cipreses, he decided to stop in at La Cabaña. Given the time of year, it would be crowded, and people would find it difficult to say at what time Johan had arrived or left if asked.

Friday, 21st December

"Boss, I'm really sorry, but it was an unfortunate set of circumstances. The battery on my mobile ran out while I was trying to reach Jorge, and Marisol had left hers at home. By the time I got to a phone in Malaga, Jorge had gone off duty. He's the only other person with the key to the DNA swab kit locker, so I agreed with him that we'd do it this morning."

Chief Inspector Diaz was angry. "Surely you knew Jorge was going off duty at two, couldn't you get to a phone earlier? Anyway you should have ordered him to collect the samples."

"The traffic was terrible, both on the ring road and in town itself, and finding parking took forever. We also need at least three of us to collect the samples just in case they are in different places."

"Ok, Ok, but get on with it. I want those samples in Madrid by six o'clock this afternoon."

Johan woke late. The adrenaline rush was long past, but he was pleased with himself; he thought he'd done a good job on Miguel. He made himself a cup of coffee and turned on his prepaid mobile; he had an SMS.

"Call me ASAP to discuss your travel plans. VM."

It was timed at three o'clock the previous day, soon after he had picked up Miguel. He rang Vicente.

"Job done. By the time they find his body, if they ever do, I'll be long gone."

"Good. Now listen, although Don Javier wants you to leave the country as soon as possible, you and I know you can't do that until Monday afternoon at the earliest."

"So what are we going to tell him?"

"That you're leaving for Belize later today. Basically it means you're going to have to keep a very low profile and remain incommunicado, i.e., mobiles and Skype off and no answering emails."

"I can stay at home today and tomorrow but on Sunday I have to be at Mrs. Nicklass' party and there are going to be a lot of people there, some of whom may know Don Javier."

"Apart from Enrique, its unlikely there will be anybody else who knows him personally and, anyway, why would they tell him you were there?"

"True, and Enrique shouldn't be a problem after Sunday. Once you reallocate the shares to me I'll drive straight to Portugal and catch the first flight to Brazil. I'll go to Belize from there."

"Perfect. Well done with Miguel; I look forward to hearing from you on Sunday afternoon."

Ramon's team of three arrived in Los Cipreses at five past eleven. When they were in place, and on Ramon's command, they rang the buzzers of Paco's, Miguel's and Alvaro's apartments simultaneously. Both Paco and Alvaro answered and let them in, but there was no response from Miguel's apartment, which Ramon had taken himself. Neither did he answer the mobile number that Ramon had for him.

Paco and Alvaro didn't object to giving saliva and hair samples, but they didn't know where Miguel was.

"Last time I saw him was on Wednesday night. We worked together at El Boqueron until about one and then had a few beers," Alvaro told Jorge. "He said he was going to have a lazy day and maybe go fishing in the evening."

Paco confirmed Alvaro's story to Ramon, who had by now arrived at Paco's apartment.

"Do you have any idea where we might find him?"

"No. He usually fishes on the rocks off Punta de Palermo until about two and then goes home. If he got up early he might be having breakfast at El Burro or Bar Marisol."

Ramon radioed Jorge and told him to go to El Burro while he went to Bar Marisol. They found no trace of Miguel and nobody had seen him that morning. After visiting a few more bars which he was known to frequent, again with no luck, they returned to the station in El Castillo to report to Chief Inspector Diaz.

"Get the samples you have to Madrid and continue looking for Miguel. See if anybody saw him fishing last night, there's usually a few people out there most nights. I'll ask Judge Bustamente for a warrant to search his apartment."

In Cayman Peter Roberts answered his mobile. It was Vicente calling to see if he had seen the press release and ordered the transfer of funds.

"Sorry old chap, you just got me out of bed – remember we are six hours behind you. Let me get showered and then I'll have a look."

"But by then it may be too late to order the transfer of funds."

"Don't worry, we still have a couple of hours and the bank is expecting my instructions. I'll get back to you shortly."

"Please call me as soon as you've seen the press release – as you can imagine, my clients would like to know when the funds are arriving," Vicente said before hanging up.

Vicente waited anxiously for Peter Roberts to call him back. If the order to transfer the funds wasn't given today it was unlikely that cleared funds would arrive in Cayman on Christmas Eve. Half an hour later his mobile rang.

"It looks like we have a deal, Vicente. I'll tell the bank to transfer the funds and Carrington Investments should receive them on Monday, although it's a half day in London and Cayman."

"That's good news; thank you Peter. My clients will be pleased to get that particular Christmas present."

"I'm sure they will, and I hope they invest it wisely. No doubt we'll be speaking again; I think my clients may require your services and connections when they come to develop the site."

"That would be my pleasure. In the meantime could you email me a copy of the transfer request?"

"It will be with you in a few minutes."

Vicente was ecstatic. After years of greasing palms, wheeling and dealing, and helping other people get rich, through legal and not-so legal means, he was going to be a very rich man in his own right.

He called Javier Urquiza as soon as he received the transfer request. "Javier, we're almost there; the money should arrive in Cayman on Monday and then I'll transfer the relevant amounts to each of the shareholder's nominated accounts, and Project Pulpo will be over."

"Great work Vicente, it was a close run thing but we got there in the end. We'll have a big celebration in St. Lucia on New Year's Eve. By the way, have you spoken with Johan? We don't want any nasty surprises."

Yes. I spoke with him this morning. Miguel has been dealt with discreetly and he should already be on his way to Portugal. From there he'll go to Brazil and then on to Belize."

"Excellent. One thing less to worry about. I'll call Fernando and Enrique with the good news."

"I'm sure they'll be delighted and looking forward to their early retirement."

"Aren't we all? Well, have a good weekend and by Monday afternoon we should all be much richer."

"No luck boss. We've been to all of his known haunts as well as trying his mobile all day. He seems to have disappeared off the face of the earth."

"Let's hope not. Maybe he is visiting friends or family elsewhere, although it is strange that he is not answering his mobile."

"So what's next?"

"I'm expecting the search warrant any minute now so get a team of three, including someone from forensics, ready and waiting to search his apartment. I'll call you as soon as it arrives and in the meantime have a couple of the lads continue to try and track him down."

Ramon nodded and left Chief Inspector Diaz's office. Chief Inspector Diaz looked pensive. Miguel's disappearance at this precise time was suspicious, but he didn't want to jump to any conclusions just yet. They would be able to get DNA samples from his apartment and hopefully he could put pressure on Madrid to produce the results by Monday afternoon in the event Paco's and Alvaro's samples failed to produce a match. In the meantime, maybe Miguel would turn up.

As soon as the search warrant arrived he went with Ramon and the search team to Miguel's apartment.

There was no sign of Miguel and his apartment was a mess, with clothes strewn all over the bedroom floor and a pile of dirty dishes in the kitchen sink. The place looked as if it had not been cleaned in weeks. The forensics operative took hair samples from the bathroom and various items of clothing, while the rest of the team searched the apartment. Chief Inspector Diaz wandered around surveying each room carefully.

Forty minutes later Ramon informed the Chief Inspector that they had found nothing suspicious.

"But don't you think it looks as if he left in a bit of a hurry?"

"Could be, but I bet he lived like this most of the time."

"Ok. I want you to get Paco and Alvaro here so they can tell us if this is the apartment's normal state, and make sure that those hair samples are in Madrid first thing Monday morning."

"Yes boss," Ramon said to Chief Inspector Diaz's back as he disappeared out of the front door.

Saturday, 22nd December

As she drove to her office Cristina decided not to tell Andy about Miguel's disappearance. After all, Chief Inspector Diaz had obtained DNA samples and they would have the results by Monday afternoon. Her immediate priority was to try and find an opportune moment to arrest all five Project Pulpo suspects.

Doug James' cooperation in delaying the arrival of the funds meant that she had until the twenty-seventh to make the arrests. However, they needed to be done simultaneously, and this would require careful planning and coordination.

"So are all the teams in place?" she asked her deputy, looking over his shoulder at the computer screen on his desk.

"Four are and we're just waiting for Team Alpha to set up around Javier Urquiza's villa. It's a bit tricky because it's quite isolated and people hanging around stick out like a sore thumb, so we're putting the team in as an emergency electricity repair unit at the end of the street. The back-up team will be in an unmarked van a few hundred yards away."

"When will they be in place?"

"Two hours at most."

"What about the other four suspects, do we know where they are?"

"No confirmed sighting of Mr. Gaards yet, but his jeep is parked outside his apartment so we're assuming he's there. Team Beta saw Vicente Maldonado drive into his underground garage last night with female company and haven't seen him since."

"And the other two?"

"Both Fernando Echevaria and Enrique Gonzalez are at home."

"Has there been any phone traffic?"

"Some, but not between the suspects themselves; just family and friends with the usual stuff."

"Anything which tells us their movements today?"

"It seems all three wives are planning to go Christmas shopping, which is no great surprise. It'll be interesting to see if they manage to drag their husbands along."

"Ok let me know when Team Alpha is in place, or if any of the suspects move. What we need first is confirmed sightings of all five of them and then we'll be able to track their movements," she said, heading for her office.

Paco and Alvaro looked round the apartment. "It's just as it always is," said Paco. "Ever since his mother died there's no one to tidy and clean up after him. He usually gets a woman from the village to come and clean the place once every couple of months."

"Have a good look around again and tell me if there's anything missing," Chief Inspector Diaz said to them.

Five minutes later they told him that the only things they couldn't see were Miguel's hunting clothes and equipment.

"That and the fishing equipment are the only things he was meticulous about keeping in order. The fishing equipment is all there in the spare bedroom but his rifle, tent, hide, hunting boots and jacket are missing."

"And do you know where he usually hunts?"

"Yes, up in the Sierra de Tejeda y Almijara off the old road to Granada."

Vicente Maldonado's prepaid mobile rang. He was barely awake, and Claudia was lying naked beside him fast asleep. He felt a stirring in his groin as he admired her almost perfect body. After the night they had had he was surprised he could still think about having sex, but then she was the most passionate lover he had ever had, and it was worth every euro he was paying her. Nevertheless, he got out of bed to answer the phone.

It was Javier Urquiza. "The police are going to search the Sierra de Tejeda hunting ground for Miguel. Is he there?"

"Yes, but Johan assured me he is well hidden in a secluded spot."

"Actually, it makes no difference if they find his body or not, they've already got DNA samples. What's important is that they don't find Johan if they manage to link him to Miguel's death. Are you sure he's left the country?"

"I haven't spoken with him since yesterday morning but I assume he has. I'll see if I can get him on his mobile and call you back."

Vicente knew that Johan was at home but that telling him this latest news might cause him to leave the country immediately, despite the lure of one and a half million euros. He moved to the kitchen, ground some coffee, placed the filter holder in the Gaggia and made himself a cappuccino before calling Javier Urquiza back.

"Don Javier, I can't raise Johan on his mobile or Skype so he must be on his way to Belize. I'll send him an email asking him to confirm his whereabouts. Anyway, the police still have to find Miguel's body and then link Johan to his death and that could take days."

"Let's hope so, and that he gets to Belize before they make any connection. As soon as you hear from him let me know."

"Will do."

He returned to the bedroom and saw that Claudia was stretching out her arms, her blue eyes slowly flickering open, just like an exotic cat.

"Hi lover boy. Up already I see!"

"I'm afraid so. A little unfinished business; but that's dealt with now, so we can relax over breakfast and then I'll take you shopping for your Christmas present."

"Hmm, sounds good, but how about a little present now?" she said, reaching out and putting her hands inside his dressing gown.

Chief Inspector Diaz instructed the two marked cars to stop at the entrance of the car park to the hunting ground.

He and Ramon drove in his unmarked vehicle to El Javeli Loco, which was a couple of kilometres further up the road. It was the only bar-restaurant in the vicinity and was the main meeting spot for hunters. There were few vehicles outside and Chief Inspector Diaz parked right next to the steps leading up to the entrance. They climbed the steps and entered the building.

Directly in front of the entrance was a long oval-shaped bar. The room containing the bar was large and dark but warm, thanks to a blazing log fire in the corner. In the far left wall were a set of double doors which Chief Inspector Diaz knew led to a large dining room.

The bar area was virtually empty. As was customary, most of the regulars would arrive in the next hour or two to have something to eat and drink before setting off for an evening's hunting. This would give Chief Inspector Diaz the opportunity to question the regulars about Miguel, but first he approached the barman, a thin, dour looking individual with dyed black hair and a matching moustache.

"Good afternoon. Can we have two beers please and I wonder if you can help us with something."

"Depends what," he answered in a surly manner, as he placed a tall glass under the beer tap.

"We're from the Policia Nacional in El Castillo and we are trying to locate a certain Miguel Martin who we think may be hunting up here," said Chief Inspector Diaz, placing a recent photo of Miguel on the counter.

The barman looked at the photo. "Why are you looking for him?"

"One of his family members has had a serious accident and Sr. Martin is not answering his mobile. His friends told us that they think he came up here on Thursday evening to hunt."

"Have you got any ID?"

Chief Inspector Diaz showed him his Policia Nacional identity card.

"Yes, I know him. He's an occasional hunter, but I haven't seen him for at least a month."

"Do you know what his favourite locations are?"

"No. You'd be better off asking Andres, they usually discuss the best spots over a beer or two before they set off."

"Is he here?"

"No, but he should be here soon."

"Good. We'll wait for him if you don't mind, and maybe you could give us some wild boar stew in the meantime."

"Why should I mind," he said, shrugging his shoulders.

As the bar slowly filled up, Chief Inspector Diaz and Ramon made discreet enquiries to see if anyone had seen Miguel since Thursday but with no joy. Andres eventually appeared and over a large brandy pointed out Miguel's favourite spots on the map.

"He tends to go for locations which are less densely wooded, because it is easier to see the boar at night and his Winchester is more effective over longer distances."

Chief Inspector Diaz thanked him, and he and Ramon left the bar with several official maps of the hunting area marked with the locations where Andres thought Miguel might be.

They drove up to the marked cars and discussed a search strategy with the rest of the team. The light would soon begin to fade, so they focused on those locations which were relatively close to the entrance. At dusk Chief Inspector Diaz called the search off.

"Let's meet here tomorrow at nine o'clock and we'll fan out further a field. Ramon, arrange for more support to be here, I want to finish the search tomorrow."

The surveillance teams confirmed that both Enrique and Fernando had accompanied their wives shopping, Fernando in Seville and Enrique in Granada. Vicente Maldonado had also been seen leaving his apartment with a rather attractive lady who looked young enough to be his daughter. However, there had still not been confirmed sightings of Johan Gaards or Javier Urquiza.

"Urquiza and Gaards must be at home," Cristina said to Iñigo. "Where else could they be?"

As she finished, the Team Alpha leader came on the line. "Visual contact established with Javier Urquiza. Look's like he's going to wash his car."

"Ok, but let me know if it looks like he's planning on leaving the house."

The rest of the day passed without incident, with Enrique, Fernando and Vicente all returning to their respective homes in the early evening. From the phone taps Cristina knew that Javier Urquiza, Enrique and Fernando were dining out with friends. Vicente and his young lady did not make another appearance, so she assumed they were having a night in.

What was concerning her was the lack of sighting of Johan Gaards. All the shutters were down and there was no hint of light or movement inside. Maybe he'd left the country, despite the fact that his 4 X 4 was parked outside his apartment.

"I was hoping to be able to make our move at dawn tomorrow, but if he doesn't make an appearance tonight I'll postpone the arrests until we've established his whereabouts," she said to her boss when she updated him on the day's events.

Sunday, 23rd December

Mrs. Nicklass' Christmas party was a "must be seen at" event and most long-established members of the expat community could expect an invitation. Nevertheless, every year there were a few surprise inclusions and exclusions, and during weeks leading up to it the guest list was subject to discussion in many homes, bars and restaurants.

Andy's parents had been regular guests, but he had rarely seen Mrs. Nicklass since they had passed away, so he'd been surprised to receive an invitation. He tended to avoid parties where retired expats were liable to harp on about the good old days but, in order to maintain contact with his parents' friends, many of whom had known him since he was young, he had decided to accept.

The invitation had specified from one o'clock so he planned to arrive just after one, stay just long enough to do his duty and leave before the real drinking and moaning began.

The house was one of the most emblematic in Los Cipreses, situated on the very crown of Cerro Grande with commanding views both east across the bay, as far as El Castillo, and west beyond Salar, ten kilometres along the coast.

Despite its isolated location there was a constant stream of visitors as Joanna Nicklass spun her web of gossip and rumours amongst the retired expat community. She was the queen bee and not someone to be crossed lightly. Her husband had long given up trying to rein her in, and spent most of the time playing golf or in the UK looking after his remaining business interests.

The road to the top of Cerro Grande was very steep and windy and in poor condition, so Andy drove slowly. At the very top he took the right-hand fork and drove past several large villas until reaching Casa Milagros at the end of the increasingly rough road. He turned his car round, parked it on the side of the road and then walked up the steep driveway to the house. This way I won't be blocked in and can leave quietly, he thought to himself. He failed to notice the silver Peugot 407 parked discreetly in a slip road just before Casa Milagros.

There were two cars and a 4 X 4 in the parking area at the top of the drive. He didn't recognise the cars but the jeep looked familiar. Joanna Nicklass greeted him effusively.

"Andy, such a long time no see and I'm so pleased you could make it. I'm sure you're very much in demand, being the most attractive single man in Los Cipreses."

"It's great to see you too Joanna and thank you for the compliment – if only it were true!"

"Oh don't be so modest. I can tell you that many of the ladies are looking forward to seeing you. Only Richard and Diana are here at the moment, but the bar is set up so go out to the pool area, get yourself a drink, and then go and say hello to them while I go and check on the caterers."

As Andy walked the length of the large kidney-shaped pool towards the bar he saw that the barman was Johan Gaards, which explained the familiar 4 X 4.

"Hello Johan, I'm surprised to see you working here."

"Hi Andy. Mrs. Nicklass is an old friend, if you know what I mean," he said with a wink, "so I'm happy to do her a favour occasionally. What can I get you?"

"I'll have a non-alcoholic beer."

"Are you sure? That's a bit tame."

"Yes thanks. They're clamping down heavily on drinking and driving this year and I'd rather not risk it."

"Fair enough; how are things with you? Are you going to take over Mike Cameron's business?"

"I don't know yet. I'm going to wait until they close the case and then decide."

"But I thought they had Carlos Maracena down for it?"

"That's what all the evidence points to, but apparently his

untimely death is delaying tying up the loose ends."

"What a way to go though – drugs and women!" exclaimed Johan, handing Andy his beer.

Andy said nothing and wandered off towards an older couple who were chatting at the far end of the pool.

Chief Inspector Diaz decided to focus the search for Miguel on the more remote locations and to actively enlist the support of the park rangers and hunters who were present in the area. At three o'clock he got an excited call on his police radio.

"Chief Inspector, we've found a body."

"Does it look like our man?"

"Yes"

"Where is it?"

"About three-quarters of the way down the valley, off the Camino del Pino."

"Who are you with?"

"One of the hunters."

"Stay where you are, don't touch anything and I'll be there as soon as I can."

He called Ramon on the police radio. "They've found a body. I'm on my way with Manuel from forensics and Juan Luis, but find another forensics operative and two more men and get down here with some spotlights."

Chief Inspector Diaz climbed down the slope. He stepped over the dead sow and stood over the body. It was definitely Miguel.

"As you can see he's off the track, and the dogs found the sow first," said the policeman who'd radioed him.

"You haven't touched anything?"

"No, but I had to turn the body over to identify him."

Chief Inspector Diaz looked down at Miguel. He turned to Juan Luis and Manuel, "Over to you. As soon as you've secured the scene check to see if he was shot from behind."

At Casa Milagros, the party was in full swing and Andy estimated that there must be nearly one hundred people there. As he was talking with one of his father's old golfing partners, Joanna Nicklass came up to them. "Andy darling, I'm sorry to interrupt but could you help with a little communication problem," she said taking his arm and leading him towards the viewing point at the far end of the terrace.

The viewing point was a semi-circular stone wall of waist height which jutted out beyond the terrace and provided spectacular views to both the east and the west. Andy could see that there were two men standing in the viewing point and as he got closer he recognised the Mayor of Los Cipreses and the large bulky one as Enrique Gonzalez, who Maria had pointed out at El Asador. They were talking animatedly but stopped as Joanna Nicklass and Andy approached them.

"Andy, let me introduce Mayor Benavente and his colleague, Enrique Gonzalez, the Urban Planning Officer for Los Cipreses." Andy shook their hands as Joanna continued, "I'm afraid my Spanish is not up to scratch so I wanted you to help me explain to Sr. Benavente and Sr. Gonzalez that I'd like to build another house on part of our land. The problem is that the current zoning does not permit the size of house I want to build, so I was wondering what I need to do to get the approval of the Town Hall."

Andy hated being put in such situations, which was made worse by the fact that he knew of Enrique Gonzalez's involvement in Project Pulpo, but he could not openly refuse to help Joanna and was comforted by the fact that Sr. Gonzalez would soon be under arrest.

"Gentlemen, Mrs. Nicklass has a dilemma which she is hoping you can help her resolve."

"Mrs. Nicklass is a valued and long-standing member of our community so I'll do whatever is in my power to help her. What precisely is her dilemma?" asked Mayor Benavente.

As Andy explained the "dilemma" Enrique Gonzalez took a sip from the glass in his hand. Suddenly the glass fell from his hand and he fell to the floor coughing and clutching his throat, spasms racking his body. Andy knelt beside him and tried to unbutton his collar.

"Call 112," he said to Joanna Nicklass who rushed off towards the house. "Do you know if he has heart problems or any other serious medical conditions?" Andy asked the Mayor, who was rooted to the ground looking on wide-eyed and speechless.

"I've no idea; he's never mentioned anything."

"What's going on here?" Johan Gaards asked, rushing over to Enrique.

"Looks like he's having a heart attack or some sort of seizure," replied Andy "and Mrs. Nicklass has gone to call 112."

Enrique's coughing had become more violent and his breathing shallower.

"Give me some space, I'm trained in resuscitation. Why don't you see if there's a first aid kit in the house," he said to Andy as he leant over Enrique, placing himself between Enrique and Mayor Benavente. As Andy ran to find Joanna Nicklass, Johan removed a pen-like object from his shirt pocket and held it close to Enrique's face, squeezing it on Enrique's next inhalation.

Andy returned quickly with Joanna Nicklass and a first aid box. A crowd had begun to gather round the prostrate Enrique, while Johan Gaards attempted a heart massage to resuscitate him. However, Enrique's breathing was becoming more laboured and his skin turning blue, and it looked as if he was slipping into a coma or might even die. Johan took an adrenaline injection from the first-aid kit and injected a small dose.

"Just in case it's an allergic reaction to a bee sting or something he's eaten," he said to no one in particular. It had no discernible effect and by the time the ambulance arrived Enrique was in a coma. The paramedics connected him to an oxygen supply and put him carefully on a stretcher and then left, followed by the Mayor, for the accident and emergency unit at El Castillo's hospital.

Once the ambulance left Andy called Cristina, "It doesn't look good. I'll be surprised if he survives, whatever it is," he told her.

"Do you suspect foul play?"

"No reason to. It looks like a seizure or allergic reaction of some sort."

"Ok. I'll get in touch with the hospital later to see what they say."

Soon after, the guests began to disappear in ever increasing numbers.

"Looks like the party's over," Johan said to Andy, as he began to pack up the bar.

"Yes, and not a great way to finish the weekend or start Christmas week for that matter. Do you think he'll survive?"

"Difficult to say without knowing what it is, but looking at him I'd give him less than a forty percent chance."

"Did you know him?"

"Not personally, no, only by sight and reputation. He was well known around here because of his position," replied Johan.

"Well I hope he does survive. Now that the new PGOU has been approved it would be a shame if he couldn't oversee its implementation."

Johan nodded, but remained silent as he continued to place clean glasses in the cardboard boxes.

Joanna Nicklass joined them but seemed more upset about the fact that the party had ended prematurely and that she hadn't been able to get the Mayor or Enrique to agree to her building project than Enrique's seizure.

"Its getting dark and I must be off," Andy said after a few minutes. "I hope you both have a good Christmas despite what's happened."

"Preliminary conclusions?" Chief Inspector Diaz asked Juan Luis and Manuel under the glare of the spot lights.

"Shot from behind but, given the way the blood has coagulated, the body was moved to where it was found," Juan Luis replied.

"It also looks like some attempt has been made to cover up any signs of activity in the immediate vicinity," said Manuel.

"So we are looking at murder?"

"More than likely, unless it was an accident but the perpetrator panicked."

"I'm sorry, I appreciate it's a Sunday afternoon and Christmas Eve tomorrow but I want you and your team to work non-stop on this and to have an initial report on my desk by tomorrow afternoon."

"Ok, we'll do our best. The autopsy will confirm the cause of death and hopefully give us the bullet, but I'll have to do that tomorrow."

Chief Inspector Diaz nodded. This was an unexpected but significant development and he wondered if Miguel's death was connected in some way to Mike Cameron's murder – but how and why was he killed and by whom?

Cristina and Iñigo watched the little green dot on the screen. "Look's like he's on his way to Granada. Just as well we were able to attach the tracker device to his vehicle," Iñigo said to her.

"But we don't want to lose sight of him in Granada. It'll be busy – the shops are still open, so get another team in place to pick him up as he enters the city – assuming that's where he's going."

Returning to her office she called Andy, "Enrique's condition is worsening and they think he is going to die. Do you think Johan Gaards could have something do with his collapse?"

"I suppose it's possible. He could have slipped something in his drink, but then he did try and resuscitate him."

"And you were with him all the time while he did that?"

Andy thought for a moment. "Actually no, he sent me to get a first-aid kit."

"So had at least two opportunities."

"I suppose so, yes. Do you know where he is now?"

"Yes, we have all the suspects under surveillance."

"So I assume you'll be making the arrests soon?"

"That's a safe assumption, but I can't say any more than that."

"Understood, but this needs to be over soon, before anybody else is killed or any of the suspects escape."

"We're doing our best," Cristina said a little curtly, the tension getting to her.

"I know you are but be careful, I don't want anything to happen to you."

"Don't worry; I'm safely ensconced at control centre in Seville, so no chance of getting a slice of the action. That's the price for being in charge of the operation."

Vicente took Javier Urquiza's call on his Bluetooth headset in the Cayenne as he was returning from a long lunch with Claudia. He'd already received an SMS from Johan: *EG in permanent coma, unlikely to survive 24 hrs.* A news flash on the local radio station had confirmed Johan's message, so Javier Urquiza call was not entirely unexpected.

"I'll call you back in ten as I'm driving and have company," he said while sliding his hand up Claudia's skirt and stroking her soft and velvety upper thigh.

When they got back to his apartment he told Claudia to go to the bedroom and that he'd join her after making his call.

"Surely it can wait half an hour, sweetie," she said to him, standing provocatively at the door to the bedroom pouting and running her fingers upwards through her hair.

"You're a very naughty girl; I'll need more than half an hour with you, so let me get it out of the way now."

He called Javier Urquiza on Skype. "Have you heard about Enrique?" Javier Urquiza asked him.

"Yes, a few minutes ago on the radio on the way back from lunch. Sounds as if he had a heart attack or some sort of seizure. He wasn't exactly the healthiest of individuals and all the stress must have got to him."

"From what they are saying it looks like he's unlikely to survive, so I need you to reallocate his shares in Carrington Investments to me. That way at least I'll recover some of the indemnity deposit I had to give up."

"Javier, I'm afraid that's not possible."

"Why not?"

"There simply isn't enough time. The funds were transferred on Friday and I've already made the share allocations and given the pay way instructions."

"Are you sure? What's going to happen to all that money if Enrique never recovers consciousness or dies?"

"I'll try to recover it from his bank account in Belize but it won't be easy so I'd write that money off to be honest."

"Well, get hold of Jim in Cayman and see what he can do, it's a lot of money."

"Will do, but don't hold your breath."

Vicente then dialled Fernando's mobile but it went straight to voicemail, so he decided to join Claudia before she fell asleep.

As he drove to Granada, Johan congratulated himself. Enrique's poisoning had gone like clockwork. No one had been suspicious and he'd even been able to administer a second dose via inhalation to guarantee that Enrique would die without regaining consciousness.

Tomorrow the last piece of the jigsaw would fall into place, and then he could get the hell out of Spain to enjoy the fruits of his labours.

On arriving in the city, he left his jeep in the Trifuno underground car park and walked to the Hostal Athenas, which was located a few hundred yards away from the Gran Via. All he had with him was five thousand euros in cash, his passport, his Apple Mac laptop, several credit cards and his two mobile phones.

He had chosen the Athenas because it was unobtrusive and because Vicente Maldonado's office was within easy walking distance. As soon as they had completed the reallocation of the shares tomorrow he would drive to Portugal.

As he walked in to the hostal's reception area, the two men following him took up positions on the opposite side of the road, where they could see the entrance, and then radioed Seville confirming his location.

"Fernando, you know better than to call me using your landline."

"I'm sorry Vicente but the batteries ran out on the mobile and the charger's in the office. I've just seen the news about Enrique on Canal Sur so I assume we're on for tomorrow."

"Yes, be at my office by one. Johan will be there also."

"Ok, see you then."

Cristina listened to the conversation five minutes later. All in all there were nearly one hundred operatives and fifteen vehicles covering various sites in Seville, Granada and Los Cipreses waiting for her order. She had planned on arresting all of them at first light, along with simultaneous raids on their respective homes and offices, but if Vicente Maldonado, Fernando Echevaria and Johan Gaards were meeting at Vicente's office tomorrow lunchtime that would make the logistics of the arrests much easier.

Monday, 24th December

Andy missed the morning news on Canal Sur, so he drove down to the paper shop, bought Ideal's Christmas Eve edition, and then went for breakfast at the Isla de Ibiza.

Enrique's seizure and coma was covered by an article on the inside page of the paper which went on to describe his achievements as Los Cipreses' Urban Planning Officer, and especially his role in preparing the recently approved, but controversial, PGOU. It finished: *"Enrique Gonzalez's condition is critical and he is not expected to regain consciousness."*

"Good morning Andy," said a familiar voice. "I see you're reading about Sr. Gonzalez. According to the news this morning his condition has deteriorated overnight."

Andy looked up. "Hi Maria, how are you? Are you going to join me for breakfast?"

"Ok, thanks; I wanted to have chat with you anyway," Maria said, pulling up a chair.

"That sounds ominous. About anything in particular?"

"You've been keeping a very low profile since we discovered the unusual option agreements and I was expecting some developments in the investigation you mentioned. But, to the contrary, nothing has happened. Instead, the golf course site has been reclassified, Carlos Maracena is dead and now Enrique Gonzalez is seriously ill. It all seems a bit odd and I was wondering if you can tell me what's going on?"

"I can understand your concern but there's really nothing I can tell you."

"Does that mean you know something but can't say; or that you know nothing?"

"I'm sorry Maria I can't even answer that," he said with an apologetic look on his face.

"Hmm. I'll take that to mean you know something but can't say, but I really hope Mike Cameron's murder, Carlos Maracena's death and Enrique Gonzalez's condition have nothing to do with those option agreements or the approval of the PGOU."

"I'm sure things will become a lot clearer very soon."

"I hope so."

They talked for a while about their plans over Christmas and when Maria finished her breakfast she left.

Andy flicked through the rest of the newspaper and on page five he noticed a headline above a short article *"Hunter's body found in Sierra de Almijara."* As required by Spanish law, the victim was only identified by his initials M.M.P. The article mentioned that he had apparently been shot and that the police were investigating the circumstances. He didn't give it a second thought.

"His kidney and liver are collapsing and he probably won't last the day. We think he's been poisoned, but haven't be able to identify with what yet," the head of the intensive care unit at the hospital told Cristina over the phone.

Cristina rang Chief Inspector Diaz's coordinator and asked him to have the Chief Inspector send a team to Mrs. Nicklass' house to search for any evidence. "I'd be surprised if they find anything – as no doubt the glasses and plates have been washed and the place cleaned – but it's worth a try."

A few minutes later, the Team Alpha leader reported that Javier Urquiza's wife had popped out, apparently to El Castillo, supposedly leaving him alone in the house. Cristina knew that Fernando was on his way to Granada from Seville, followed by an unmarked car, while Johan Gaards had had breakfast at a nearby bar and then returned to the hostal. She had been advised that Vicente Maldonado had not emerged from his apartment.

So all the suspects were accounted for and all the arrest and search teams were in place. There was nothing more she could do except wait, but she was calm and confident.

At quarter past twelve, as Fernando was approaching the outskirts of Granada, Vicente Maldonado emerged from the underground car park in his Cayenne. He was alone; a member of Team Beta followed him on a scooter to his office in Calle Tejeiro. A short while later, Johan Gaards left the hostal, walked briskly to the building in Calle Tejeiro and pushed a button on the entry phone. He entered the building and walked up the stairs to the first floor.

"Have you seen the news today?" Vicente Maldonado asked him.

"Yes, I saw on Canal Sur that Enrique remains in a coma and that his condition is worsening."

"And that's why we're here, but have you read Ideal?"

"No. Why?"

Vicente showed Johan the article on page five of Ideal. "Although they haven't publicly stated it yet, Don Javier's source says they are treating it as murder."

"Shit. I didn't think they would find him so quickly."

"Actually, it shouldn't matter provided you can get out of the country before they identify you as a suspect. Are you leaving this afternoon?"

"Yes."

"Good. As soon as Fernando arrives we'll call the lawyer in Cayman, who's expecting my call, and then you should go. In the meantime here's the paperwork relating to the reallocation of the shares and the transfer of the money to your account in Belize."

Once Fernando had parked in the Neptune Centre's underground car park, he walked halfway up Calle Recogidas and then turned into Calle Tejeiro.

"Target has entered the building," she heard over the secure radio.

This is it, thought Cristina, the sense of excitement and tension palpable in the ops centre. After months of hard work, and a little bit of luck, we should have all four in custody very soon. She checked her watch. It said 12.45.

She radioed the Team Alpha and Team Beta leaders, "Confirm you're in position and ready to move."

"Confirmed," they both replied.

"Good. I want you to enter both premises and arrest the suspects in exactly five minutes."

Fernando shook Johan's hand and then sat down on the sofa next to Vicente. "Job well done Johan. From what I gather, Enrique is not expected to regain consciousness and you fully deserve your bonus."

"Thanks, but let's get this final step out of the way and then we can all relax."

"Before we call the lawyer I want you to check the paperwork. Johan's already been through it and is happy with it," Vicente said to Fernando, handing him some documents.

"I'll go to the loo while you do that," Johan said.

As he headed down the marble-floored hallway towards the small lavatory next to the front door, five special unit operatives entered the building via the main entrance. They had two hand-held metal battering rams to break down the front door to Vicente Maldonado's office.

As soon as he heard the three loud thuds in rapid succession followed by the noise of the front door breaking open, Vicente realised what was going on. He got up from the sofa and began to move quickly towards his desk on the other side of the room.

Several armed police stormed down the hallway, the sound of their boots resonating throughout the apartment, and burst into the room. "Police. Stay right where you are and keep your hands where we can see them," one of them shouted.

He and Fernando offered no resistance while they were handcuffed and two of the policemen searched the other rooms.

"Where is Johan Gaards? We know he entered the building," demanded the one who appeared to be the leader.

"I think he went to the bathroom and then left just after you arrived," Vicente replied, smiling and looking towards the open front door.

The leader turned round and ran back down the hallway, stopping at the part open door on the left, just before the front door. The bathroom was empty. He radioed his number two who was meant to be coordinating the rest of the unit.

"Johan Gaards has escaped. Have you seen him leave the building?"

"Yes, three operatives are chasing him on foot. I'll keep you posted."

Cristina was furious. "How the hell did you let him escape? Why was no one posted at the front door to the office?"

"There was a misunderstanding, I thought my deputy was going to send someone up after us to secure the landing and he thought one of my team was going to secure the front door and landing until the suspects were in custody."

"Fantastic, with all the experience you've got a misunderstanding is all we needed. So where's Johan Gaards now?"

There was awkward silence for a few seconds.

"We've lost him."

"Marvellous, it gets better. Not only do you let him leave the building but then you lose him. What was the street unit doing – their Christmas shopping?"

"They saw him late, so he got a good head start on them. He ran down a number of side streets and they weren't able to keep up with him because of the pedestrian traffic. It looks like he was heading for the Neptune Centre."

Cristina was familiar with Granada's main shopping centre, which was located just inside the ring road on the western edge of the city. It covered two blocks, excluding the adjacent Corte Ingles department store, and had several entrances. It would be extremely busy and she knew that, even if they did manage to spot Johan Gaards, being able to arrest him discreetly would be very difficult. He might also be armed.

"So what action are you taking?"

"I've split the unit into teams of two. Five teams are monitoring all the exits on a rotating basis and three are sweeping the area, both inside and outside the centre. I've also sent a team to watch his car and one to the railway station. That's all I've got left as the others are tied up searching Vicente Maldonado's office and apartment."

"Put a call in to all the local taxi firms to keep an eye out for him. I'll notify the airlines and ask the Civil Guard at the airport to watch out for him. For your sake I hope you find him soon. Where are Vicente Maldonado and Fernando Echevaria?"

"They're being taken to the police station as we speak."

"Let's hope they don't manage to escape too."

"Ma'am, there is some good news."

"And what might that be?"

"Mr. Maldonado's computer was on and he was logged on to his email and Skype accounts. If we disconnect the machine from the ADSL line we'll lose access to email and Skype records so forensics are sending over a technician to start examining the machine in situ."

"That is good news and at least you've had one lucky break. I want regular updates on how the search for Johan Gaards is going and let me know as soon as the technician arrives."

"Yes Ma'am."

The dogs started barking furiously so Javier Urquiza turned to check the CCTV screen – it was suspiciously blank. He looked out of the window and saw several armed men dressed in black and wearing helmets standing on top of the wall by the front gate. The three Doberman were running up and down at the bottom of wall, barking continuously and occasionally leaping up, jaws snapping, to try and reach the men.

Javier Urquiza thought quickly. He opened the drawer to his desk, took out his loaded Browning Hi-Power 9-mm semi-automatic pistol, rushed downstairs and through the door onto the rear patio. As he ran across the patio, onto the grass lawn, he heard an electronically magnified voice shout: "Police, the house is surrounded, please come out with your hands up."

There was no one in sight and he continued to run, heading to the right of the infinity pool at the far end of the garden towards the steps in the cliff face which would take him to the tender of his Rodman.

Suddenly two Special Forces policemen emerged thirty yards ahead of him, cutting off his escape to the steps. They were pointing what looked like assault rifles at him and shouted at him to stop. He swerved to his left, pointing the Browning at them and pulling the trigger several times. Both policemen dropped down onto one knee, took aim and fired. The first bullet hit him in the calf and the second one caught him in the chest. As he fell he knew it was all over – but at least he hadn't given up without a fight.

The dogs having been tranquilised, the Team Alpha leader called in the medical team and then radioed Cristina.

Johan wandered around the edges of Parque Federico Garcia Lorca, keeping a close eye out for any police and always staying close to an exit. The park was a block north of the Neptune Centre and he figured the cops would be focusing their efforts there. Using his car was out of the question, so he made two calls and then went to the far north exit on the junction of Camino de Purchil and Calle Arabial and waited.

After a few minutes a white Renault Clio stopped close to the exit on Calle Arabial. Johan took one last look along the street and then walked slowly over to the car and got in the passenger side.

"Hi Luis, I really appreciate this."

"No problem. I was dying to get away from the girlfriend; she's on a shopping mission today. So what's the problem?"

"My car's broken down and I need to get to the airport. Getting a taxi is impossible so I thought I'd give you a call on the off chance – it's been a while."

"Too right. So to the airport then?"

"Yes. I'm off to Amsterdam to see the kids."

Luis pulled out, turned right then left into Camino de Ronda. A few minutes later they took the exit signposted A92 Seville. Granada airport, a compact one-terminal facility, lay ten kilometres along this motorway to the west of the city.

"No need to park; just drop me off outside," Johan said to Luis as they drove down the approach road to the airport ten minutes later.

"Are you sure?"

"Yes, I'm going to have to rush, so there's no point in you parking and hanging around."

The access road ran the full length of the only terminal building. About a third of the way along Luis stopped outside the sliding glass doors of the main entrance. Johan shook Luis' hand and thanked him for the lift.

"No problem, but try and give me more notice next time and we can have a few beers."

"Yes, sorry about that. I'll give you a call in the New Year," Johan said getting out of the car.

He waited for Luis to drive off before entering the terminal. Almost directly in front of him was the check-in area. Departures occupied most of the right-hand side of the terminal while the arrivals area was to the left of the check-in desks.

It was just gone three. Perfect timing, he thought, as they'd said between three and four. He looked around slowly. There were one or two people checking in. Other than that the airport was deserted.

He could see nothing untoward but instead of heading for the check-in desk he turned left and walked towards the Avis car hire counter, which was directly in front of the arrivals area. A bored-looking man wearing glasses was sitting at a desk behind the counter doing a Sudoku puzzle. He looked up as Johan leant on the counter.

"Good afternoon. I'm Mr. Gaards and I rang earlier to hire a car."

"Hello Mr. Gaards, we've been expecting you," said the man. "It's a bit short notice but the car's ready. All I need is your credit card and driving licence and for you to sign the contract in the places indicated, and then she's all yours."

"Actually, I'm going to pay cash."

"That's fine but since you made the reservation at such short notice we've already charged your card with the deposit. Also, as I'm sure you are aware, it's standard practice to keep a signed credit card authorisation on file to cover any additional costs when you return the car.

"Of course, I understand." said Johan, reluctantly passing a credit card and his driving licence over to the man.

The clerk completed some boxes on the rental contract and put it on the counter in front of Johan, who scanned it quickly then signed it where marked. The man gave Johan the key to the car and explained where it was parked. Johan left the building, crossed the access road to the car park and got into a BMW 320.

"It doesn't look good boss. He took a bullet in the chest and he's bleeding profusely and barely breathing. The medics are with him now and I've called in the helicopter to get him to hospital as quickly as possible."

"We really need him alive."

"I know, but he fired several shots at my men and was determined to escape. They had no choice but to return fire, not only to protect themselves but also to try and stop him."

"I appreciate that but …"

"Hang on a second, shit, it looks as if he's just died."

"Damn," exclaimed Cristina.

The news of Javier Urquiza's death was a severe disappointment, and with Johan still on the loose Cristina felt Operation Palmera might be disintegrating before her very eyes. Nevertheless, she took some consolation in the fact that they had Vicente Maldonado and Fernando Echeveria safely in custody.

Back in Los Cipreses, Chief Inspector Diaz was reviewing the forensics and autopsy reports on Miguel Martin. The autopsy report confirmed what he already knew – that Miguel had died as a result of being shot from behind. It concluded:

"Lack of rigor mortis means that death occurred at least 48 hours before the body was found. The evidence suggests that a third party moved the body from its original resting place and moved it to where it was found while at the same time trying to cover their movements and presence. This, together with the fact the victim was shot from behind, leads me to conclude that this was not an accident. As yet we have no indication of who this third party might be. A priority is to find the gun from which the bullet was fired in order to identify its owner."

Aside from the bullet removed from the body, the evidence gathered by forensics comprised fresh tyre marks, partial footprints and some pieces of fabric in the branches, as well as two mobile phones, both with dead batteries.

"So nothing which identifies the murderer?" he asked Manuel, who was seated in front of him.

"Unfortunately not; but if we can access the phones and find the gun, then that would be a start."

"Ramon's searching the surrounding area for the gun and I'll see if I can get UDYCO to use their special software on the phones to see what that throws up. In the meantime, see if you can match the tyre treads to a particular vehicle model."

"The lab's already onto it and they're also analysing the bullet and the fabric."

"Good. Sounds like everything is under control; why don't you go and help Ramon?"

Just as Manuel was leaving the office Jorge walked in.

"Did you find anything?" Chief Inspector Diaz asked him.

"A few shards of broken glass in the viewing area, which may come from the glass Sr. Gonzalez was using; they've been sent to the lab."

"Well done. Anything else?"

"No, that's all, but there's been a bit of action in Los Cipreses."

"What sort of action?"

Jorge described how he had seen the Police Nacional helicopter hover over and then land at a house on the Punta.

"I was up on Cerro Grande so I couldn't see much but I'd say the house belongs to Javier Urquiza. Trouble is no one at HQ seems to know what it's about, or else they don't want to say."

"I'll make some enquiries," Chief Inspector Diaz told him.

A few minutes later his boss confirmed that UDYCO had arrested Javier Urquiza and that they had also arrested a number of other suspects in Granada.

"Can you tell me who?"

"Officially, no, but off the record it was Fernando Echevaria, the Chairman of the Junta's Environmental Planning Committee and Vicente Maldonado, a lawyer based in Granada. A third suspect, Johan Gaards, has escaped but is expected to be in custody shortly."

"Very interesting. Looks like a planning-related issue then?"

"Yes. My sources in UDYCO say it's to do with the reclassification of some land under the new PGOU for Los Cipreses."

"Which would explain why Sr. Gonzalez's collapse is being looked at more closely."

"Yes, they think he's been poisoned. Anyway, leave that to UDYCO, they seem to have it under control. How are you getting on with your two murder investigations?"

"The autopsy report on Miguel Martin confirms he died after being shot from behind. On the Mike Cameron case I'm still waiting for the results of the DNA tests to see if the hairs found on his fleece belong to Miguel."

"When are you expecting them?"

"They only received Miguel's DNA samples this morning, but

they're going to try and get me the results later this afternoon."

"Good. Keep me posted of any developments. I'll be available on my mobile for the rest of the day and also tomorrow."

Chief Inspector Diaz put the phone down and thought carefully about what he'd just been told. It was now a possibility that, somehow, Mike Cameron's murder was connected to the UDYCO investigation; after all, he had been working on a deal involving the reclassification of land in Los Cipreses. And, if the hairs found on Mike Cameron's fleece belonged to Miguel then, in all probability, Miguel, not Carlos, had murdered him.

But why? Was is it to do with the land deal, or had he actually been acting for Carlos? And who had killed Miguel and why?

He felt increasingly certain that some of the answers lay with UDYCO, and hopefully today's arrests and Miguel's murder would be the catalyst for them to reveal details of their investigation to him. If not, he'd have to continue with his own investigations and hope that he and his team could come up with the answers. It was not an ideal situation and he cursed UDYCO's intransigence.

Johan drove out of Granada airport and joined the A92 in the direction of Seville. He breathed a sigh of relief – at least he'd got out of Granada without being spotted. Now he needed to get to the Portuguese border fast. It would take him about three hours, although most of it would be under the cover of darkness.

He looked in his rear-view mirror and noticed two Policia Nacional cars about seventy metres behind him. They were behind another vehicle and maintaining their distance. He kept to the speed limit and kept an eye on the cars behind for a few kilometres. The presence of the police cars made most drivers cautious, and everybody kept to the speed limit creating a steady, but well-spaced, stream of traffic behind him.

Suddenly, a Mercedes S class came screaming up in the outside lane and overtook him, the Policia Nacional cars pulled out and followed it. Fool, thought Johan, as he watched the two police cars chase the Mercedes, but at least it'll rid me of the escort. A couple of minutes later he checked his rear mirror and saw two more police cars fast approaching in the outside lane – both had their blue lights flashing and sirens wailing.

Something didn't feel right; looking ahead, he saw that the Mercedes and the two police cars had formed a barrier across the motorway. The cars in front of him were slowing to a halt with their emergency lights flashing. The first police car pulled level with the BMW and then slowed to maintain pace with him. The second car tucked in directly behind him. The policeman in the car on his left indicated he should pull over.

Johan looked to his right: the hard shoulder was free. He swerved into it and accelerated. The police car behind him followed and the second police car moved into the inside lane, but had to slow down to avoid the slowing traffic ahead. Johan could see the back end of the Mercedes sticking out slightly into the hard shoulder but reckoned he could squeeze the BMW between it and the crash barrier.

He continued to accelerate and the BMW was doing 160 km per hour as Johan steered it into the narrow gap. Just as he thought he was clear there was a tremendous bang, as the rear left wing hit the Mercedes.

The car rebounded against the crash barrier and yawed violently as it broke free. Johan was unable to bring it under control. It hit the crash barrier again, flipping over and rolling two or three times until coming to rest on its roof.

Johan's capture brought a collective sigh of relief from the UDYCO team in Seville. Although Operation Palmera had not exactly gone as planned, at least three of the leading suspects were under arrest.

Cristina called Judge Bustamente to give him the latest news.

"How did you know Johan Gaards was on the A92 in a hired car?"

"He used his credit card to pay the deposit and we traced it. We nearly got him at the airport, but the Guardia were airside and we couldn't give them enough notice before he left. The team was already on the way, so they waited until he joined the A92 to implement the stop strategy."

"Well that's very good work; I hope no one was injured?"

"No, fortunately not, only Gaards himself."

"What's his condition?"

"He's conscious but concussed and on his way to La Señora de la

Nieves for a checkup."

"And the others?"

"Maldonado and Echevaria are in separate cells at the main police station in Granada. As you know, Gonzalez is on a life support unit at La Señora de la Nieves."

"Ok, I want you to transfer Maldonado and Echevaria to Seville prison this evening. Keep them separate and don't let them communicate. Take Gaards there as soon as the doctors give him the all clear."

"Will do."

"Have the search teams finished collecting all the physical evidence?"

"Not yet. They're searching Javier Urquiza's house and grounds and removing items from Fernando Echevaria's office. Also, Vicente Maldonado's computer was on and connected to the Internet so we are waiting for a technician to review his Skype account and web-based email account before taking it to the lab."

"That's excellent news and should save us a lot of time. Have you found any mobile phones?"

"Yes. From what I've been told, each suspect had at least two and they're already on their way to Madrid for analysis. I've asked them to initially concentrate on identifying calls and SMSs on and around key dates."

"Good, and when can we expect a summary of the phone and computer evidence?"

"Probably the day after tomorrow at the earliest. I have a team working on it 24/7 but it really depends on how easy the computer data is to access and how much phone traffic there is. When are you planning on interviewing them?"

"Tomorrow morning, so I suggest we meet at your office at eight to review the evidence before going to the prison."

"That's fine. I'll see you then."

Cristina put the phone down and called a team meeting in half an hour in order to get an update on the evidence gathered to date and to assign priorities. Then she closed the door to her office and picked up the phone.

From his terrace Andy had seen and heard the Police helicopter hovering over the Punta and assumed Cristina was making her move. He knew it wouldn't hit the news immediately so he decided to have lunch at Luque's. A couple of hours later he got home and, as turned the television on to watch the news, his phone rang.

"Hi Andy, it's Cristina. As you've probably heard, we've arrested a number of people a couple of hours ago. Unfortunately, not every-thing went according to plan and I wanted to give you the real version before the media place their own interpretation on events."

"I'd prefer if you were here in person but I suppose I'll just have to wait a bit longer for that," he replied. "Actually, I've been out to lunch and was just about to watch the news so, aside from one of your helicopters hovering over the Punta earlier on, I'm in the dark. Tell me what's been going on."

"I'll be brief because I need to go to a meeting, but we arrested Vicente Maldonado and Fernando Echevaria a couple of hours ago in Granada. Johan Gaards was captured a few minutes ago on the A92 after a car chase. He's hurt, but not seriously. Unfortunately, Javier Urquiza decided to make a fight of it and has been fatally shot – however, we're saying publicly that he's badly injured."

"Certainly sounds like an action-packed morning; I'm sorry about Javier Urquiza, it would be nice to see him behind bars, but at least you have the others."

"Yes, it's very disappointing about him. By the way, we are not releasing the names of those arrested or of Javier Urquiza until Judge Bustamente has interviewed them and we've gathered more evidence. Listen, I have to go. I'll call you when I get a chance but, as you can imagine, I'm rather busy."

"Ok, but try and save some energy for me!"

"I'll see what I can do."

Andy put on an Astrid Gilberto CD and lay on the sofa listening to the melodious sound of The Girl from Ipanema. He was soon asleep, the effects of the wine at lunchtime and stress of the last few days taking their toll.

When the team meeting finished, Cristina walked across the open plan operations centre back to her glass fronted office. She was tired.

Today had been a long day and tomorrow would be no different. There was still a lot to do, but at least the principal suspects were in custody, and they appeared to have all of their mobile phones as well as, unexpectedly, access to Vicente Maldonado's Skype and anonymous email accounts.

She checked her emails and saw that she had received two during the course of the team meeting. The first was from Chief Inspector Diaz's coordinator passing on the Chief Inspector's request if they could analyse the two mobile phones found on Miguel's body. It also confirmed that they had found shards of glass at the scene of Enrique Gonzalez's collapse.

The second was from the lab in Madrid saying that they had matched the hairs on Mike Cameron's fleece to Miguel's DNA. In the excitement of the day she had forgotten all about this. She sat back down at her desk and called Judge Bustamente with the news.

"So if Miguel, not Carlos Maracena, killed Mike Cameron then perhaps both their murders are related to Project Pulpo," she said to him.

"Not necessarily. There's no evidence that Miguel knew about Project Pulpo."

"So why would Miguel kill Mike Cameron?"

"Maybe they had a dispute about money. Maybe Carlos Maracena put him up to it. Maybe Javier Urquiza put him up to it. They're all possibilities."

"So finding Miguel's murderer is key. I'd place money on Johan Gaards, but we need to know what evidence Chief Inspector Diaz has in order to try and confirm that."

"Yes, and we also need to establish whether or not Mike Cameron's death was related to Project Pulpo."

"Then we can't give Chief Inspector Diaz the DNA results until we have confirmed whether or not Miguel's murder was related to Project Pulpo."

"Agreed, so don't release the results to him; arrange for him to be here on Thursday morning, when you and I can bring him up to speed with the status of our investigation."

Cristina emailed Chief Inspector Diaz's coordinator to confirm that they would analyse Miguel's mobiles and asking him to invite the Chief Inspector to a meeting with UDYCO in Seville to discuss matters "of mutual interest" related to their respective investigations. *"Please ask him to come alone and to bring all the evidence he has collected related to Mike Cameron's and Miguel Martin's murders."* the email ended.

She then told the lab that they were not to release the DNA results to Chief Inspector Diaz. "Tell him you're overloaded with work on Operation Palmera and that they won't be ready until Thursday afternoon."

Cristina pushed open the door of her office and called for her team's attention. She told them about the DNA match and the fact that Miguel's mobile phones were on their way to Madrid.

"So we're looking for anything which links him to Project Pulpo and/or the death of Mike Cameron. It also looks as if we have some physical evidence from the scene of Enrique Gonzalez's collapse which forensics are examining. Ok, thanks for all your hard work and I'm afraid I'll be seeing some of you tomorrow. The rest of you enjoy Christmas Day and see you on the twenty-sixth."

Christmas Day

Cristina slept well and woke feeling refreshed. She put on a two-piece black trouser suit with plain white sea island cotton blouse and arrived at her office at eight o'clock, followed shortly afterwards by Judge Bustamente. They were joined by Iñigo.

"It's a real shame about Javier Urquiza," the judge commented "he was the one behind Project Pulpo, and now we may never get to the bottom of all his dealings."

"I know, but my men had no choice, he was firing at them and trying to evade capture. Anyway, I'm sure Vicente Maldonado will be a mine of information into Urquiza's financial dealings."

"Talking of which, the documents we found at Vicente Maldonado's office, along with his emails, prove that all four of the big guns were involved in Project Pulpo," interjected Iñigo, as he passed Cristina and the judge a sheath of documents.

Cristina and Judge Bustamente flicked through the documents, focusing on the items highlighted with a yellow marker pen.

"I see. We've even got details of the bank accounts where the money received by Carrington Investments was going to be transferred to – which just about ties up the tax evasion charges," she said.

"Yes, but there's a twist. Have a look at these."

Cristina took more documents from Iñigo. While she studied them he continued: "As you can see, it also appears that Sr. Maldonado, Sr. Echevaria and Johan Gaards were planning to reallocate Enrique Gonzalez's shares in Carrington Investments to themselves before issuing the final instructions to transfer the funds out of Cayman."

"Interesting; that's a very strong motive for killing Enrique Gonzalez," remarked Cristina.

"Have you found any evidence of bribery or their involvement in the murders of Mr. Cameron and Miguel Martin?" asked Judge Bustamente.

"Not yet. Most of the files on the hard drives are encrypted. The techies are confident they'll be able to access them, but as yet we've nothing to prove that anybody has been bribed or that any of them are involved in the murders."

Cristina thought about this for a second. "How are they doing with the mobile phone analysis?"

"Slowly. They had skeleton staff yesterday and they're bringing in more people this morning. I hope that they'll have some of the key date analysis by mid-morning tomorrow."

"Good, keep them at it; we've already got more than enough here to charge them with tax evasion at the very least. That being the case, I am going to keep the interviews as short as possible. We can spend more time questioning them tomorrow, when hopefully we'll have some evidence of bribery and possibly even murder. Come on let's go," Judge Bustamente said, standing up.

When they arrived at the prison they were taken to the interview room they would be using. Cristina watched the judge and Iñigo conduct the interviews through a one-way glass screen in the adjacent observation room.

Vicente Maldonado was first. He had decided not have a lawyer present and when confronted with the Reservation Deposit and Share Purchase Agreements found in his office he did not deny involvement in Project Pulpo.

"But it's perfectly legal since it does not involve the sale of physical assets in Spain, so I'm not sure what I'm doing here." Cristina smiled wryly to herself. He was trying to be clever.

"Not so I'm afraid. As you know, all Spanish residents must declare any income they receive outside of Spain to the Spanish tax authorities. In your case, you would be liable to declare and pay tax on the proceeds of the shares in Carrington Investments that you were about to sell," replied Judge Bustamente.

Vicente Maldonado stroked his neatly trimmed beard for a few seconds before replying. "I can assure you that I was going to declare the income had I received the proceeds."

"What once the proceeds had been transferred to your bank account in Lichtenstein?" the judge rejoined. "Ok, let's assume you would've declared the income, however unlikely that seems; can you tell me why you were in the process of reallocating Enrique Gonzalez's shares between you, Sr. Echevaria and Johan Gaards?"

"Of course. We heard about Enrique's unfortunate collapse and decided it was better for his share of the proceeds not to be lost in an inaccessible offshore bank account. We'd have returned the money to him if he recovered."

"How very thoughtful of you, but Sr. Gonzalez's collapse is being treated as attempted murder and I think there's more to this than meets the eye. Anyway, let's see what else our investigation into your computer files, emails and phone records throws up, shall we?" said the judge, standing up.

Vicente looked on despondently as Judge Bustamente and Iñigo left the interview room.

Fernando readily accepted that he was involved in Project Pulpo but denied that he had influenced the planning process.

"I merely gave the project my wholehearted support and tried to persuade other committee members of its merit. I only stood to gain if the land was reclassified and that decision was down to the entire committee."

"Unlikely don't you think? Much more likely that money was paid to you and various committee members to buy their vote. Don't worry, we'll find the evidence, so you might want to re-consider your story for the next time we meet," replied Judge Bustamente.

"Ok, take him back to his cell."

As Fernando reached the door, Iñigo asked him:

"By the way Sr. Echevaria, can you tell us why you were in the process of reallocating Enrique Gonzalez's shares between you, Sr. Maldonado and Johan Gaards?"

Fernando turned round to face them.

"Yes, I got a call on Sunday night from Vicente Maldonado suggesting that in light of Enrique's unfortunate condition we should reallocate his shares, as he was unlikely to be able to benefit from their sale."

"So it was a last-minute decision and one driven by Sr. Maldonado?"

"Yes, that's right."

"So why would he include you and Johan Gaards in the reallocation. He could have kept it all himself and you would have been none the wiser."

"I've no idea, but Vicente is basically a fair man so I assume he thought I deserved it."

"To the tune of nearly five million euros?"

"Why not? I helped get the result they wanted."

"You certainly did, but look where you are now. Anyway, we'll have another chat tomorrow after you have had time to reflect on what we have discussed."

Johan Gaards was due to arrive from the hospital at any moment so Cristina, Judge Bustamente and Iñigo grabbed a sandwich from the staff canteen and went over the morning's interviews.

"I think we've planted enough seeds in their heads for them to have a sleepless night. As far as Johan Gaards is concerned, as it stands, the only evidence we have of wrongdoing is the intention to reallocate some of Enrique's shares to him; there's nothing connecting him to any of the murders. Is that correct?" asked the judge.

"Yes, the evidence of his involvement in Sr. Gonzalez's collapse is circumstantial. Basically he had motive and opportunity and I am confident that the physical evidence will prove that he was intimately involved in Enrique Gonzalez's collapse, as well as the deaths of Mike Cameron and Miguel Martin," replied Cristina. "Also Fernando lied – it was him that called Vicente Maldonado on Sunday night and we have the transcript," she continued.

They left the canteen and returned to the interview room. Cristina went to the observation room to watch the proceedings. She knew Johan was arrogant and self-confident but wondered how much more so he would be if he realised how little evidence they currently had against him.

Johan walked in to the interview room with his lawyer at his side – a rather shabby-looking individual dressed in jeans, a brown corduroy shirt and worn leather jacket. Johan's right arm was in a plastic half-cast and was supported by a sling. Other than that he did not appear to be suffering any physical ill-effects from his car accident. He looked at Judge Bustamente and Iñigo defiantly.

"Please sit down Mr. Gaards. My name is Judge Bustamente and this is Officer Velasco, and we wish to talk to you about your involvement in Project Pulpo."

Johan sat down but said nothing.

"Mr. Gaards, we have evidence which proves you were familiar with Project Pulpo and that you intended to benefit from the reallocation of some of Sr. Gonzalez's shares to yourself. Is that correct?"

"Yes."

"And you knew that if carried out as planned this transaction would constitute tax evasion?"

"No, because I'm not a Spanish resident."

Judge Bustamente considered this. "Anybody who spends more than one hundred and eighty days a year in Spain is automatically deemed to be resident for tax purposes and I'm sure this applies to you."

"I travel a lot, so it'll be difficult for you to prove how long I have spent in Spain this year."

"We'll see about that; our tax authorities are very thorough. Putting that to one side for the moment, I think we also have a few other things to talk about. For example, what do you know about Enrique Gonzalez's collapse?"

Johan shook his head, "Nothing. I was there serving drinks and he suddenly collapsed. I tried to do everything to help him."

"So I understand. Quite the model citizen."

"I like to think so."

"What can you tell us about the deaths of Mike Cameron and Miguel Martin?"

Johan feigned shock. "Is Miguel dead? When did that happen?"

"Come on Mr. Gaards surely you knew. He was killed a few days ago."

"That's news to me. How did he die?"

"I'm not at liberty to discuss that but can you tell me where you were between Thursday afternoon and the time you arrived at Mrs. Nicklass party on Sunday?"

"Yes – I was at home."

Judge Bustamente considered this. He knew from UDYCO's surveillance that he'd certainly been at home from the Saturday morning.

"And what about Mike Cameron's murder?"

"Why should I know anything about that? Didn't Carlos Maracena do it for the money?"

"Well, we have new evidence which suggests Miguel Martin, not Carlos Maracena, murdered Mr. Cameron, and now he's been murdered too. All a bit strange, wouldn't you say?"

"Los Cipreses is a strange place; there is a lot of jealousy and feuds going on under the surface."

"So you're denying any involvement in their deaths and in Enrique Gonzalez's collapse?"

"Absolutely."

"Ok, thank you Mr. Gaards. That will be all for now."

"Since you have no evidence of any wrongdoing I assume you're going to release my client?" Johan's lawyer said.

"Your client was an accomplice to a much larger planned tax evasion involving Spanish residents, and we're still gathering evidence about this and his involvement in other related matters, so he'll be staying with us for at least another forty-eight hours," replied the judge.

On their way back to the office, the hospital rang Cristina to tell her that Enrique Gonzalez had died. "They're still waiting for the results of the toxicology tests from a lab in Barcelona specialising in poisons and hopefully they should get those soon," she told Judge Bustamente.

Back at the office the IT geeks had not yet deciphered any of the files recovered from the various hard drives they had seized.

"But we've been able to identify a number of anonymous email addresses and Skype accounts that Vicente Maldonado was in regular correspondence with. If we can access those then we'll discover a lot more."

"Give me a list of the accounts and we'll ask Skype and the relevant service providers first thing tomorrow to see if they'll cooperate with us voluntarily before asking for disclosure warrants. When do you expect you'll be able to access the encrypted files?"

"We're close. Probably in the next few hours; but there's a lot of them, so it's going to be quite a job going through them."

"Once you've decrypted them, catalogue them by computer, with the name of the file, the type of file, the date it was created, by whom and the date it was last accessed. Then we can prioritise them."

She left the office at seven o'clock, shortly after the geeks had begun to decipher some of the computer files. She knew they had a long night ahead of them but there was nothing she could do to help.

When she got home she had a long soak in the bath. She considered calling Andy but decided against it, not because she didn't want to speak with him but because she knew how dangerous that could be; she needed to stay focused on the investigation.

Wednesday, 26th December

After several hectic days, Christmas Day had proved a brief, but welcome, relief. But now, only one day later, Chief Inspector Diaz was back at his desk in El Castillo.

He had been annoyed that the results of the tests on Miguel's DNA had not been available on Monday as promised, but not too surprised to receive what was effectively a summons to UDYCO's headquarters in Seville. "Matters of mutual interest" and being asked to bring evidence were sure signs that, as he suspected, Mike Cameron's and/or Miguel's deaths had something to do with Operation Palmera. He was happy to admit he might be wrong about Carlos Maracena, but the evidence pointed to him and UDYCO may have misled him or even withheld vital evidence.

In the meantime, he was continuing his investigation into Miguel's murder – Ramon was back up in the Sierra de Tejeda searching for the weapon used to kill Miguel while, acting on a hunch, he'd asked Jorge to find Johan Gaards' 4 X 4. To date, neither had been successful.

Cristina was delighted with the progress her team had made in cataloguing the hundreds of files they had found on the computers they'd seized on Christmas Eve. It was a laborious, painstaking, but essential task and Iñigo told her that they would be finished by the end of the day. Then they could start cross-referencing files and look at individual files themselves in detail.

"Have you been able to find anything which would confirm bribery was used to influence the reclassification of the land?" she asked him.

"We think so – have a look at this spreadsheet which was on both Vicente Maldonado's and Javier Urquiza's computers."

Cristina looked at the spreadsheet. It was a landscape document with five headed columns reading: Beneficiary, Amount, Paid To, By and Date, from left to right. She counted fourteen separate entries in total. The entries in the Beneficiary column looked like initials while the Paid To column contained the names of cities, mainly Seville, Malaga and Antequera or what looked like bank account numbers. The By column also contained initials, usually VM but DG in three cases.

The total of the Amount column was five million euros with a series of payments totalling three million euros having been made on the seventh and thirteenth of the current month.

"Certainly looks like a record of payments and some of these initials in the Beneficiary column look familiar. Have you checked them against members of the Environmental and Urban Planning Committees?"

"Yes."

"And?"

"Both committees have members with these initials and they all voted for the reclassification of the land."

"Excellent. That should be enough to get arrest warrants for these individuals and search and seize ones for their property. Have you seen Judge Bustamente? He should be here by now."

"He rang to say he was caught up in traffic, but he's due any minute now."

"Ok, what else have you got that we can use today? Has the key dates analysis come in from Madrid?"

"No, but it should be with us by early afternoon. By the way, have you had any joy with getting Skype, Hotmail and Gmail to give us access to the accounts Vicente Maldonado was communicating with?"

"I've talked with Skype's legal officer in Luxembourg and they'll be sending us passwords for the accounts in question before eleven. Both Gmail and Hotmail require warrants so when Judge Bustamente arrives we'll ask him for them. In the meantime, have you found anything that links Mike Cameron's or Miguel's murders to Project Pulpo?"

"I'm afraid not, and there's nothing from the lab on Enrique Gonzalez yet but we do have more spreadsheets similar to this one. The problem is I don't recognise any of the Beneficiary initials. The Paid To and From entries look like bank account numbers."

Cristina looked at the spreadsheet. "They could be drug-related payments. Have you found details of any offshore bank accounts, apart from those we already know about?"

"No, we're snowed under cataloguing and haven't had a chance to electronically index all the files yet. Once we do we should be able to search across them using keywords."

"Do you need more resources?"

"Yes, it would help speed things up if we had more people to examine the financial documents in order to identify the bank accounts and start tracking the money flows."

"I know just the man – leave it to me."

At that moment, Judge Bustamente knocked on the glass door of her office and walked purposefully in. "Good morning. So what further evidence have you uncovered?" he asked them. Cristina handed him the spreadsheets Iñigo had showed her and explained what they thought they were.

He reviewed them carefully. "I agree, but I'd like to wait until we have the key date phone traffic analysis before re-interviewing them. In the meantime, I'll issue the arrest and search warrants for the committee members and get my secretary to prepare ones for the email accounts."

The mid-morning news had no new information about Operation Palmera and Andy was becoming increasingly curious to see if UDYCO had managed to find any evidence linking Johan Gaards to Enrique Gonzalez's death or if they had found any evidence of bribery.

He had not spoken with Cristina since she'd called two days ago to briefly update him on the arrests, and he was missing the sound of her voice, her green eyes, ash-blond hair and much else besides. He imagined how busy she must be and so far had resisted the temptation to call her, but now he decided to send her an email asking her to call him when she had time.

Just as he was composing the email his phone rang.

"Andy, hi; it's Cristina."

"I'd recognise that voice anywhere! Perfect timing – I was just about to email you. How are you?"

"Very busy, but beginning to make good progress. And you?"

"Bored and frustrated!"

"Good, I'd like to take advantage of you."

"Sounds like fun, I'm all yours."

"Don't get too excited until you know what I'm proposing," Cristina replied laughing.

"I'm listening."

"You are still retained by us on a consultancy basis so I'd like to tap into your expertise in moving money around the world. Are you available to help us? We have a lot of documents to go through."

"I'd be delighted. When do I start?"

"How about this afternoon?

"Perfect. I'll be there as soon as I can."

"Excellent. I must be off now; Judge Bustamente is waiting to go through more evidence with me. I'll see you later."

Ramon was continuing the search for the gun that killed Miguel with a growing sense of unease, as rumours about Operation Palmera, along with the names of those involved, circulated within the force. He'd known that Javier Urquiza was involved in illegal activities, but had assumed it was drug related. However, now it appeared much more was at stake.

As yet, there had been no confirmation that Mike Cameron's or Miguel's murders had anything to do with Operation Palmera but, whether they did or didn't, Ramon was increasingly certain Javier Urquiza was behind them, as well as the death of Enrique Gonzalez, and he realised that his information and actions had played an important role in contributing to at least one death.

So he was in a quandary. He knew that Javier Urquiza was dead, but did UDYCO have any evidence that he had been receiving inside information? If so, did they know the source and were they aware of the role this information played in the events since Mike Cameron's murder?

As far as he was aware nobody knew of his relationship with Javier Urquiza and all communication had been through prepaid mobiles so, now he was dead, he reasoned that it would be virtually impossible for UDYCO to identify him as the source of any inside information. They may suspect but they could not prove. He decided to continue as if nothing was amiss but, as a precaution, smashed his prepaid mobile into hundreds of pieces and threw them into the Beznar reservoir. All he could do now was wait.

Just before two o'clock, Iñigo advised Cristina and Judge Bustamente that the key date mobile phone analysis had arrived. "It's clear that they were under instructions to delete all SMSs and call logs. Nevertheless, that fancy Scotland Yard software was able to recover all deleted items."

"And?"

"Firstly, the cross-referencing of the times and dates of calls made to and from the various mobiles clearly show certain individuals were in touch with one another around key events. I expect the cross-referencing of the Skype calls to show the same. As you know, it was this type of evidence which helped convict the Brinks Mats robbers in England. However, there is one problem."

Judge Bustamente and Cristina looked at him expectantly.

"Two of the mobile phones involved in certain calls are missing. From the analysis, we're working on the assumption one of them belonged to Carlos Maracena; but as for the other one, we have no idea who it might be."

"What are the call patterns for this unidentified phone?" asked Cristina.

"The communication is only with Javier Urquiza, so we think it may be a drug supplier."

"Ok, keep working on it. Maybe Vicente Maldonado can enlighten us. Have they found any incriminating SMSs?" asked the judge.

"Yes, and you are going to love this. Johan Gaards called Miguel early in the evening of the fourteenth of November and then at quarter past eleven sent him an SMS saying: *Send agreed SMS anonymously to MC before 11.30 and proceed to his office.*"

At 11.27 there is an outgoing SMS from Miguel's phone to Mike

Cameron's mobile which says: *"Arriving tomorrow. Need pick up from airport if poss. Sending email now with full details. Apologies for short notice."*

Then there is an SMS from Johan Gaards' phone to Miguel's phone timed at eleven forty-six. This one says: *"MC should be at office shortly after 12.00."*

Cristina gave Judge Bustamente a knowing look. "Got him! Johan Gaards set up Mike Cameron to be killed by Miguel. The question is why. Have they found any SMSs connecting any of the others to Mike Cameron's or Miguel's murder?" Cristina asked Iñigo.

"No. But in the early morning of sixth of December, the night Carlos Maracena drowned, Miguel sent Johan Gaards an SMS stating, and I quote: *"CM no longer a threat. Clean job. Leave cash in usual place."*

"So Miguel also killed Carlos for Johan Gaards," Judge Bustamente said with a puzzled look on his face, "but what on earth for?"

"Maybe to try and get the police to close the Mike Cameron case?" replied Cristina.

"Yes, Carlos' accidental death would probably have achieved that had forensics not found Miguel's hairs on Mike Cameron's fleece," Iñigo chipped in.

Judge Bustamente looked thoughtful. "The plot thickens, and I think Mr. Gaards has a lot of questions to answer. What else have they found, Iñigo?"

"That's it for now. We're still waiting to get access to voicemails from the servers; the warrants were only served this morning. In the meantime, they're going to extend the analysis beyond the key dates."

"Excellent work; I think we've more than enough to convict Johan Gaards of conspiracy to murder Mike Cameron and probably Carlos Maracena," Judge Bustamente said to both of them.

"When are lab results on Enrique Gonzalez due?" Cristina asked Iñigo.

"Tomorrow, apparently."

"Ok, we'll re-interview Mr. Gaards tomorrow when we've finished with Chief Inspector Diaz. Let's see who else he implicates in any of the murders," Judge Bustamente said.

Andy arrived in Seville mid-afternoon and, after checking in at the Alfonso XIII, made his way to the address Cristina had given him. It was a restored building in the historic party of the city and the nameplate announced: Seville Exportaciones y Importaciones S.A., or Sexi for short, he thought to himself!

As he was escorted to Cristina's office he could see that the operations centre was a hive of activity. There were groups of people poring over documents, and others glued to computer screens clicking, scrolling and typing; printers were whirring and there was a strong sense of purpose.

Cristina introduced him to Judge Bustamente and Iñigo.

"It's a pleasure to meet you Mr. Montalvo. I hear you've been of tremendous assistance in helping us progress our investigation," Judge Bustamente said to him.

Andy looked suitably embarrassed. "That's very kind, but most of the credit should go to Ms. Ibañez who runs a first-class operation. I'm just one of many cogs."

"You are too modest; we're delighted to have you as part of the team."

Cristina called in the members of the forensic accounting team and they spent the next hour showing Andy the financial evidence they had found so far.

"As soon as the geeks finish indexing all of the deciphered computer files we should be able to do keyword searches across all the files and hopefully find details of all offshore bank accounts and funds transfers. That's when the fun will start," Iñigo told Andy.

"We also need you to liaise with Doug James at CIMA to ensure he has all the evidence he needs to retain the two hundred and twenty-five million euros transferred by the investors. Remember the deadline for providing supporting evidence is tomorrow," Cristina interjected.

"I'll make that my first priority."

"Ok, I think we're done here. Let's catch up later."

A few hours later Andy knocked on Cristina's door. She was alone and beckoned him in.

"Business first," he said to her, sitting in the chair in front of her desk. "Doug James is happy and we've started to track down details of the offshore bank accounts, so tomorrow we can make a start on identifying the flow of funds to and from these."

"That's great. I knew you would add value."

"Thanks, but this afternoon I heard that Miguel has been murdered. Can you tell me all about that and the DNA results?"

Cristina looked at him. She enjoyed his company immensely and wanted to get to know him better but tomorrow, he would discover that his friend had probably been killed as a result of his forced involvement in Project Pulpo, and it would be reasonable for him to blame her.

"Andy, I'm sorry, I really am, but I'm not authorised to tell you anything about that until I've met with Chief Inspector Diaz tomorrow morning."

"Not even a sneak preview for an old friend?"

"I'm afraid not."

"Fair enough. It's been a long day; do you fancy grabbing something to eat?"

"That would be very nice, but it's late and tomorrow's going to be a big day."

"I understand; I guess I can wait a day or two longer."

"By the weekend the pace should have slowed down considerably, so maybe we can arrange something then."

"You don't sound very enthusiastic," Andy said looking at her carefully.

"I'm sorry but I'm tired and there's a lot going on in my head at the moment."

"No worries, I understand. I'll see you here tomorrow morning then. I'll be here at eight."

"Me too, and thanks again for all your help."

Thursday, 27th December

It was Chief Inspector Diaz's first visit to UDYCO's Seville HQ and he'd been taken directly to a private dining room on the third floor. The room contained a round table set for four in the middle and a buffet breakfast set out on a side table along the far wall.

He helped himself to coffee and waited. A few minutes later, a slim, attractive woman who looked vaguely familiar walked in, followed by Judge Bustamente and another man.

"Good morning Chief Inspector and thank you for joining us. My name is Cristina Ibañez; I think you know Judge Bustamente, and this is my colleague Iñigo Velasaco. I'm sure you're hungry, so why don't we help ourselves to some food and talk over breakfast."

As he was spooning the fruit salad into his bowl, Chief Inspector Diaz remembered where he had seen Cristina Ibañez before – she was Samesa's representative in Los Cipreses. A good cover, he thought. When they'd all sat down Cristina explained the origins of Operation Palmera and how they'd recruited Mike Cameron to help them.

"Initially we suspected his death was linked to the operation, but we had no evidence other than the mystery SMS. Your own investigations seemed to point clearly at Carlos Maracena, being the culprit so we had to let you run with that. Now you know about Operation Palmera, you will understand the need for utmost secrecy about our investigation and why nobody but you could know we were running an undercover operation."

Chief Inspector Diaz nodded without saying anything. Cristina continued.

"On Monday afternoon forensics matched the hairs found on Mr.

Cameron's fleece to Miguel Martin's DNA, which makes it likely that he, and not Carlos Maracena, killed Mr. Cameron. However, we needed a couple of days to study the evidence we'd seized to confirm that and to establish if Mr. Cameron's murder was linked to Project Pulpo."

"And I assume I'm here because you have found such evidence?"

"Yes and no," replied Judge Bustamente. "We have evidence that Miguel Martin killed Mike Cameron in collusion with Johan Gaards. What we don't have yet is any evidence linking his murder to Project Pulpo or to Javier Urquiza or any of his associates."

"So if Miguel did kill Mike Cameron on the instructions of Johan Gaards, then Carlos Maracena was innocent all along," declared Chief Inspector Diaz.

"Yes, and we believe he was set up to be the fall guy to deflect attention from Miguel."

"Why do you think that?"

"Because we also have strong evidence to suggest Miguel killed Carlos Maracena on the instructions of Johan Gaards."

Chief Inspector Diaz looked stunned.

"But forensics and the pathologist were convinced that Carlos' death was an accident."

"A very timely one don't you think. If your main suspect dies accidentally then you can close the case."

"Which I very nearly did," said the Chief Inspector, pensively.

"Well we're very grateful you insisted on re-examining Mr. Cameron's clothes and for your perseverance in trying to identify who the hairs belonged to," replied Cristina. "They've provided a major breakthrough."

"So how can I help now?"

"To identify Miguel's killer. We believe Johan Gaards killed Miguel to stop him spilling the beans on his involvement in Mike Cameron's and Carlos Maracena's deaths once we'd identified the hairs as being his."

"I must admit Johan Gaards is my main suspect as Miguel's murderer, and my team is searching for the weapon and clothing used, as well as his car, to see if they provide any evidence linking him to the crime. The problem is we've found nothing so far."

"We can't help you with the weapon or clothes, other than what he was wearing when we captured him, but we do have his car and it's currently being processed by forensics. What do you need?"

"I have a mould of tyre tracks and footprints found at the scene; if we can match either of those to Mr. Gaards car or shoes then we can place him at the scene. If there are any soil samples in the car that we can match then that will strengthen our case further. Of course, finding the weapon and clothing would be the icing on the cake."

"Excellent. When we've finished I'll take you to forensics and you can go through the evidence you have with them. Judge Bustamente will be re-interviewing Johan Gaards later this morning, and we'd like to be able to charge him with at least one murder."

"I've one more question," Chief Inspector Diaz said, putting down his cup of coffee. "Is there anything suspicious about Enrique Gonzalez's death?"

Cristina looked at Judge Bustamente. He turned to Chief Inspector Diaz, "Yes, we're ninety-nine percent certain he was poisoned by Johan Gaards as part of a double-crossing plot but the lab still hasn't been able to identify the substance used. They hope to have something for us later today."

"I must say, this is all rather complicated, but it looks like you've just about got everything sorted out."

"We hope so, but there are still a few loose ends to tie up, some with your help," Cristina said rising from the table. "Shall we go to forensics?"

By half past nine they had matched the tyre moulds and soil Chief Inspector Diaz had brought with him to Johan Gaards' jeep.

"It's time we paid Mr. Gaards another visit," said Judge Bustamente "and I think you should present the evidence regarding Miguel to him, Chief Inspector."

"With pleasure."

Johan Gaards looked sullen and tired as he was brought into the interview room, his usual air of arrogance and nonchalance no longer present.

"Good morning Mr. Gaards, I trust you slept well. We've quite a lot of questions for you today and Chief Inspector Diaz has also joined us as he'd like to ask you some questions about Miguel Martin's death. But first let's start with Mike Cameron's murder shall we?"

"I've already told you, I know nothing about that."

"So why did you send Miguel Martin two SMSs on the evening of Mr. Cameron's murder giving him instructions with regard to Mr. Cameron?"

Johan swallowed nervously. "Can I have a word with my lawyer in private?" he asked after a few moments.

"As you wish. Let's reconvene in quarter of an hour shall we. Maybe then you'll have more to tell us."

Judge Bustamente, the Chief Inspector and Iñigo joined Cristina in the observation room. While they waited Cristina's mobile rang. It was the lab.

"The poison used to kill Enrique Gonzalez was ricin and it looks as if he ingested and inhaled it – a double whammy and the way to a certain death."

"And have you found traces on the glass shards recovered from the scene?"

"Yes."

"Fantastic. Just to wrap it up can you see if you can find any traces on Johan Gaards' clothes and in his car?"

"We're already on the case."

"That's the final nail in the coffin. When we've finished questioning him about Mike Cameron and Miguel's deaths we'll move on to Carlos Maracena's and Enrique's."

Johan Gaards and his lawyer were escorted back into the interview room.

"Interview with Johan Gaards recommencing at eleven-thirty on Thursday the twenty-seventh of December," Judge Bustamente said into the tape machine on the desk.

"Mr. Gaards, more evidence has just come to light but we'll get to that a little later. So where were we? Oh yes, here's a copy of the SMSs you sent to Miguel Martin on the night of Mike Cameron's murder," he continued, placing a piece of paper in front of Johan.

"As you can see they clearly give instructions to Mr. Martin about luring Mr. Cameron to his office. Quite compelling evidence wouldn't you say?"

"No, I didn't send any SMS to Miguel Martin so I'm not sure where you got these from."

"From the mobile phone in your possession when we arrested you."

"That phone isn't mine. It actually belongs to Javier Urquiza."

"Oh come on, there's plenty of other calls and SMSs we've identified on that phone which prove beyond reasonable doubt that the phone was yours. Anyway, we already have Senor Urquiza's mobile."

There was a long silence. Johan Gaards looked at his lawyer, who nodded virtually imperceptibly.

"Ok, Ok, I admit that I arranged for Miguel to kill Mike Cameron but I was only the middleman. It was Javier Urquiza who asked me to organise it."

"Good, we're finally getting somewhere. Tell me why?"

"Because Javier Urquiza had found out he was about to inform you lot of his involvement in Project Pulpo."

"And how did Sr. Urquiza find that out?"

"Mike Cameron told me one night when he was drunk that he was involved in a large property transaction and that once he had more details he was going to inform the authorities."

In the observation room, Cristina took a deep breath. So here was the confirmation that Mike Cameron's murder was not only directly related to his involvement in Project Pulpo but also his reluctant cooperation with UDYCO.

"I see and I suppose you realise that your actions make you an accessory to murder," said Judge Bustamente. "Now tell us about the SMS you received from Miguel on the morning of sixth of December concerning Carlos Maracena," he continued, taking a piece of paper from the file in front of him. "Something about '*no longer being a threat*' and '*leave cash in usual place*' it says here."

Johan looked at his lawyer again and then back to the judge. "Can I have another word with my lawyer in private?"

"Why not, but this is the last time so make sure you are ready to cooperate fully when you return."

"So Mike Cameron let slip his intention to inform the authorities and that was his downfall," Cristina said to the others while they waited in the observation room.

"Yes, it looks that way. Well he's on the slippery slope now so with luck we'll get a full confession out of him by the end of the morning, even if we have to prompt him with a few more bits of evidence," Judge Bustamente replied.

When Johan returned he told them he didn't know why Miguel had sent him that SMS. "I assumed it was sent to me in error and was meant for Don Javier or someone else."

"Oh please, don't take us for fools Mr. Gaards, but why don't we set that to one side for a moment – the Chief Inspector has some questions for you about your whereabouts last Thursday evening."

"I already told you, I was at home."

"Unfortunately for you we have evidence which puts you at the scene of Miguel's murder," Chief Inspector Diaz.

Johan denied he was there, claiming that was a spot he had visited regularly and had actually been there a few days before. "It's just a coincidence. I told Miguel about it and I assume he went up there on my recommendation."

"So who pulled the trigger?"

"Beats me," he said shrugging his shoulders.

"So if you know nothing about Carlos Maracena's or Miguel Martin's deaths what can you tell us about your involvement in the death of Enrique Gonzalez?" asked Judge Bustamente.

"We've been through this already. Nothing. I tried to help him."

"Tell me have you ever handled ricin? It's very dangerous you know."

"No, never."

"Wrong answer. There are traces of it, along with your finger-prints, on the glass you gave Enrique Gonzalez at Mrs. Nicklass' party, as well as in your car and on your clothes. I'm afraid that's one murder you cannot deny."

A look of resignation appeared on Johan's face. "Ok, Ok, what's the deal if I tell you all I know?"

Three hours later they had full details of the murders, his involve-ment in Javier Urquiza's drug-running operation and Vicente Maldonado's role in Javier Urquiza's activities.

"Tell me, how did you get the ricin?" asked Cristina, as they led him away to his cell.

"Vicente got it from a contact of his at the University of Granada's Medical Research Faculty."

Judge Bustamente decided to delay re-interviewing Vicente and Fernando until the following day, when they had had time to review Johan's confession against the evidence they had, and were continuing to uncover.

Back at Cristina's office, after the four of them had reviewed Johan Gaards' confession in detail, they were ecstatic.

"It's a fantastic result. Not only are they going away for tax evasion, money laundering, bribery and a host of other related charges, we can also charge Johan Gaards with all four murders and Vicente Maldonado and Fernando Echeveria with that of Enrique Gonzalez. It would be nice to be able to pin Mike Cameron, Carlos Maracena and Miguel's on Vicente Maldonado too, but the evidence is circumstantial. It's just a shame Javier Urquiza is dead. I'd love to see him spend the rest of his life behind bars," said Judge Bustamente.

"I think the only unanswered question is who in the Policia Nacional was keeping Javier Urquiza informed as to the status of the murder enquiries," said Cristina. "Who do you think it might be Chief Inspector?"

"We had a lot of people working the cases so it could be one of several people but I'd say it would have to be Ramon or Jorge as they were pretty much aware of everything that was going on. I'll ask internal affairs to start an investigation straight away."

Before updating the rest of the team Cristina knew she had the difficult task of telling Andy about Javier Urquiza's involvement in Mike Cameron's murder.

"Can you give me five minutes alone with Andy Montalvo before we tell the rest of the team about Johan Gaards' confession. I think I owe it to him to tell him what happened to Mike Cameron personally."

"I'll stay with you if it'll make it any easier," Judge Bustamente volunteered.

"Thank you, but I prefer to do it alone. We've worked closely together over the last three weeks and I think we understand each other."

Cristina called Andy on his mobile and asked him if he wanted to grab a coffee in the bar round the corner from the office.

"Sounds ominous, do I need to bring a lawyer?" he asked, trying a light-hearted approach.

"Of course not, I think we can manage on our own. I'll see you there in five."

Andy ordered two coffees and then listened attentively as Cristina explained the events leading to Mike Cameron's murder as described by Johan Gaards. When she finished there was a long silence between them. Eventually Andy asked, "Whose decision was it to coerce him into working for you?"

Cristina looked him straight in the eyes. "It was my idea and my boss agreed to it. It was the only way we could see of catching Javier Urquiza after months of surveillance. We told Mike not to tell anyone but clearly he let it slip to Johan before we had the evidence we needed."

Andy considered this information. "I don't think he should ever have been put in that situation," he said, tight lipped.

"Andy, I realise that this is very difficult for you but I also hope you realise we had little choice. Mike was already dealing with Javier Urquiza. We just used the leverage we had to have him keep us informed about Project Pulpo."

Andy shook his head. His mind was in turmoil. "I need time to think about this. In the meantime, you'd better tell your team the good news. It'll mean they can take it a bit easier and also know where to focus their efforts," he said getting up and walking out into the street.

Friday, 28th December

Cristina had had a restless night. She had tried to call Andy the previous evening after updating the team, but his mobile was off and he wasn't at his hotel, so she'd reluctantly gone for celebratory drinks and tapas with her team.

When she awoke the next morning, later than intended, she was disappointed not to find a message or missed call from Andy on her mobile. She rang Iñigo.

"I'm running late so I'll see you all at the prison in an hour. Is that Ok?"

"Of course, everything is under control and the judge is straining at the leash."

"Good. I'll see you there then. By the way, have you seen Andy Montalvo?"

"Not yet. From what you said last night, he wasn't too happy about our involvement in Mike Cameron's death."

"Yes, he looked angry and I suppose that's understandable. Ok, I'll see you in an hour."

The fact they had obtained a full confession from Johan Gaards and that the evidence to support his version of events was compelling, meant Vicente and Fernando offered little by way of resistance. Unfortunately, neither was able to tell them who Javier Urquiza's source in the Policia Nacional was.

"My money's on Ramon," Chief Inspector Diaz said to Cristina in the observation room "he's a pushy little bugger and always wanting to know about every undercover investigation. He's also been trying to join UDYCO, but I think we'll need to find that missing mobile in order to prove anything and somehow I doubt we'll find it. Whatever happens, at the very least he's being posted to some backwater in Extremadura for a very long time."

By three o'clock they had finished the interviews and so headed back to the office. Andy was not there and nobody had heard from him, and Cristina wondered if she should call him. She decided against it; he'd get in touch in his own time, she thought to herself.

It had been a long week and they had achieved a lot in the last two days and so, after updating the team on the new information obtained from Vicente Maldonado and Fernando Echeveria, she told them to go home. As she was turning the lights to her office off, Iñigo came in looking rather excited.

"What's happened?" she asked.

"A very interesting development which we all, but I think Chief Inspector Diaz in particular, need to hear. Both he and the judge are on their way back here so, if you don't mind, I'll wait until they arrive before revealing all."

The judge arrived first and shortly afterwards Chief Inspector Diaz walked into the office. "What's going on, I thought we'd finished for the weekend?"

"Apparently there's been a very interesting development which Iñigo is just about to tell us about," said Cristina. Iñigo had their full attention.

"As you know we've been going through the anonymous email and Skype accounts to gather information and tie up who was communicating with whom, about what, etc. Given that we did not think Carlos Maracena was involved in Project Pulpo, his emails were given a low priority.

However, today one of my team has been focusing on his email accounts and found the following email to his anonymous Hotmail address," Iñigo said, handing each of them a printed email.

Hi gorgeous,
Arrived safely but going to be in and out of phone and Internet coverage during my Patagonian and Andean jaunt so drop me an email about the plans for Mr. C – the window of opportunity will be brief if he starts formal divorce proceedings.
All my love,
B

After they had read the email Iñigo continued. "As you can see it's from another anonymous Hotmail address and dated the seventh of November, a week before Mike Cameron's murder."

Carlos responded on the eleventh of November with this," he said handing out 'another printed email:

My love,
I'm sorry we've not been able to speak the last few days and I hope you are enjoying the wilds of Patagonia. FYI, the Mr. C issue should be resolved soon. Once A has her inheritance it should be easy to get access to the money. Let me know when you're back in BA so we can talk.
All my love and looking forward to being with you when this is over. C.

"And now look at this email which, as you can see, is dated the fifteenth of November."

Darling,
All going smoothly. Mr. C passed away in unfortunate accident last night. A will be sorting Wills in next few days and I expect to get log in details to offshore account soon. Not long to go now! Email me when you are back in BA so we can talk.
Love.
C.

"Wow, it looks as if Carlos was planning to kill Mike Cameron all along," Cristina said raising her eyebrows.

"Not much doubt in my mind," replied Iñigo. "There's a last email from B dated the twentieth of November confirming she's back in Buenos Aires. After that there's a fair amount of Skype traffic but, unsurprisingly, it all goes quiet after Carlos' death."

"Hmm, the question is, did Miguel and Johan Gaards beat him to it or was Miguel also working for Carlos?" asked Chief Inspector Diaz.

"From the last email it would seem Carlos believed Mr. Cameron's death was part of his plan, so I guess Miguel was double-dipping. Unfortunately, we'll never really know, but it seems clear that Carlos was planning to kill Mr. Cameron to get his hands on Ann's inheritance."

"I agree," said Judge Bustamente "so now we need to try and find this mysterious B, as she was clearly an accomplice."

"We've been checking the H and Skype accounts for B and they're all in fictitious names. It also seems they were only ever accessed from Internet cafés in Marbella and Argentina and they've been inactive since Carlos' death."

"Actually, she might have been the brains behind Carlos' plan to get his hands on Mike's money, but somehow I doubt if we'll ever find out. Anyway, we need to tell Andy Montalvo – at least then he might not hold us fully responsible for Mike Cameron's death," Cristina said.

"Has anybody heard from him since yesterday?" asked the Judge.

Both Cristina and Iñigo shook their heads.

"I'll call him when we're finished up here," Cristina said.

Andy switched on his mobile for the first time in nearly twenty-four hours. He saw he had several missed calls from Cristina, but he wasn't ready to talk to her yet. He knew UDYCO could manage their investigation into the various money transfers without him now that most of the key bank accounts had been identified. So he switched off the phone and went to the check-in gate to board his flight.